I TATTI STUDIES IN
ITALIAN RENAISSANCE HISTORY

Sponsored by Villa I Tatti
Harvard University Center for Italian Renaissance Studies
Florence, Italy

THE PRINCE'S BODY

Vincenzo Gonzaga and Renaissance Medicine

VALERIA FINUCCI

Harvard University Press

Cambridge, Massachusetts
London, England
2015

Copyright © 2015 by the President and Fellows of Harvard College
All rights reserved
Printed in the United States of America

First printing

Library of Congress Cataloging-in-Publication Data

Finucci, Valeria.
  The prince's body : Vincenzo Gonzaga and Renaissance medicine / Valeria Finucci.
      pages cm — (I Tatti studies in Italian Renaissance history)
  Includes bibliographical references and index.
  ISBN 978-0-674-72545-4 (alkaline paper)   1. Vincenzo I Gonzaga, Duke of Mantua, 1562–1612—Health.   2. Medicine, Medieval—Italy.   3. Renaissance—Italy—Biography.   4. Medicine—Italy—History—16th century.   5. Medicine—Italy—History—17th century.   6. Human body—Social aspects—Italy—History.   7. Aging—Social aspects—Italy—History.   8. Beauty, Personal—Social aspects—Italy—History.   9. Human reproduction—Social aspects—Italy—History.   10. Rejuvenation—Social aspects—Italy—History.   I. Title.
  DG975.M32F46 2015
  610.945—dc23
                                                                              2014014549

Contents

List of Illustrations vii

Introduction
Staging the Body 1

1. *The Virgin Cure*
Manual Exams and Early Modern Surgeons 28

2. *The Aesthetic Cure*
Skin Disease, Noses, and the Invention of Plastic Surgery 62

3. *The Comfort Cure*
Managing Pain and Catarrh at the Spa 96

4. *The Sexual Cure*
Searching for a Viagra in the New World 121

Epilogue
Unwrapping the Body 150

Notes 157
Selected Bibliography 237
Acknowledgments 263
Index 267

Illustrations

1. Jacopo da Empoli and Workshop, *Marriage of Eleonora de' Medici and Vincenzo Gonzaga*, ca. 1584. 11
2. Frans Pourbus the Younger, *Family Portrait of Eleonora de' Medici with Her Children*, ca. 1596. 12
3. Peter Paul Rubens, *The Gonzaga Family Adoring the (Holy) Trinity*, 1605. 14
4. Girolamo Fabrici d'Acquapendente, "Speculum Uteri," in *Opera chirurgica in duas partes divisas*, 1619. 37
5. Girolamo Fabrici d'Acquapendente, "Rari 117.25," in *De anatomia abdominis et partium in eo contentarum*. 39
6. Girolamo Fabrici d'Acquapendente, "Rari 117.26," in *De anatomia abdominis et partium in eo contentarum*. 40
7. Gaspare Tagliacozzi, frontispiece dedicated to Vincenzo Gonzaga, in *De curtorum chirurgia per insitionem*, 1597. 67
8. Giacomo Franco, "Vincentio Gonzaga Duca de Mantua," Plate 23 in *Effigie naturali dei maggior principi et più valorosi capitani di questa età con l'arme loro*, 1596 69
9. Gaspare Tagliacozzi, "Icon Tertia," in *De curtorum chirurgia per insitionem*, 1597 79
10. Gaspare Tagliacozzi, "Icon Quinta," in *De curtorum chirurgia per insitionem*, 1597 80
11. Gaspare Tagliacozzi, "Icon Octava," in *De curtorum chirurgia per insitionem*, 1597 81
12. Gaspare Tagliacozzi, "Icon Decimaquinta," in *De curtorum chirurgia per insitionem*, 1597 82
13. Gaspare Tagliacozzi, Surgical Instruments, in *De curtorum chirurgia per insitionem*, 1597 83
14. Domenico Vandelli, "Bagni de Abano," in *Tractatus de thermis agri patavini*, 1761. 109
15. Lucas Cranach the Elder, *Fountain of Youth*, 1546 119
16. Frans Pourbus the Younger, *Vincenzo Gonzaga*, ca. 1605 124
17. "Forse che sì forse che no," Ceiling of the Hall of the Labyrinth, Palazzo Ducale, Mantua 151

THE PRINCE'S BODY

Introduction

Staging the Body

> Is man no more than this? Consider him well.
> —William Shakespeare, *King Lear*, 3.4.93

> For you have but mistook me all this while:
> I live with bread like you, feel want,
> Taste grief, need friends—subjected thus,
>   How can you say to me, I am a king?
> —William Shakespeare, *King Richard II*, 3.2.171ff.

EARLY IN THE YEAR 1612, Vincenzo Gonzaga I (1562–1612), fourth duke of Mantua and Monferrato (Montferrat) and munificent sponsor of art, music, and theater—a Renaissance prince in every sense of the word—realized that he had a physical problem that required some urgent addressing: he had been lying in bed for a while with an intermittent fever accompanied by excruciating pain on his side and a sense of utter fatigue. Among his doctors, fear had recently garroted hope, as no remedy they administered seemed to work: he had been bled; he had been purged; he had been given enemas; he had been administered, in fact, all the pills, balsamic oils, paps, gelatins, shavings, herbs, and narcotics that the myriad apothecaries, distillers, and aromatists currently employed at the Gonzaga court felt necessary to recommend. This time, however, the duke's body was refusing to respond and heal.

Vincenzo was not yet fifty years old. Lately he had been feeling unhinged and oddly pensive. The stability that his wife of twenty-seven years, Eleonora de' Medici, had brought to his life had seemingly evaporated after her death a few months earlier.[1] And so Vincenzo called to his bedside his children presently at court—three grown-up boys, a girl, and a cherished illegitimate son (another daughter was away in France, an illegitimate daughter was in a nunnery, and a second illegitimate son was in Naples)—and also, feeling in need of redemption, solicited visits from confessors. Then he asked that some items of the priceless and sophisticated art collection he had indefatigably put together through the years—for many in the art world, Vincenzo was a collector par excellence of the last two decades of the sixteenth century and the first of the seventeenth—be brought to his bed, where he lovingly caressed and cried over them. It was arduous for this aesthete to let go of the bibelots, the little carvings, the polished statuettes, that had so gratified his finely tuned aesthetic sensibilities, but they too were in the end transitory possessions. Finally, on February 3, just six days before he expired, Vincenzo dictated his last will:

> He willed and ordered that the body (*quidem cadaver*) be buried and that it be buried not as is the custom lying down, but sitting up with his sword placed at his side on a marble chair prepared for this purpose; that it should in no way (*nullo modo*) be put in a wooden coffin, but that it be placed in the little room where lies the body of Domina Eleonora, Duchess of Mantua, his most beloved wife.[2]

Although one can safely assume that last wills, especially last wills of princes, are faithfully executed, we do not know whether Vincenzo got his desire to be buried enthroned and with a bejeweled sword at his side, as this would have been an extraordinary form of burial.[3] We do not know in fact where the duke's body lies. According to official documents, Vincenzo should be buried in a secret chamber inside the crypt of his treasured Church of Sant'Andrea, next to his wife and to the relic of the Most Precious Blood—the hugely significant religious remains that he cherished throughout his life and even brought along to his battlefields in Hungary. This crypt, however, has not been found. Over the years the area has been minutely explored and the walls have been perforated in search of a chamber, but nothing has emerged. In December 2007, however, during routine maintenance work on the floor of the Church of Santa Barbara—a church also used for burial of Gonzaga family members and now integrated within the precincts of the Ducal Palace—a hidden crypt divided into two rooms was discovered. In one room were scattered bones of female bodies; in the other, remains of male bodies, such as those of Vincenzo's father, Duke Guglielmo I (the founder of the church), and grandfather, Duke Federico II, as well as those of Federico II's son, Duke Francesco III, and of two of Vincenzo's own sons, Duke Francesco IV, who died a few months after his father, and the infant Guglielmo Domenico (Lungaspada), who had died twenty years earlier.[4] Essentially all Gonzaga dukes from 1540 to 1612 were either buried there or transferred there from their original burial ground, as Vincenzo had specified in his will, with the apparent exception of the duke's own body. The crypt had been violated more than once in the past four centuries, and the bones scattered over the area.[5] Duke Guglielmo (or at least so says the stone engraving near the body) was found in the exact manner in which documents attest he was laid to rest: lying on a marble bed, without crown or emblems of his ranks—a burial practice that had become common by the early modern period. Could Vincenzo, then, have been buried sitting on a marble throne as he had wished, just like the emperor Charlemagne was rumored to have been entombed, thus figuratively fulfilling his lifelong dream of being perceived as the latest embodiment of a chivalrous paladin defending Christendom?[6]

That Vincenzo would have liked his funeral to have an appropriate pomp, similar to the ones he had meticulously showcased through the years for his father, mother, wife, and toddler son, is consistent with his narcissistic and flamboyant personality. Here, however, I am interested in the psychological reasons why Vincenzo felt his embalmed cadaver needed to sit on a throne rather than lie flat, and why he wanted a sword at his side when princes were usually buried in modest, indeed often penitential, garments. That during his lifetime Vincenzo wanted a throne, everybody knew: there had been hushed negotiations a few years before his death for him to become king of Poland; he had also been approached for the throne of Albania, which it was understood could be his following an adequate disbursement of money.[7] Nothing serious came of either transaction. Earlier Vincenzo had proposed to King Philip III of Spain that he be named governor of Flanders and Portugal, and he had sent Peter Paul Rubens—the Flemish painter he discovered during one of his trips abroad and employed at court—to solicit the king with appropriate artistic gifts, but this request fizzled out. What's more, his desire to be named generalissimo of the Mediterranean, for which he had embarked on a visit to the reign of Naples, had been crushed as soon as he landed. And so now he was going to give himself a throne of his own, by fiat. But the sword? Why did Vincenzo Gonzaga need to appear so phallically alive at the time of his death, when nobody could care less whether he was phallically challenged? What bothered the Duke of Mantua till the very end?

This is a book on the body; more precisely, it concentrates on a few carefully chosen moments in the life of a Renaissance prince when disturbing or periodically festering physical problems came to control and define not only his self-esteem and body image, but also his strategic alliances and political leanings. It is true that at times princes use their corporeal troubles as diplomatic tools to discreetly surmount intractable political impasses—we know, for example, that Vincenzo's great-grandfather, Francesco Gonzaga, used his syphilitic flare-ups to bow out of diplomatic meetings that required him to act contrary to his wishes. Either way, a prince's body allows us to enter into the culture, fears, and preoccupations of his time, for in my reading, history attaches itself to everything, and an individual life, particularly one well documented in archives, can discreetly flesh out the world it inhabits. As Bernardino Ramazzini, the inventor of the branch of medicine now called occupational, wrote in *La salute dei principi,* "The public well-being depends through and through on the health of princes; and therefore nothing should be left untried to defend it." When a prince is sick, Ramazzini added, "the welfare of all citizens is at stake," and there will be "those who in the name of change take advantage of such moments to subvert the social order and set off civil wars."[8] Needless to say, my focus is not on Vincenzo's body politic, "a Body that cannot be seen or handled, consisting of Policy and Government, and constituted for the Direction of the People, and the Management of the public weal," as Edmund Plowden formulated in his *Reports,* written under Queen Elizabeth.[9] Rather, I focus on Vincenzo's body natural, that is, "a Body mortal, subject to all Infirmities that come by Nature or Accident, to the Imbecility of Infancy or old Age, and to the like Defects that happen in the natural Bodies of other People."[10] Vincenzo lends himself to such an examination because he lived precisely in the decades now often referred to as being at the origin of modernity, when scientific and medical inroads revolutionized the ways in which human beings related to the surrounding world. As Galileo with his telescope directed heavenward poked holes into man's relationship to the universe and God, so anatomists poked holes with their scissors, scalpels, and knives into man's relationship with his own body. A desire to know *how* things work and *who* is the "other" (or whether there is a "there" somewhere) translated into a thirst for biological inspections and geographical discoveries. This was an era when interconnected global ecological and economic enterprises brought massive, at times bewildering, changes in the life of plants, animals, men, and microorganisms. A longing to take charge of one's life rather than leaving the care exclusively to God's grace provided the urgency for doctors to address disabilities and confront the array of diseases that were ravaging the body, from syphilis and tuberculosis to malaria and parasites—even though current medicine was often just a palliative. This longing also fostered a culture in which patients began to expect a fair relationship with their healers: sick people felt that their bodily issue (pain, fever, insomnia, fatigue, skin eruptions, disfigurations) required not just the consolation of faith but the specific care of doctors whom they were willing to pay for a fair shot to a cure.[11] More to the point, Vincenzo Gonzaga left a treasure trove of documents concerning his physical difficulties that cracks open the world of gentility with which noblemen surround themselves at court, thus tantalizing researchers to dig deeper and find associations relatable to our modern sensibilities and aspirations.

In the end, this is neither a book about Duke Vincenzo Gonzaga nor a book in which a string of documents unfolds the bursting dimensionality of a life lived to the fullest. It is rather a book that examines some surprisingly modern-day medical problems that one way or the other afflicted Gonzaga, although none were fatal, as I follow key moments in the life of a man struggling with the burdens—and pleasures—of manhood, money, and honor. My aim is to participate in the current debate among historians of medicine, cultural studies theorists, psychohistorians, and literary critics regarding key interrelated preoccupations of the early modern period (or indeed of any period): sexuality, beauty, pain management, and aging. I will use four pathophysiological and well-recorded moments in the life of Vincenzo as my guide, for as Roy Porter and G. S. Rousseau put it, "Decoding disease is integral to the understanding of culture, society and biography."[12] By examining documents in the Gonzaga and Medici archives in loosely chronological order—letters, doctors' advice, reports, receipts, travelogues—together with (and against) medical, herbal, theological, and even legal publications of the period, I flesh out an early modern cultural history of the physiopathology of human reproduction, the science of rejuvenation by way of aesthetic medicine, the luxury pursuit of wellness care addressing impairments and fatigue, and the therapeutics of antiaging that confronted the decline in quality of life as each impacted a prince with a large ego and an even larger purse. The questions I address as I oscillate between the personal and the medical in looking at the tribulations affecting the identity of a hyperactive prince are wide ranging: How did the discovery of new body parts translate into political disempowerment? When did the worshiping of beauty motivate radical experimentations with cosmetic surgery? Why were comfort cures in alternative places like spas so fashionable? And why did provincial herbalists fight to do fieldwork in newly discovered lands?

Biography

Vincenzo Gonzaga was born on September 21, 1562, the only son of Duke Guglielmo Gonzaga (1538–1587) and his archduchess wife, Leonora of Austria (1534–1594), daughter of Emperor Ferdinand I von Habsburg. From the start it was clear that this blue-eyed, red-haired infant with attractive facial features and an exquisite bone structure was surprisingly healthy. I say surprisingly, because there had been a disease ominously plaguing the Gonzaga line for many (too many) generations that he did not seem to carry, a disease that was famously disfiguring the profile of his father's body, for Duke Guglielmo was a hunchback. The tuberculosis of the bone that Guglielmo's spine defect announced (Pott's disease and probably rickets) and that through the years had made some members of the family objects of pity, or alternatively of ridicule, had seemed finally to escape the current duke's offspring, since neither Vincenzo nor his two sisters—Anna Caterina (1566–1621), later married to her uncle, Archduke Ferdinand II of Austria-Tyrol, and Margherita (1564–1618), the bride child of Duke Alfonso II d'Este of Ferrara (and ultimately dowager-in-chief, scheming her path at the Mantuan court)—were showing any vertebral collapse or spinal curvature (kyphosis) that would spell its presence to the eyes of contemporaries. But, alas, bone tuberculosis can manifest itself in many ways, and Vincenzo's array of autoimmune and metabolic disorders—arthritis, persistent fevers, knee pain, gout (or goutlike) flare-ups, skin lesions, abdominal disorders, and occasional difficulty in ambulating—as well as his sisters' obesity, could be read today as likely manifestations of their father's extrapulmonary TB syndrome. This diagnosis is of course tentative, since it is not confirmed by any DNA finding. There will be more on this later.

Vincenzo's youth was unremarkable. To his credit, Duke Guglielmo took special care to educate his son well and searched attentively inside Italian universities to find the best tutors. He eventually chose those teaching in the most famous place of learning at the time, Padua, in whose "Studio," tightly controlled by Venice's *provveditori,* members of the Gonzaga nobility and cadet branches have often been educated.[13] Guglielmo recruited professors of mathematics such as Giuseppe Moletti (1531–1588), Galileo's predecessor in that chair in Padua; Gian Paolo Branca, a doctor; and Marcello Donati (1538–1602), a physician and humanist, who later became Vincenzo's most appreciated counselor at court. Vincenzo loved sports, especially hunting and fishing but also the new sport of soccer (*palla*), and indeed later in life he tried to recruit a foreign soccer player, much as national soccer teams do today. He also enjoyed swimming, despite the fact that this activity was discouraged at court, not only because the still-influential dictates of Galenic medicine did not welcome the opening of man's pores to outside air for the sake of keeping the body in good health but because one of his uncles, Francesco III (1533–1550), had died at seventeen of pneumonia after falling into the cold waters of one of the lakes surrounding Mantua while hunting.

For Duke Guglielmo, his brother's untimely death had been fortunate, since he was second in line to the succession to the duchy. He immediately manifested his desire to be inaugurated as the next duke, even though his yearning to rule (he was still under age at the time of Francesco III's death) was contested within his own family. Many Gonzaga members regarded Guglielmo's physical disability—and perhaps the supercilious, stiff, and scornful personality that the disease had reactively promoted—as hardly embodying the condottiere image that often personified the Gonzaga stock to outsiders. But Guglielmo got the upper hand and became Duke of Mantua and Marquess (later Duke) of Monferrato at seventeen (1550–1587). His athletic cadet brother, Luigi (1539–1595), whom many had wanted to succeed Federico II to the duchy, chose to move to France to inherit the assets that the family had acquired through their grandmother, Anne d'Alençon. Then through marriage to Henriette of Cleves, Luigi became Duke of Nevers, a circumstance that fifty years later would be of capital importance to the destiny of the Gonzaga family and especially of Mantua. The city's tragic, indeed heartrending, historical destiny was in fact set in motion when Luigi's son, Carlo (1580–1637), marrying back into the main line in Mantua, took as his bride Guglielmo's great-granddaughter, Maria Gonzaga (1609–1660), and became Duke of Mantua (1627–1637). This event upset the balance of power of half of Europe and spurred a war of succession in 1629–1631 that saw imperial troops rush to Mantua to subjugate the duchy, an epochal invasion and siege that traumatized and paralyzed northern Italy, eventually canceling Mantua forever from historical significance. It also put in motion an ecological disaster of epic proportions: the wiping out through plague (the second or third largest plague ever to hit the peninsula) of two million Italians.[14]

Vincenzo was barely out of childhood when he experienced a physical problem seemingly coming out of nowhere: he developed a fistula near his anus, which required drainage and cauterization. Retrospectively we may assume that his doctors were not actually treating a fistula but a psoas abscess, which presents itself as a lump in the groin area resembling a hernia and is often associated with bone tuberculosis.[15] In any case the fistula was left partially open to allow for fluids to seep out, as was usual at the time, and nobody showed any concern about it for years, until it became an object of investigation in the days following his first marriage. In the meantime Vincenzo was finding it somewhat traumatic to abandon his adolescent ways, for his personality was diametrically at odds with that of his father. The clashing of wills of these two Gonzaga males has often been recorded: on the one hand Duke Guglielmo, an inveterate and disdainful miser (in the negative view of many), who ducat after ducat left in the Gonzaga's vaults a fortune nobody had previously heard of or thought possible (in the positive view of many), and on the other Vincenzo, an extroverted lover of beauty, art, and display, who adored luxurious items, refined clothes, and a glitzy lifestyle—all mixed with a warm, infectious, high-voltage charm. The fact that Guglielmo was very short, awkward socially, and unbecoming physically, and that he carried his disability on his back for all to see, may have contributed to his need to regularly affirm his authority, apply overarching force, and be vindictive, even though these actions contributed to making him more hated or despised. And the fact that he was barely "alive" may have contributed to a pietism that directed him to found a number of churches in Mantua and even to marry a very pious woman, Leonora, of whom it has been said that she wedded the physically repugnant Gonzaga specifically because this allowed her to punish and chastise herself.[16] Between a headstrong father, whom some historians claim was jealous of his son's energetic and buoyant character, let alone his fine physique, and a thoroughly self-absorbed and attention-seeking son stood the mother, who understood Vincenzo but felt unable to negotiate better terms between her offspring and his father.

Vincenzo was thus left with too little money to fit his view of his status and was given no real participation in the government of the duchy that he was going to inherit. And so began the winter of his discontent. Why was his father treating him like a child (*da putto*), he complained to the ducal secretary, Aurelio Pomponazzi, when he was nineteen, and why was he denied the chance to dress and live as his rank would require? He had tried hard to be humble and obedient.[17] Out of frustration, time and again he left Mantua to visit his sister Margherita, then residing at the entertainment-obsessed Este court in Ferrara. Now and then his lack of prudence and his hypersensitive personality got the best of him. One day he killed in an ambush his father's young English savant, Lord James Crichton (1560–1582), who was said to be able to beat anyone at philosophical debates and mathematical pyrotechnics and may have played, unwillingly perhaps, the part of the dutiful son to the unloving father, Guglielmo. Vincenzo's direct involvement in the killing of this well-educated, foreign "encyclopedist" has never been established, but even his tutor, Marcello Donati, expressed his concern at the time—or perhaps one should say his despair—that his pupil had entered a downward spiral, occupying himself too much with "what one should not do than with what one should rather do."[18] Vincenzo was an alpha male in search of a cause.

To be sure, Vincenzo's mind was quite occupied at the time with the aftereffects of an event that had originally provided him the sought-after way to (at least partial) freedom from his father's grip but later turned into a handicap that forever defined, through hearsay and innuendo, the early years of his life and notoriously stamped his personality with a profound, if ostensibly hidden, psychological trauma. The event was his wedding to a princess of the neighboring Farnese duchy of Parma, Margherita (1567–1643). The marriage was soon in deep trouble, as Chapter 1 will document, because of a medical problem affecting Margherita's sexual reproductive system. As a result, the union was deemed unconsummated and a new noble bride was found for the Gonzaga prince. By 1584 Vincenzo was married to the Florentine Eleonora de' Medici (1567–1611), the daughter of Grand Duke Francesco and his first wife, Johanna of Austria (the newlyweds were thus first cousins) (Fig. 1).

Vincenzo and Eleonora soon produced children. Francesco, the firstborn (1586–1612), married into the Savoy family and became briefly Duke of Mantua upon the death of his father, but he himself died within a year of smallpox, leaving an infant daughter, Maria, who was not in line to succeed him because the Mantuan duchy followed Salic laws of inheritance. Vincenzo's second-born son, Ferdinando (1587–1626), was destined to the church, and indeed he was made a cardinal at twenty, but upon his brother's death the red hat came off and he became Duke of Mantua. He married Caterina de' Medici (1593–1629) and had no children from her.[19] Vincenzo (1594–1627), the third son, had been left to lead a life of leisure, as often happens to scions not immediately implicated in the line of succession, but found himself on call when upon the ascension of Ferdinando to the duchy's helm he inherited his cardinal's hat. But then he fell in love, left the ecclesiastical career in dishonor, and became Duke of Mantua as Vincenzo II upon the death of Ferdinando in 1626. He had no legitimate children. A fourth son, Guglielmo Domenico (1589–1591), rumored to be his father's favorite, died in infancy. And then there were two daughters, both placed in international, advantageous marriages.[20] The first, Margherita (1591–1632), was married to Henry II, Duke of Lorraine, in a trendsetting luxurious ceremony. She had four children, two of whom survived infancy and were married to their cousins, who were both to become Dukes of Lorraine. The other daughter, Eleonora (1598–1655), was married to Ferdinand II, the Holy Roman emperor, but this extraordinarily valuable connection to the imperial household proved problematic for the Gonzaga, since some counselors rejected the marriage. It did not help that she was childless (Fig. 2).

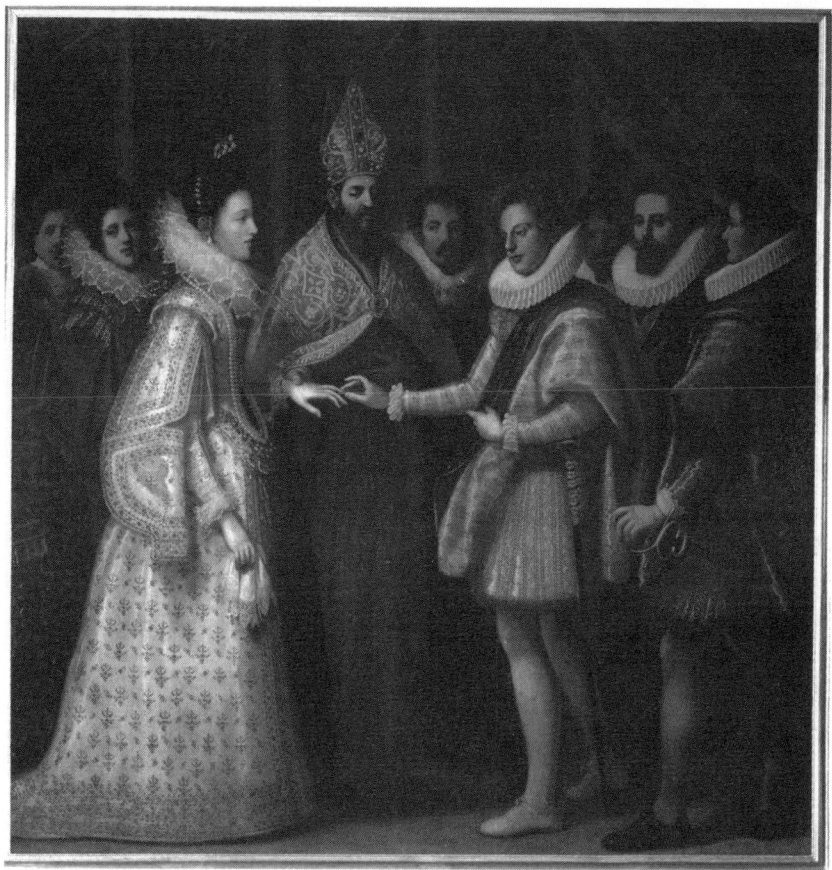

Fig. 1. Jacopo da Empoli and Workshop, *Marriage of Eleonora de' Medici and Vincenzo Gonzaga,* ca. 1584. ("Depositi," Galleria degli Uffizi, Florence. Photo: Polo Museale della città di Firenze, Florence.)

In the meantime, because of Guglielmo's debilitating illnesses Vincenzo did not have to wait too many years to become a duke. He seemed hardly willing to hang around much longer and had publicly begun to assert that because of his father's disrespect, he had good reason to move to France, an unacceptable pronouncement in a duchy that would lose its independence if there were no male heirs to succeed Guglielmo.[21] Vincenzo's painstakingly orchestrated inauguration ceremony on September 22, 1587, was the most lavish that Mantua—or any nearby states for that matter—had ever seen. Nothing was sober, diminutive, or

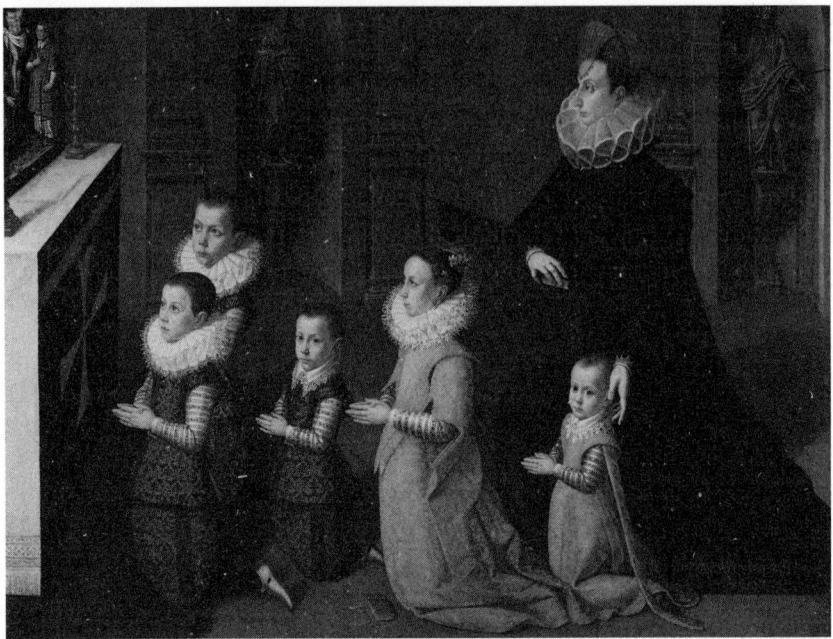

Fig. 2. Frans Pourbus the Younger, *Family Portrait of Eleonora de' Medici with Her Children*, ca. 1596. (Palazzo Ducale, Mantua. Photo: Bridgeman Art Library.)

understated. As an awed contemporary historian described it, a white ermine mantel covered the young duke's pearl and gold embroidered silk jacket, heavily jewel-encrusted arms and a ceremonial baton of rule were at his sides, and a massive crown sat on his head; this was a man wholly aware of his charisma, political aptitude, and birth-given status.[22] As the poet Torquato Tasso enthusiastically proclaimed for the occasion, "Here there was a prince in whose breast bloomed all that is good or liked on earth" (A cui fiorisce in seno / tutto quello che ne giova in terra o piace).[23] Vincenzo had found his calling.

The investiture ceremony inaugurated the beginning of a previously unheard of spending spree in the Mantuan duchy. Immediately seizing an opportunity to shine, Vincenzo started to spend *alla grande* the money his father had left hidden in the duchy's coffer, and thus in the space of a few years Mantua moved from parochial to international. The first 300,000 ducats were used to get a knightly decoration that would proclaim to all Italian princes Vincenzo's new status, the Order of the

Golden Fleece (*Toson d'oro*), which the new duke acquired in 1589 by lending money to the king of Spain, Philip II, in a deal that was not supposed to be repaid. As the Venetian ambassador Francesco Contarini reported, mentioning in malign sympathy the duke's full bells-and-whistles largesse, Vincenzo's gesture indeed gained him some leeway with the Spanish court, to which the Gonzaga had traditionally been tied politically (the nearby duchy of Milan had been annexed to the Spanish crown since 1540), but which the Venetians viewed with suspicion.[24] Militarily speaking, Vincenzo authorized and punctiliously followed the building of the supersized fortress of Casale—a magnificent engineering feat he commissioned in 1590 and for which he employed major military architects in order to protect his eastern possession, the Monferrato region, which was not contiguous to the duchy of Mantua, at a cost of 1,000,000 ducats.[25] Within the space of six years he embarked in three crusades against the Turks—all abandoned before achieving any tangible results yet all extremely expensive, not so much due to the size of the army Vincenzo brought along but to the princely accoutrements that he felt he needed to surround himself with in the field. Vincenzo was also an indulgent, inveterate gambler, losing so much money in places like Genoa and Brussels—trips he undertook with the outward purpose of curing his physical ailments with lengthy sojourns to the baths—that he once had to leave behind in Flanders a heavily jewel-encrusted sword and a box with eight diamonds, as an amused Peter Paul Rubens revealed in a letter.[26]

Vincenzo was also a very refined collector, summoning painters such as Rubens, Van Dyck, and Pourbus the Younger to his court, and collecting works by Raphael, Titian, Mantegna, Correggio, and Tintoretto, to name a few (Fig. 3). In fact, he had so many works of art in his palaces that when Vincenzo II found it necessary to sell some to the English king, Charles I, to pay for his heavily indebted duchy, the pieces listed numbered in the hundreds.[27] Vincenzo traveled widely with the purpose of adding to his collection: in Milan he bought clothes, jewels, arms, and cut glass; in Venice he acquired precious stones; in Rome, statues and drawings; in Naples, textiles.[28] And then there were artifacts coming from the East and the New World: pearls, unicorns, furs, exotic animals.[29] By all contemporary accounts, Vincenzo's personal style was extremely refined, his clothes the most fashionable, as every ducat that could be spared in his duchy (as well as many of the ducats that

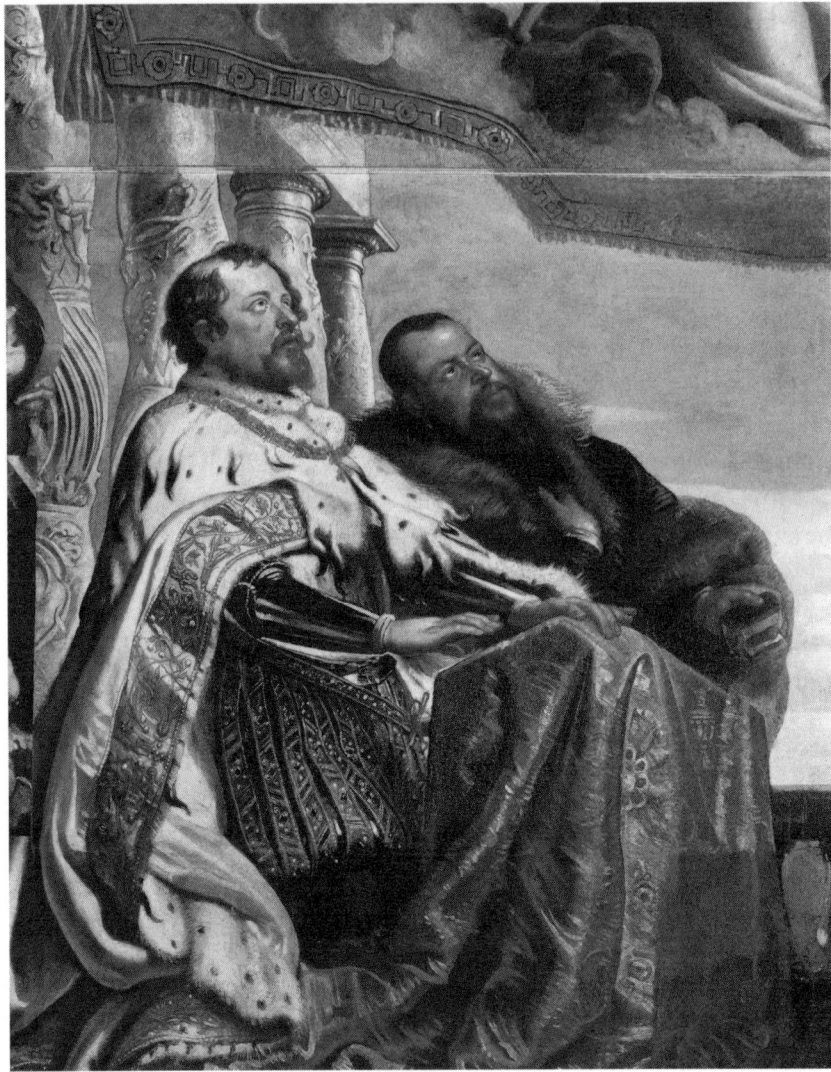

Fig. 3. Peter Paul Rubens, *The Gonzaga Family Adoring the (Holy) Trinity,* 1605. (Palazzo Ducale, Mantua. Photo: Bridgeman Art Library.)

could not) was used to bankroll his glitzy self-indulgence, carousing needs, and aesthetic sensibility.[30]

And although he was not known for either his eloquence or his erudition, luckily for us Vincenzo possessed the most sensible ear of any prince at the time: not only did he sponsor the extensive and groundbreaking musical work of Claudio Monteverdi (1567–1643) by hiring him for a quarter of a century as his chief musician—*maestro et de la camera et de la chiesa sopra la musica* (master of chamber and church music)—but thanks to him, opera as a musical genre was virtually created at his court out of the original *intermedi* (the musical sequence between acts in staged plays) with the lavish performance of *Orfeo* in 1607. When tenor Francesco Rasi in the title role and castrato Giovanni Gualberto Magli in a mythological role went onstage in February of that year, the musical theater took a leap forward that forever changed Western music. Under the most benign sponsorship of Vincenzo and with the coffers of the duchy always unlocked for anything that had the potential for being spectacular, Monteverdi repeated his musical feast in May 1608 with the stunning performance of *Arianna,* in which actress-turned-singer Virginia Ramponi, modulating in the title role her "Let me die" lament ("Lasciatemi morire!"), inaugurated the most popular fixture of Italian opera for the next two generations.[31] Vincenzo also fostered the apprenticeship of a number of singers, both male and female, and heavily recruited them for either the new genre of *recitar cantando* or their instrumental skills.[32] He embraced the work of Salamone de' Rossi, the leading Jewish composer of the late Italian Renaissance, who wrote madrigals and pioneered the trio sonata and suite at court. (Traditionally, during many years of Vincenzo's reign, there were palace performances on Friday nights).[33]

In addition, Vincenzo paid for the lavish staging of the much-awaited pastoral drama *Il pastor fido* (*The Faithful Shepherd*), by Giovanni Battista Guarini (1538–1612), which he had wanted performed in Mantua at the time of his wedding to Eleonora in April 1584 but which would have to wait until 1598, when it was staged with elaborate intermezzi, dance, singing, and an up-to-date theatrical apparatus. This performance too was of great historical importance because it constituted the beginning of a remarkable triumph for the new genre of pastoral theater. Moving away from realistic actions, shepherds, shepherdesses, satyrs, and nymphs now expressed their angst over their (often) unrequited love in accents that all actors in Europe soon appropriated to great, long-lasting success.[34] And the new theatrical genre of commedia dell'arte would not by any means have reached the heights that it reached in Italy (and France) if Vincenzo had not felt sufficiently titillated by live performances to sponsor and pay all expenses of such companies as the

Fedeli—directed by Giovan Battista Andreini, noted playwright, actor, and stage director (and son of the most famous Italian Renaissance actress of her time, Isabella Andreini)—which every court, especially the French, wanted to host.[35] In this, Vincenzo was fully hands-on, and perhaps it was inevitable, given his performance-oriented personality and self-promotional skills, that "often he personally mimed, danced, sang, and recited masked on stage."[36]

Vincenzo also protected poets, many of whose books were dedicated to him. He was able to free the "mad" poet Torquato Tasso (1544–1595) from his prison at the Este court in Ferrara, then brought him to Mantua. He sponsored later poets, such as Gabriello Chiabrera (1552–1638), and an array of authors writing in the Marinisti vein. He approved the creation of a new university in Mantua to educate the children of the nobility, the Peaceful University of Mantua, which his son Ferdinando actualized a few years after Vincenzo's death.[37] Lastly, Vincenzo was a protoscientist, not so much because he personally performed experiments but because he sponsored the creation of a botanical garden, the second ever established in Italy. There he tried the new medicinal herbs coming from the New World, in addition to the known ones from the East. He also hired numerous chemists, who were given the task not only of producing all sorts of medical and alchemical concoctions needed at court but also of solving his persistent financial needs through the production of potable gold (*aurum potabile*) and silver and of aiding his military campaigns by producing gunpowder and noxious fumes. He earnestly tried to hire Galileo for the position of military architect after he had heard him in Padua explain the use of a military compass. Although the two men did not agree in the end on a yearly wage, Vincenzo was well aware of the importance of the mathematician's work, having had Galileo's predecessor in Padua as his tutor.[38] Money was never an issue. Whatever Vincenzo wanted, Vincenzo would have—and thus he inevitably fed the uncorrectable cash drain that plagued the Mantuan duchy until its demise.

Posterity has not been too kind to Vincenzo, and he has often been reproached for being an impulsive megalomaniac and a foolish squanderer.[39] But this fashioning *a ritroso*—essentially asking, since the duchy of Mantua underwent plunder and sack less than a quarter century after Vincenzo's death, could this loss have been avoided if he had left his state financially sound?—does not match the view of him held by his contemporaries. Let's take, for example, the report of the ambassador to the Venetian senate, Francesco Morosini, in 1608. Official reports to the Serenissima were customarily dry, factual, and perceptive, for their purpose was to assess issues by seeing their positive and negative sides, not to glorify or undercut them. In this vein Morosini stated:

> It can really be understood as most true what the Granduke of Tuscany goes around saying that his Lordship's [Vincenzo] youth is long lasting, since he is not slowing down in any of the tastes and pleasures that he used to enjoy when younger. He is a prince of large spirit and generous thoughts and so large in spending that he always finds himself in wants and needs; he is affable, benign and clement with his subjects, whose souls he has so much conciliated with his kindness that even though at times he weights down on them more than usual, they accept the burden willingly, thanks to the affection they have for him.[40]

Morosini's words seem to reflect what others also saw and remarked on: no matter how profligate the hedonistic Vincenzo was or seemed to be, and no matter how many new taxes he had to institute from time to time to cover the duchy's debts, by all accounts he had a cross generational appeal and was liked and trusted by his subjects. It could be that his flamboyant persona rubbed off on his constituency by making people in Mantua feel worldly too (the city had 40,000–45,000 inhabitants at the time and produced an income of around 20,000 ducats per year). It may be that where it mattered—the protection of the most indigent members of the Mantuan society—Duke Vincenzo was solicitous, a go-to savior with a common touch: he intervened efficiently during floods, weather-connected agricultural crises, and food shortages; he protected the production of gloves and lacework, chief industries in the duchy; and fostered local artisanal offerings. At the time of the flooding of the Po River in 1588 and later, following the drought that swept through Italy in 1591, he was politically efficacious and helped his subjects by improving the duchy's infrastructure through the creation of jobs in the new arsenal of Catena, a port built on one of the lakes surrounding Mantua. When necessary, he distributed bread by mixing the scarce wheat with rice.[41] He often provided free medicine to his subjects, as when he was described as being out of ointment for treating epilepsy because so many people were asking for it.[42] He also solicited medications and new remedies from outside Mantua for people at court.[43] He commissioned and richly decorated churches, donated relics of many saints, and introduced in Mantua the religious orders of the Theatine and the Hospitallers.[44] At the same time he did not let religious issues get the upper hand, even under papal pressure, much unlike his father, who had been brutal with those whom he believed to be creepy religious plotters. Vincenzo was able to keep as neutral as possible even at the shifty times of Pope Paul V's Venetian interdict—the result of a religious controversy involving church revenues—when he nimbly navigated muddled political waters that alternately rendered him crypto-French (his sister-in-law, Maria de' Medici, had married the King of France and Navarre, Henri IV), proto-Spanish (and how could he be otherwise in the fragile system of political alliances in Italy, with the Spaniards in the duchy's western border of Milan?), or make-believe neutral (as with Venice, from which most of the goods needed in Mantua came by waterways and where many of the exports went). Attentive to the political ramifications of his gestures, Vincenzo tried to conquer by charm and often got what was impossible for his father—who was much too aggressive and greedy—to be given.

Vincenzo even became the de facto master of style at the imperial court in Prague, where his recommendations on what fine art to buy and who was "in" artistically were continually sought by an eager and moneyed collector, Emperor Rudolph II. And although Vincenzo did order the creation of a ghetto in Mantua on November 7, 1602, following pressure from Pope Clement VIII (the gates were closed on January 30, 1610), he was nevertheless reproached more than once for being too tolerant with the Jewish community as a whole. He employed Jews (such as Salamone de' Rossi for musical entertainment and Leon Ebreo for staged plays), but forbade Jewish physicians to treat Christians and allowed for the burning of a Jewish octogenarian, Giuditta Franchetti, accused of witchcraft.[45] In the end, perhaps Vincenzo was just lucky, for he often left the burden of the state to his wife, Eleonora, who proved to be smart, resourceful, and skilled, and an impressive administrator, calmly able to smooth her husband's impulsive personality with good doses of Florentine levelheadedness.

On the other side of the coin, Vincenzo clearly did not seem to possess the military skills for which his ancestors were often praised, although he had stated that the dream of his life was "to show the world that he wanted to live and die as a soldier as my forebears did."[46] Although this may have been his ambition, he was hardly a fierce warlord. He never dazzled in the field, he was at times wrongheaded, and his three campaigns in Hungary terminated abruptly. Ingenious as Vincenzo was (he once used the very modern technology of biological warfare to end a siege) and even courageous in his sorties, he was not an attentive tactician. In fact, he could hardly keep his attention focused on a specific issue for any length of time. What inspired him was the yearning to be a savior of the faith, like the rabble army of crusaders populating his most beloved book, Torquato Tasso's *Jerusalem Delivered* (*Gerusalemme Liberata*, 1581), which rushed toward Palestine to reclaim Christian control over the "infidels" in the first "holy" war.[47] Looking at the issue under such a lens, it becomes easier to understand why Vincenzo took so much time before each departure to make sure he had the colors right for the uniforms of his tight coterie of fellow paladins and soldiers, and for the flag they were going to display. With dubious reliability, Vincenzo's crusades were triumphantly glossed by anonymous Mantuan historians as successful, even if their accomplishments were limited in scope. The international powers knew better, however, and Vincenzo never got any military recognition.

I quoted earlier Morosini's assessment of Vincenzo's extended youthfulness (*gioventù*). What Morosini precisely meant was well known to every courtier and gazetteer in Italy and perhaps Europe at the time: at whatever age, Duke Vincenzo behaved as a sexual profligate, a philanderer, and a rake, and was known both inside and outside his court for his many paramours, chosen from the nobility as well as from the lower classes. Vincenzo had no communication handicap with women and had children out of wedlock spread throughout Italy, from Mantua to Naples, and perhaps also abroad. In fact, he so enjoyed going out at night to visit the women he fancied that his wife's uncle, Grand Duke Ferdinando, writing from Florence, had to beg him to be prudent because he had heard of a man who was saying that he could sell the duke's life at will, since Vincenzo "was coming at night surreptitiously to his house to lay often with his stepdaughter."[48] The grand duke was not alone; even Vincenzo's own bishop in Mantua, Friar Francesco Gonzaga, found it necessary to write two letters scolding the duke for his scandalous sexual romps.[49] Vincenzo's dizzying array of feminine conquests knew no age boundary: he was just as happy with older women, such as Barbara Sanseverino, Countess of Sala, as he was with younger ones; with rich as well as poor. The list of women is long. As for his best-known liaisons, he was for years attached to Agnese del Carretto, who gave him a son,

Silvio, whom he recognized and moved to court to live with his legitimate children. Later in life Adriana Basile, a famous singer of the early opera, occupied his thoughts, and he lured her to Mantua from Naples together with her husband. He was rumored to have had a child with her. Less is known about the other women, such as one named Elena in Mantua and the unnamed Neapolitan noblewoman with whom he had a son, Francesco.[50]

Others knew of Vincenzo's fame as a heartbreaker and protected themselves or simply monetized that knowledge when it counted. For example, when Vincenzo called to his court the barely thirteen-year-old budding Roman soprano singer Caterina Martinelli, called La Romanina, who was scheduled to sing the title role in *Arianna* (she died before opening night), her father wrote that he was certifying through a doctor his daughter's virginity at departure and therefore would not allow her to stay at court. She ended up living under the protection of Claudio Monteverdi's wife in her lodgings, with Vincenzo's approval of the terms of the contract.[51] Even more telling is another episode from those years: Pope Paul V's response to Vincenzo's petition in 1607 to approve, give a pension, and confer indulgences to a knightly order that he desperately wanted to create in Mantua for the protection of the Catholic faith, the Order of the Redeemer (Ordine del Redentore), had a seemingly insurmountable codicil. The pope wished all knights to swear to keep their conjugal chastity before wearing the insignia of the new order. Vincenzo was taken aback: how could he make such a promise? As he explained, "In no way he would accept this obligation of promising conjugal chastity with a solemn vow and by swearing on it, knowing so well . . . how much worse would be the sin in case of transgression."[52] The creation of a Christian order could constitute for Vincenzo the ultimate redemption he was seeking (like many men of his time he had a deep religious bent, and he often mentioned his plan of ending his days in seclusion in the monastery of Camaldoli). Or perhaps it was just the ultimate display of his splashy, high-energy, self-assured exercise of power, as his portraits at the time by Frans Pourbus the Younger make evident. Either way, he could not agree to tie his hands with a vow that required monogamy and sexual restraint.

Vincenzo's connection to unbridled, licentious sexuality had become so taken for granted in the following centuries that when Giuseppe Verdi needed to Italianize the main character of his opera *Rigoletto*, because the original French model was proving politically dangerous, he found it natural to mold the figure of his lustful Duke on Vincenzo. He knew his man, for as in Victor Hugo's *The King Has Fun* on which the opera is based, for Vincenzo too "L'amour, c'est le soleil de l'ame" (Love is the sun of the soul).[53] Along the same lines, when the opera was staged in London under the direction of David McVicar in the late 1990s, the tenor Marcelo Álvarez played the duke in full frontal nudity. "Women are fickle like a feather in the wind" (La donna è mobile qual piuma al vento), the Duke callously sings in *Rigoletto*. Everyone in the audience knows, as every person who was acquainted with Vincenzo in his time also knew, that the feelings evoked must be those of the duke himself. As in *Rigoletto*, Vincenzo never felt as happy as when he could drink love on women's bosom ("Pur mai non sentesi felice appieno chi su quel seno non liba amore").[54]

As the years went by, no matter how restive and mischievous Vincenzo felt in spirit his body started to give up, an inconvenient reminder of a life lived to the fullest. There were recurrent fevers plaguing his days (fever was understood at that time to be a disease rather than a symptom of diseases), epic headaches, excruciating arthritic fits, violent coughing bouts, and disfiguring skin lesions. And as happens to many, including his contemporary Michel de Montaigne, Vincenzo was increasingly finding that his authority could now be contested more by his disobedient body than by his courtiers, and that his will could be flatly refused by the unwelcome vagaries of his sexual organ.[55] Unwilling to let go of his youthful ways, he fearlessly and proactively fought the passing of the years. In his make-believe world, he valiantly addressed ways to improve his skin going haywire with infections by asking renowned doctors for topical creams, and he sought immersion in water—mineral water and seawater, that is—as a way to tackle the (perhaps) parasitic pathogens that were making his immune system nonfunctional. Three chapters of this book will be concerned with the array of remedies that Vincenzo sought to stop the passing of time and get relief from what may have been constant pain or a low-grade fever plaguing his days.

Structure and Organization

I start Chapter 1 with a youthful episode, in fact a shocking one that spelled trouble—big trouble—for Vincenzo's self-esteem and could very well have set the stage for his future profligate ways. I examine Vincenzo's marriage at nineteen to Margherita Farnese, which had to be annulled within the customary three years of probation, as per church requirement, because it could not be consummated. Margherita was a rich, young, and appropriately chaste princess. Yet just a few days after the marriage ceremony, her body came to be perceived as deviant and anomalous. Doctors from various courts were asked to speedily converge on Mantua and Parma to give their opinion on what makes a female body typical, for Margherita's was not, due to a rebellious hymen that was making a joke of Vincenzo's marital caresses. In working through the problematics of normal/subversive, typical/monstrous, as applied to the female body, I address the medical discovery (actually, recovery) in the Renaissance of precise information about the constitutive elements of the female sexual apparatus and the emergence of a technical discourse on women's virginity that coexisted, and in fact complemented, the theological discussion that figured women's chastity euphemistically in terms of sealed entries, locked doors, and fenced gardens. As history tells us, a princess's body belongs to the state, because issues of succession hinge on its being potentially able to conceive. The reports of surgeons called on at the time to examine Margherita's unyielding body (and that of four other virgins used for anatomical comparison) thus constitute a windfall for scientific research into female anatomy—besides feeding political discourses on subjectification and control. In this context I examine the church's take on what makes a marriage valid, the politicians' schemes to guarantee an ordered succession, and the cultural hysteria coming from a woman's inconvenient "hyster."

Barely now twenty-one years old and his manly reputation scathed by the drama of the incomplete nuptials, Vincenzo sought to marry again, but the parents of his bride-to-be unexpectedly asked for proof of his virility. Vincenzo's supervised congress with a certified virgin to corroborate the proper functioning of his genitalia delivered so many juicy angles to an eager public looking for gossip that it is no surprise that it became the most famous sexual scandal of the Italian Renaissance—or so many cultural historians claim. I scrutinize it in this chapter not for its erotic frisson, nor because it perfectly fits a Foucauldian panoptic logic, but because it addresses the issue of female desire from a physical rather than a psychological point of view. The astonishingly detailed exit interviews of Vincenzo's virgin-for-hire could very well have served sexologist Alfred Kinsey and his later colleagues William Masters and Virginia Johnson, I argue, in understanding the nature of instinctive body reaction and the physiology of sexual response. This endlessly discussed event (was it staged in defiance or was it delirium?) shriveled Vincenzo's credibility in Italian courts. It made him an object of ridicule, and yet, needless to say, it paved the way for his subsequent well-deserved reputation as a ladies' man with a promiscuous agenda.

In Chapter 2, with Duke Vincenzo now in his thirties, an array of health problems—facial erysipelas, arthritis, and acute nasal catarrh—required the intervention of the famous Bolognese doctor Gaspare Tagliacozzi, known today as the father of plastic surgery (his book, the first ever on the subject, was dedicated to Vincenzo). "Beauty surgery" can very well be a modern preoccupation involving mostly women, but beauty culture was very much part of Renaissance philosophy, art, music, and literature. I address the novel use of plastic surgery for the repair and reconstruction of men's noses through an examination of its theological implications (is the surgeon imitating God in remaking man?), moral predicaments (can a slave provide missing parts?), political ramifications (does cosmetic surgery enable a ruler's personal transformation?) and medical shortcomings (is the pain worth it?). The cutting off of noses as punishment for adultery, prostitution, betrayal, unorthodox sexual choices, or just plain old malice and jealousy was not unusual in the early modern period, just as the so-called saddle nose visually testified to the presence in the bearer of a disease such as syphilis, lupus, or scrofula. In a society often described as increasingly violent, a missing nose was a mark of retribution: slashing off the enemy's nose in a duel rather than killing him outright was a choice too common, in township after township, to keep it under wraps. For aesthetic reasons, literature has often avoided talk of noses. Petrarch did not like them and repeatedly (or purposely) forgot to mention Laura's nose in his precise catalog of her beauties, unlike Shakespeare, who was quite taken by Cleopatra's nose. We do not have to wait for Freud to establish the double meaning of the nose in culture (as in the movie *Roxanne:* "With that nose you can satisfy two women at the same time!"). Already in his book on physiognomy, Giambattista della Porta had implied that one's nose was sufficient to understand not only character and disposition but also sexual attributes.[56] At a time when artists were emphasizing the importance of harmony and décor, it is not surprising that doctors began to put their skills into beautifying facial features—historically facial operations may have been the first case of elective surgery—even though the operation could be excruciatingly painful and the risk of subsequent infection high.

In Chapter 3 I look at why comfort cures were so important at a time when most diseases were chronic and most medicines, even if they worked somewhat, often had only palliative effects. Famously affected for generations by chronic ailments, the Gonzaga of Mantua were aficionados of thermal spas, from Porretta, near Bologna, known for curing gastric disorders, to Villa, near Lucca, which they used to address digestive troubles. Not satisfied with Italian baths, Duke Vincenzo made a point of traveling all over Europe to cure his various morbidities, which ranged from tuberculosis and arthritis to laryngeal catarrh and bacterial skin infections. By examining an assortment of letters and documents, this chapter retraces the duke's repeated, customized visits to spas and geothermal mineral waters in Italy and abroad, such as Spa in Flanders, Innsbruck in Tyrol, and Pozzuoli in Italy. Hot or cold healing springs were Vincenzo's favorite place to detoxify, enjoy life, live large, pause for some peccadillo—whether it was wine, gourmet delicacies, or sex—act on his fantasies, and gamble fortunes, all in the hope, perhaps, of finding a miraculous fountain of youth.

Although it is generally understood that most baths were shut down in Italy during the early modern period—often as a result of hygienic measures taken by local governments in the aftermath of the diffusion of syphilis and of pernicious contact dermatitis—this chapter argues that the culture of baths as therapeutic places addressing both the need for leisure and the care regimes of the middle to upper classes (although poor people also used baths) was very much alive. Like today, in the early modern period thermal spas welcomed patients with an assortment of personalized treatments, such as scrubs, mud baths, herb therapies, moisturizing oils, stress-relieving steams, and body balms. Most of all, it was mineral water, whether the prescription was to drink it early in the morning on an empty stomach directly from bubbling fountains or to bathe in springs, that drove health-seeking pilgrims to various locations in Italy and abroad and created a long-lasting philosophy of relaxation, festivity, and occasionally political intrigue. Such was the case of Vincenzo's repeated visits to the spas.

In Chapter 4 I follow Duke Vincenzo's search for a biostimulator to cure his legendary restlessness, for he was now in his late forties and was experiencing amatory difficulties, despite a surfeit of opportunities. It is true that his early troubles at the time of the wedding to Margherita Farnese had been powerfully vindicated by the robust and salacious sexual reputation he had constructed throughout the years, but aging was not making Vincenzo aware of the virtues of abstinence either. His was an operatic life consumed at the edge of scandal alerts, one not exactly to be parsed under the covers of discretion or inhabited by the reality of restraint. I will look at the events that surrounded the duke's hunt for a remedy to counter his andropause (or perhaps simply to indulge his hedonism), which made him send an unknown apothecary, Evangelista Marcobruno, on a secret two-year journey by coach, boat, galleon, mule, llama, and foot from Italy to Spain, and then to the New World, all the way down to Ecuador, Peru, and Bolivia, to find a Viagra-like remedy. What Vincenzo wanted had a simple name: *gusano*. It was a Spanish word with the widest meaning: worm, vermin, earthworm, spider worm, caterpillar. Years earlier, following his (false) voyage along the coast of Brazil, Amerigo Vespucci had described a nature-enhancing bug that shameless local women used to invigorate their men's genitals. The quest for this "bug" is at the center of the chapter, for Vincenzo Gonzaga was notoriously a Don Juan on the loose, all appetite and imagination, a man for whom it was psychologically imperative to keep demonstrating that he could successfully exercise his libido even as age was advancing. Thus Vincenzo sent his apothecary to the Andes in the hope of addressing for good the physical limitations imposed by his andropause. Ravishment fantasies inform both the apothecary's penetration into the virgin's territory of Peru and the prince's narcissistic desire for youthful exploits.

Vincenzo Gonzaga's final illness did not last long. As a contemporary historian wrote, the duke

> fell ill in February with a fever so acute accompanied by pain on his side and such an obstinate mass of catarrh that in less than four days he was already reduced to the extreme. The entire city humbly sent public and deeply felt prayers to God for the health of its excellent ruler, and indeed he improved so much that his doctors, judging him no longer in danger, allowed the convalescent to drink and eat his usual dinner. . . .

> But then a new fever assaulted him and in brief he again was reduced to the extreme. He then . . . disposed of his temporal things; after that, he prepared himself to the eternal ones.[57]

We do not have a catalog of the therapies or holistic cures that Vincenzo underwent in those final days to address his lethal puzzle of maladies, but if we can take as guidance the list of remedies tried out to succor his wife, Eleonora de' Medici, when one year earlier she suffered an apoplectic fit that left her stuttering and with a distorted mouth, we know that they were bewilderingly many. In week one and after the usual treatment with purging and massaging, Eleonora was given, for example, salted cinnamon water and nut pastes applied to the root of her tongue and palate. Then she had to imbibe rosemary water with liquid theriac, the nape of her neck was seared, and heated cups were placed on her left side. Next she was administered oil and shavings of human skulls, shaved horns of rhinoceros and unicorn, shaved bones of deer, grated nail of elk, coral-derived salts, and a set of "ordinary and extraordinary" anointments. All this not being enough, Eleonora had a "sneezer" placed over her head and again underwent enemas and cupping. This is not even a full inventory.[58]

So what bothered the Duke of Mantua to the very end? Let's recap. In terms of personality, Vincenzo Gonzaga was a most restless and hyperactive man, cramming his days so full that he had no time left to reflect on his mortality. If Ritalin had been invented in the sixteenth century, I would have no story to tell. Vincenzo was not a dexterous politician, but he was not a dunce either. In fact, he was often wise and, when he wasn't, was able to select smart bureaucrats to guide him away from questionable political strategies. He had the emotional intelligence and gentle grin that made him connect suavely with women and respond with compassion to his subjects' smarts and grievances. He followed intuitively his heart and was not known for being capricious. He loved to live, and indeed he lived fully, obsessively fully. His exquisite patronage of all artistic forms, from music and painting to theater and literature; his aspiration to systematize nature through acquisition of *mirabilia* (marvels) and, more constructively, through botanical investigations; his intellectual curiosity; and his emotional generosity made him already legendary in his lifetime.

In the end, what bothered Vincenzo was essentially that he had to let go. Although he prepared himself for the darkness that was to engulf him, as the procession of priests and friars before his deathbed testify, and although he had the time to tell his loved ones, legitimate and illegitimate, one last time how much he cherished them, it was difficult for a man with the outsized personality of a duke who loved to behave like a king ("Duca Re") to abandon a world constructed as an orchestrated denial of death. At fifty Vincenzo was not yet broken down, still embedded in the world he had created of artifice and illusion. Betting on God's help, he vowed to go on a pilgrimage to Jerusalem to visit the Holy Sepulchre.[59]

Thus, I surmise, he chose to define himself for posterity with a last bravado choice, a sword. It had been the icon of salvation and retribution that had saturated his youth when, confident and self-aware, he had immersed himself in chivalric stories idolizing crusaders splitting the skulls of the infidels with their avenging blades. And yes, there was also that other matter informing the theatrics of his early life and for which he had been endlessly teased, even by his own father—the proper functioning of his more personal "sword," which had to be checked and rechecked by doctors of more than four Italian courts and two Italian universities, not for natural but for pseudopolitical reasons, thus compromising forever his sense of manhood. True to his aesthetic sensibilities, it had to be a jewel-encrusted sword that would accompany him now to his resting place. Facing his death uncertainly and with his body shutting down, in the end Vincenzo seems to have chosen to channel his psychic energies, his libido, his anxiety, and indeed his aggression—one last time—into a self-aggrandizing, megalomaniac emblem of the man he wanted to be: the duke who has it all. He, the inveterate pleasure seeker, was the last of the entire Gonzaga line to personify how erotic the allure of power can be.

1

The Virgin Cure

Manual Exams and Early Modern Surgeons

> It is one of the superstitions of the human mind
> To have imagined that virginity could be a virtue.
> —Voltaire, *La pucelle d'Orleans*

> A husband will be a wife's best doctor.
> —Poggio Bracciolini, *Facezie*

SOMETIME IN MARCH 1581, Vincenzo Gonzaga I, future fourth Duke of Mantua and Monferrato and munificent sponsor of art, music, and theater—a Renaissance prince in every sense of the word—realized that he had a physical difficulty that required secrecy or, alternatively, a creative and perhaps radical solution. Historians are in agreement today that this particular ducal predicament came out of the blue. The nineteen-year-old Vincenzo had just married in Parma the not yet fourteen-year-old Margherita Farnese (1567–1643) and was looking forward to bringing his bride to the duchy that he would eventually inherit from Duke Guglielmo as his only son. The bride was the daughter of Maria d'Aviz of Portugal (1541–1577), whose early death caused her child to be placed under the care of her paternal grandmother, Margaret of Habsburg, the illegitimate daughter of Charles V. Margherita's father, Alessandro Farnese (1545–1592), was a renowned military man who had fought for the Holy League at Lepanto and had become a successful governor-general of Flanders under Philip II of Spain. Once the day of marriage was set, Margherita was allowed to leave her home in Namur, Flanders, where she was living, for the Farnese fiefdom of Parma, where her grandfather Ottavio, the current Farnese duke, was ready to give her in marriage to the future Gonzaga duke.[1]

On his part, Vincenzo liked the idea of marrying and felt that the event would mark his way out from under his father's iron fist and from his father's unforgiving attitude toward him and all-over miserly predisposition—his ticket to adulthood. By all accounts he had been smitten by Margherita's loveliness. At their first encounter at a dinner party in nearby Piacenza one month before the wedding ceremony, he had judged her beauty superior to that of the portrait he had been sent, or so was reported by the ducal counselor, Aurelio Zibramonti, to Duke Guglielmo back in Mantua: "His Highness called me while he was eating and whispered in my ear that he was very much satisfied with his lady bride, for he liked her very much and loved her enormously, because in person she is even better than in the portrait."[2] The wedding was lavish.[3] Later that evening Margherita could not refrain from mentioning to her lady-in-waiting how pleased she was with such a noble groom: "as she entered her bed and while she waited for her prince, she called Signora Bianca . . . and told her that she thanked God infinitely for having been given such a suitable husband and so much to her liking."[4] Given the pair's expectations, everything led to the assumption that this marriage would reasonably endure—and not just in political and dynastic terms. Yet days went by, and the couple was unable to get Duke Guglielmo's permission to come to Mantua.

There was in fact a predicament in the couple's bedroom that from the start seemed to border on the tragicomic, so much so that Vincenzo soon found the courage to tell Marcello Donati—his preceptor, court physician, and future ducal counselor—that he had been unable to make a wife of his bride after repeated attempts. This could have been a case of psychogenic impotence affecting young newlyweds, one that could be resolved, as Michel de Montaigne had recently recommended, with patience and relaxation.[5] Donati soon realized, however, that the couple's problem was more complicated than that and found it proper to inform Margherita's grandfather and ad hoc tutor, Duke Ottavio.[6] No official explanation in the meantime was given for Vincenzo's uncommon stay in his bride's duchy, even though courtiers all over Italy were whispering that some unexpected health issues had abruptly surfaced. Soon it became known that Duke Ottavio had asked the most renowned surgeon of the day, Girolamo Fabrici d'Acquapendente (Hieronymus Fabricius ab Aquapendente), professor of surgery and anatomy at the University of Padua and by all accounts a most sedentary surgeon, to please rush to Parma for a consult. The impasse, everybody presumed from the start (and why not, given the male-friendly bent of such a report), was coming from Margherita, for Vincenzo, no matter his young age, had already launched for himself a solid reputation as a sexual profligate and womanizer, a reputation that in the coming decades would establish him as a true lothario.

At the time of her marriage on March 2, "May had not yet bloomed in her," Marcello Donati had remarked metaphorically on the subject of Margherita's childish physical appearance and physiological status in a letter to Duke Guglielmo, to whom he began to explain after first interviewing Vincenzo what was going on (or rather, what was not going on) in the newlyweds' bedroom.[7] Although consummation of marriage in the early modern period in Italy was usually allowed only when a girl had reached the age of menarche, this was not necessarily the case for noble families, whose dynastic alliances were often officially sealed soon after heirs—male or female—were born or, in any case, by the time they reached their teens. In instances in which a wedding was to take place before the girl had attained physical maturation, her parents would often request that she be kept within the paternal household until the time was deemed appropriate for consummation, which in the middle and upper classes meant the bride's physical passage from the father's to the husband's household. Margherita had thus been joined in marriage before she was technically out of childhood. Being a physician, Donati knew that a menstrual discharge signified that the woman's genitals were wholly formed; lack of it could be understood by him as natural at the present time due to the bride's age, as his letter hints, but abnormal if it lasted.

To be sure, Donati did not find Vincenzo's inability to conquer his child bride's hymen worrisome. From the start, he was confident that the problem was caused neither by a lack of desire on the part of the young prince to perform his conjugal duty nor by some physiological impossibility on his part. Still, just to be reassured, Vincenzo's sexual organ was examined in a state of both repose and performance, and although Donati with a perfect masculinist spirit (or perhaps with a faultless courtesan mien) did not fail to note on paper the notable dimension of the prince's apparatus, he concluded that size per se was not a problem in successfully performing the act, even though in the best of all worlds, he stated, it would have been better for the prince to possess a more contained instrument ("*cotale*," as he puts it). On March 15, less than two weeks after the wedding ceremony and following a lengthy vaginal exam of Margherita, at which other unnamed doctors were also present, Donati felt ready to send his conclusions to Duke Guglielmo.[8] As he explained in his matter-of-fact letter, "Although many are the reasons why a man's member cannot come close to a woman, still, leaving aside all that, I will concern myself with the problem that in our case has been deemed appropriate. The eye be my witness that there is a fleshy excrescence and this, my Lord, has to be cut off because, being punctured, all our doctors conclude that it wholly impedes the entry of a man's member."[9] Some methods to enlarge the opening of the vulva were tried right away, and we know from other letters to Guglielmo that screams could be heard coming from Margherita's bedroom. Then pessaries were tried.[10] It is at this point that Fabrici was called in by Duke Ottavio for a consultation.

In this chapter I use the issues exposed by the very articulated hymen of Princess Margherita Farnese to work through the critical imbrications of tangible virginity, cultural chastity, and married sexuality when political necessity demands accurate observation and fitting answers. First, though, I will trace the emergence of a scientific discourse on women's virginity in Italy in the early modern period and focus on the work of some professors of anatomy, such as the previously mentioned Fabrici and his predecessors at the University of Padua, whose research has since set standards in the field of human physiology, particularly female. I will then turn to the case of Margherita, because here an exception to conventions surrounding the duo of chastity/virginity helps explain its significance for culture. The events that surrounded the couple's relationship expose a set of interrelated issues central to the Italian family, church, and polity, as well as some medical concerns on how to categorize and define physical virginity in the first place. The intent of course was to read the body of women independently of women—that is, as a commodity meant for heterosexual use, whose objective scrutiny could bypass any female performance of chastity.

Locating Virginity

First, then, let's define the issue. As Mozart has it sung in *Così fan tutte*, "The faith of women is like the phoenix from Arabia. That it exists, everyone says; where, nobody knows."[11] For "faith" presumably Mozart had in mind female chastity, although his desire to know where such a faith resides makes us think that he believed there to be a location to this secret. And indeed in culture, virginity and chastity are often confused with each other, even though the first is a physical condition that only experts can read in the female body, and the second is a psychological state that anybody can decipher or interrogate, making it impossible to trust. For church canonists, such as John Chrysostom, virgins should not talk to men or sit next to them or laugh in their presence, because the veil of chastity does not need a physical contact to be destroyed; the verbal one suffices. As does the visual, since a woman seen is a woman who belongs to everybody.[12] Chrysostom identified virginity with a behavior rather than a physical state: the veil to which he referred (others will talk of a seal, cloister, sign, lock, enclosed garden) is a moral one. For the church fathers as well as for many self-appointed moralists through the ages, the boundary between the physical and the moral are never well established when a woman is at issue.

Spying on the female body has always been a well-practiced activity. For the natural philosopher and playwright Giambattista della Porta, for example, it was easy to recognize whether a girl was a virgin by having her drink a concoction of black amber and wine. If she was intact, she could keep the liquid for a long while; if not, she had to evacuate it immediately.[13] Likewise, uroscopists in the Middle Ages claimed left and right to be able to discover whether a girl was a virgin based on a urine test. According to Albertus Magnus in *De secretis mulierum*, the urine of virgins is clear and brilliant; if it is clear but golden, the woman will not remain so for long, since the yellow color is an indication of heat in her body and thus of a strong sexual desire. The urine of nonvirgins is turbid, and were one to look closely, he wrote, male seed is visible at the bottom.[14] To be sure, uroscopy as a diagnostic or prognostic tool was already waning in the early modern period, although not in popular medicine; doctors were still being presented in the woodcuts of the period as holding glass flasks.[15] According to the Roman doctor Giulio Mancini, virginity could be ascertained in a much simpler way by checking the color of a woman's labia, allowing simulated virginity to be mercifully unmasked by any prying eye.[16] The most popular way of checking virginity—the nipple, people believed, changed color when a maiden was deflowered—"is absurd in the extreme," wrote Laurent Joubert, chancellor of the medical school of Montpellier, whose book, translated into Italian, was a popular one in pharmacies. Likewise, he snickered at the notion that a woman was no longer chaste when her nose's tip opened slightly or when a string around her neck did not have the same span as one measuring the face lengthwise.[17] In short, although virginity can only be confirmed when it is no longer there, it has to be investigated, because its unchecked absence threatens patriarchal control over a woman's body. But virginity also has to be ephemeral, once it has signified the male fantasy of first, and hopefully definitive, possession.

Given that until very recently it was culturally important to be a virgin or to appear like one, it is not surprising that women knew many secrets to simulate a material virginity and to act out a behavior in front of doctors, fathers, brothers, husbands, tutors, and priests that reflected what was convenient, or necessary, for them to show.[18] Women also knew how to repair their lack of chastity, if necessary, through the construction of a new virgin body, and there were plenty of doctors, midwives, female healers, *materculae,* herbalists, and charlatans ready to offer hymenoplasty procedures suitable to any case. A medieval recipe from the School of Salerno, for example, recommended putting a leech the day before a bride's wedding in the external part of her sexual organ, taking care not to let the animal penetrate too deeply ("vulvam ne forte subintret"). In the hours preceding the consummation a crust would form; the subsequent friction during sexual contact would assure that blood would flow out, creating a notion of virginity sufficient to satisfy any peering eye.[19] Jacopo Berengario da Carpi argued, however, that only stupid men do not know the difference and denounced "some shrewd women who corrugate the neck of the matrix [womb] with astringents, and then through fraudulent means let the blood out so that they appear virgin to the dim-witted."[20] The herbalist Caterina Sforza, writing arguably on the side of women, offered another technique to renew the intimate parts of a "corrupted" woman, teaching her how to both behave like a virgin and intervene with potions to make "what we women prefer to call nature" so tight that everyone, including experts, would have no doubt regarding her virginal status.[21] Guglielmo da Saliceto's advice was to insert in the vaginal canal a kind of primitive condom made of a dove's entrails filled with blood. Upon contact with the male organ, the condom would break and blood would pour out to the general satisfaction of everybody involved.[22] In other words, the ocular proof had to be simulated in every which way because in Western culture, the woman to admire, and therefore to marry—the future *mater familiae*—was required to have a legible body: impenetrable before the marriage and penetrable at leisure after, and this impenetrability had to be demonstrated in a visual manner, independent of women's will, for use both personal—the case of the husband—and social—the case of the extended household clan—because issues of legitimacy, property, and propriety required a continuous monitoring of her material purity.[23] A problem of *hyster*, whether perceived or real, was cause, to say it appropriately, of hysterics.

That there was a tangible seal—a physical mark to shut the passage from the before to the after in the female body and thus to mark the difference between a child and an adult, a maiden and a wife—had surprisingly been of scarce importance in culture until the early modern period. The hymen, in fact, had been a concern, a "sign," only for Arab physicians. With the exception of the Roman doctor Soranus of Ephesus (A.D. 98–138), who in any case denied its existence, Western medicine had not yet talked about it. Indeed, the female anatomy of the pelvic area in all its constituents—sacrum, coccyx, uterus, mons veneris, frenulum clitoridis, vulva clitoridis, urethra, nymphae, and hymen—was hardly common knowledge. Rhazes (end of the ninth and beginning of the tenth century), Avicenna (eleventh century), and Averroes (twelfth century) spoke of the hymen without naming it. In *De animalibus*, Albertus Magnus (thirteenth century) noticed a membrane at the mouth of the womb in virgins, which could be destroyed in the sexual act, he wrote, with the result that a small amount of blood is lost.[24] For Mondino de' Luzzi (fourteenth century), there were two enclosures within the female organ: "the small labia to protect from cold, and a bit more inside, at the height of the cervix, a thin veil."[25]

We have to wait for the fifteenth-century doctor Michele Savonarola, professor of medicine in Padua and Ferrara, to leave aside euphemisms and speak directly and for the first time of a hymen. The neck of the uterus, he argued, is covered by a thin membrane called a hymen, which is broken when defloration occurs to allow for the blood to flow out.[26] *Pace* Savonarola, the general tendency of medical practitioners was to remain imprecise as to what effectively one could see in the vaginal orifice until the 1540s, when public anatomy lessons took off as (occasionally) theatrical events (often reserved for the Carnival season and accompanied by music), and exploring the body inch by inch became an honorable activity, one often eagerly sponsored by local administrations because it attracted students as well as visitors.[27] Andreas Vesalius, professor of anatomy and surgery at the University of Padua, wrote of having found the hymen of two virgins during a trip to Tuscany: that of a nun, who thanks to her status one presumed to be a virgin and whom he dissected in Florence, and that of a seventeen-year-old girl, whose cadaver had been stolen from the cemetery in Pisa so that he could analyze it. She was surely a virgin, the anatomist offered, because she was a hunchback, and thus it was improbable that any man would have wanted to take her "virtue."[28] His desire to see specifically virgins must have been longstanding, however, because he also reports that one of his students had earlier stolen the cadaver of a six-year-old girl from a Paduan cemetery so that he could study it.[29] Still, although he recognized the hymen, Vesalius was unwilling to state that all women had it, since it could not be found in animals and because two examples were not sufficient in his judgment to generalize a principle.[30] Indeed, his often reproduced illustrations of the female pudendum do not show a hymen. Gabriele Falloppio (or Falloppia), also a professor of anatomy and surgery in Padua from 1551, recognized the hymen as well and spoke of a fibrous membrane placed transversally, immediately after the urethra, which closes the vaginal canal and breaks upon sexual contact.[31] Later in the century, Joubert offered a remarkably precise description of this anatomical part:

> I find that behind the conduit of the bladder, through which the urine empties into the large canal, there is on each side of it a fleshly membrane in the shape of a half-circle, and that both of them join to close the large canal. Their conjunction is aided by a certain viscosity resembling the gowl that collects and sticks the eyelids together. It is not a continuous membrane, as several have believed, but two contiguous ones joined with some sort of glue, and by means of which the large canal is slightly closed so that when the menses happen along, a small passageway is made in the very center, through which the menstrual blood beads and drips out.[32]

But even after the authoritative intervention on the subject of a number of anatomists, the hymen continued to be a phantom anatomical attribute for many in the medical profession, although midwives—by profession and gender more attuned to the particularities of the female body, even though their knowledge was willingly excluded from the academic world—never had any doubt about its presence.[33] Orazio Augenio, professor of theoretical medicine at Padua, denied that it could be empirically observed: "Nullo certo signo distingui possunt virgines a mulieribus."[34] Realdo Colombo, who briefly succeeded Vesalius in the post of surgery at Padua, doubted that every woman had a vaginal "flap," and when one had it, he hypothesized, carnal knowledge could not occur.[35] Girolamo Mercurio, a Dominican priest and obstetrician who had studied in Padua with the renowned physician Ercole Sassonia, admitted that many doctors were not sure of the hymen's presence in all women, but he was convinced that it did exist, because many midwives were saying so and because he had personally seen "that hymen so celebrated, so beautiful, so well done, so polished" (quell'imeneo tanto celebrato, così bello, ben fatto e compito) by doing the autopsy of a virgin in Bologna. But when he described it, calling to his aid the animal world in order to come up with a convincing parallel ("like the crest of chicks"), he surprisingly confounded it with the small labia.[36] Ambroise Paré, first surgeon and chamberlain to the French king Charles IX, wrote that he had once fortuitously found the hymen in a seventeen-year-old virgin, but he had searched long for it, without ever finding one, in women "of all ages from three to twelve, of all that I had under my hands in the Hospital of Paris."[37] Even as late as 1651 Nicholas Culpeper, a most prolific physician and botanist in London, was unwilling to declare that all women had a hymen and preferred to "suspend my own judgment till more years brings me more experience."[38]

No matter the confusion surrounding the presence of a film, lid, or flap in all virginal women, in their practice many surgeons had occasionally seen cases of imperforate hymens and had in fact intervened with the knife to permit sexual relations or, in more problematic and urgent cases, to allow the outflow of menstrual blood. Even though men's digital examination of female pudenda was frowned on until well into the nineteenth century, when the need arose we know that women, often urged by their male relatives, solicited and welcomed the searching eye and speculum of surgeons (Fig. 4). As Joubert offers,

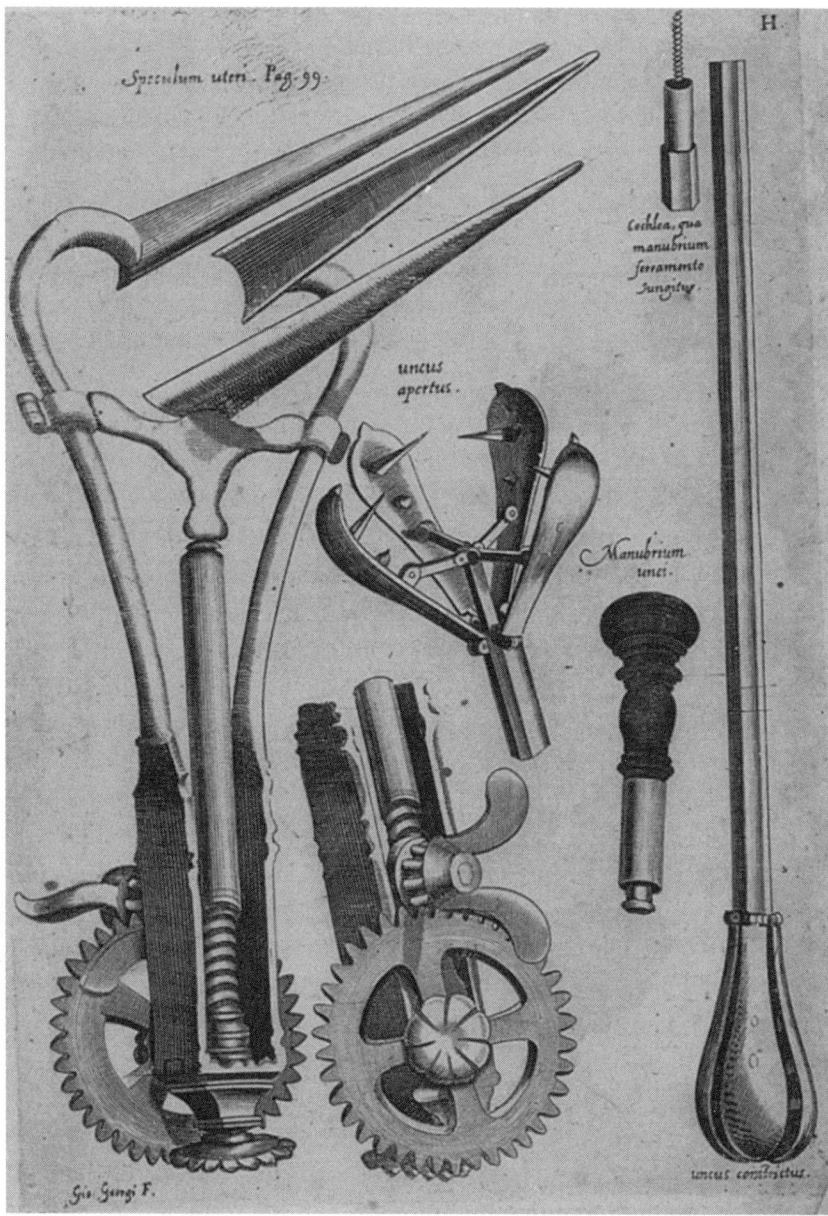

Fig. 4. Girolamo Fabrici d'Acquapendente, "Speculum Uteri," in *Opera chirurgica in duas partes divisas,* 1619. (Photo: Biblioteca Vincenzo Pinali, Sezione Antica, Università di Padova, Padua.)

there are many proper and decent women who, in order for some ailments or condition of their womb to be more precisely recognized, will indeed allow surgeons (for a reason that convinces them to do so) to uncover their shameful parts and, in the presence of a physician, examine them closely with a speculum, which permits us to see right to the bottom of the passageway.[39]

In some circumstances, vaginal occlusion could be resolved without a surgical intervention, as in the case of a servant girl recounted almost facetiously by Girolamo Fabrici, who had succeeded Falloppio in 1562 as professor of anatomy and surgery at Padua, a position that he kept for almost fifty years: "many students tried to make love to her, but I told her that when she wanted to get married, it was better for her to come to me, for I would have made it possible. She did not come, however, because I believe that she found somebody else more anatomical than me to break her hymen."[40] Notice the winking and hardly scientific style with which the famous professor, a recognized father of embryology and "almost" discoverer of the circulation of the blood, recounted this anecdote.[41]

Later in his career Fabrici had an artist painstakingly illustrate in color and in detail the "thin skin that is called hymen" by juxtaposing the pudendum of a virgin (the drawing—the first I know of on the subject—shows the hymen with the prepuce above and the small labia below) with that of an older woman who had given birth to many children (the drawing shows the typical opening of the uterus in such cases) (Fig. 5, upper and lower illustration). He also had the image of a hypertrophic hymen drawn, in which case the vagina would clearly need reconstruction for the woman to be able to engage in sex (Fig. 6).[42] In his printed work, unlike the earlier case I just cited, Fabrici used appropriate technical language in describing the complicated case history of "an imperforate virgin, called by the vulgar people one with a lid" (coperchiata), a case that, he confessed, was so unusual that he had seen it only once in his forty-three years as a surgeon. Many doctors had tried to treat this woman in every possible way, thinking that her symptoms and pain meant problems with her articulations, Fabrici wrote, but only he was able to address that vaginal malformation with a precise cut of the membrane, when it looked as though nothing else would work:

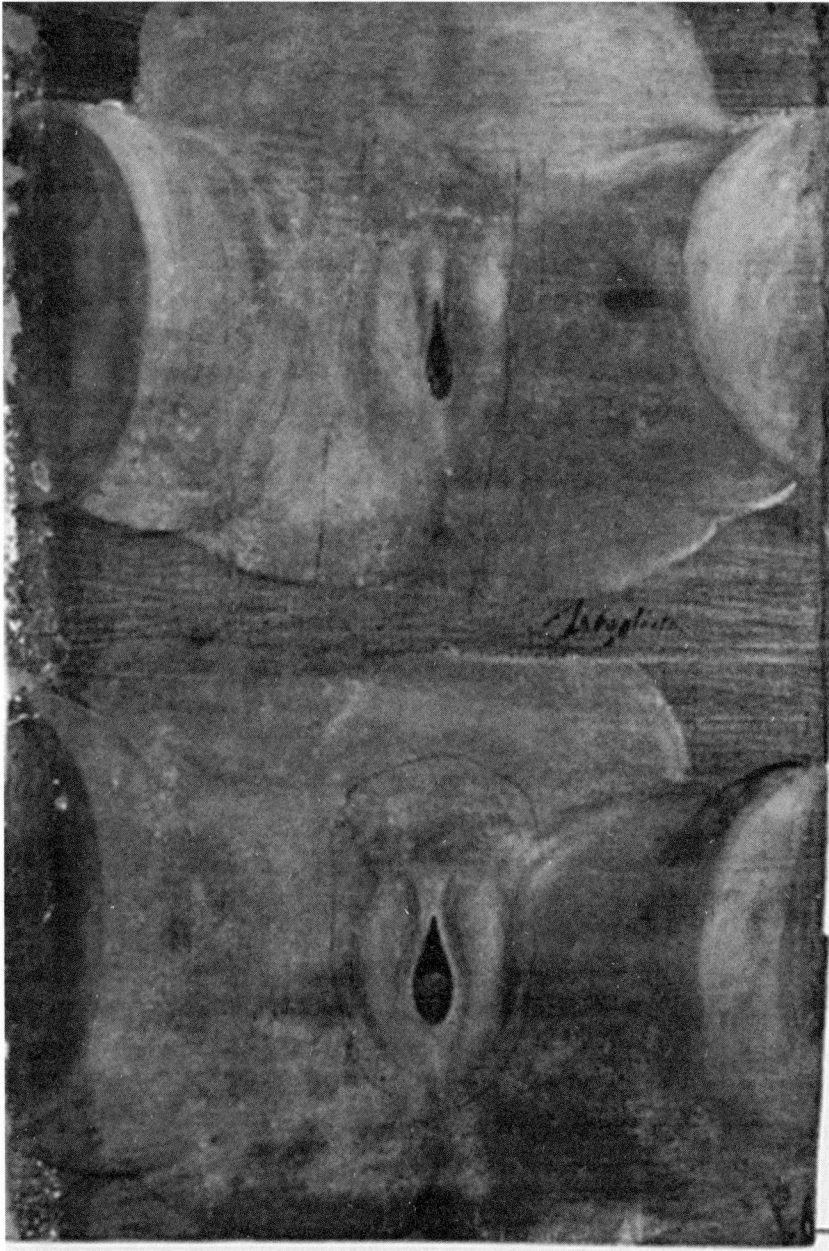

Fig. 3. Girolamo Fabrici d'Acquapendente, "Rari 117.25," in *De anatomia abdominis et partium in eo contentarum*. (Photo: Biblioteca Nazionale Marciana, Venice.)

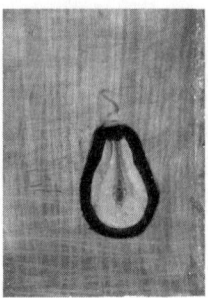

Fig. 6. Girolamo Fabrici d'Acquapendente, "Rari 117.26," in *De anatomia abdominis et partium in eo contentarum*. (Photo: Biblioteca Nazionale Marciana, Venice.)

I went to her finally, when it seemed that she was already close to death. I saw the problem with my own eyes, and with a simple cut I separated the membrane. Immediately a large amount of thick, viscous, rusty-colored, and fetid blood flowed out, and almost by miracle she found herself freed of all pain.... This is the surgery which—skillfully and with huge success—I used on that virgin, and on her imperforate hymen.[43]

Examining a Princess's Pudendum

Fabrici's skill had been sorely tested just a few years earlier by the case involving his most prestigious clients, the dukes of the Gonzaga family in Mantua and of the Farnese family in Parma. He had not yet published his observations on the hymen then (his *Opera omnia* would come out only at the end of his career, in 1617), but it was clear that his studies in embryology and obstetrics were leading him in that direction. It was with a sure sense of his expertise, therefore, that he accepted Ottavio Farnese's call to uncover the reasons behind Margherita's unbreakable hymen. Fabrici arrived in haste in Parma on April 3.[44] After careful examination of the princess's pudendum, he found that there was a kind of veil in her private parts that prevented penetration, a problem exacerbated by the fact that, he surmised, the patient was so young: "that membrane called hymen, which all virgins have, ... in this one is inordinately fleshy, and besides her nature is small because of her young age."[45] He decided to forgo surgery and prescribed, more conservatively, dilation of Margherita's vaginal canal. Just to be sure, the chair of surgery at the University of Bologna, Giulio Cesare Aranzi (or Aranzio), was called in to give his opinion. In agreement with Fabrici, he performed some cuts on the vaginal opening, but the unfortunate result, as it was later lamented, was to make it callous and in a sense more intractable.[46] In the end, Margherita was left with a thoroughly inflamed vagina, whereas her hymen remained unconquered.[47] Thus the issue became political.

In Western culture the possession of a hymen has typically given worth to a girl and has facilitated family and dynastic alliances, but a married woman with a hymen has been deemed a thorough aberration, because in canon law a marriage is invalid unless it is consummated.[48] Margherita's virginity, "such that no virile member, even one made of iron, could penetrate it," as the Mantuan physician Cesare Pendasio remarked in his scientific opinion on the case, soon ended up signifying nothing.[49] As with the Virgin Queen, Elizabeth—like Margherita, she was rumored to have had a physical abnormality—when "patriarchy creates a need for virgins, the perspective shifts when virgins themselves theorize the process."[50] With Margherita, the prized virgin's intact body turns into the abnormal body of the spouse, for the battle continuously lost by the prince of Mantua with a fourteen-year-old hymen ridicules his virility and sense of masculinity; more importantly, it exposes the Mantuan duchy to political calculations. It is impossible to determine a posteriori whether the source of the problem was Margherita's lack of a vaginal canal or whether it was an inadequate vaginal development (vaginal atresia or aplasia). The fear on the part of the Gonzaga was that the congenital malformation was hiding a deeper ovarian syndrome, which could portend a lack of pregnancies for Margherita.[51] The duchy of Mantua, lacking a second heir (succession in the Mantua duchy was exclusively along the male line), would have been at risk of passing to the Gonzaga Nevers, the French side of the family, or to the cadet side of the Gonzaga of Guastalla.[52] The Gonzaga began rethinking their end of the deal: to be sure, the bride had brought a formidable dowry to the marriage, and the idea of giving it back (or partially back) to the Farnese as per contract was unpalatable in Mantua, but the crisis had to be tackled.[53] More to the point, it was necessary to regain control over a woman's body that was refusing to be "stamped," because the issue was calling undue attention to other well-known physical disabilities circulating among the Gonzaga—some, embarrassingly visible, such as Duke Guglielmo's hunchback.

We have arrived at this point at stage three of our family saga. Let me briefly summarize how we got here. In the days immediately following the wedding ceremony, courtiers and doctors were aware of the trouble in the prince's bedroom but judged that the marriage remained unconsummated because of the bride's extremely young age and because the predicament could be psychological: one could think of a form of vaginismus on the part of Margherita and of clumsiness or immaturity on the part of Vincenzo. Within two weeks, however, the crisis had entered stage two, as the case of the *intacta virgo* began to be redefined as physiological. The impediment was real, the physicians of both the Farnese and the Gonzaga now agreed, the bride needed to be examined, and Fabrici and Aranzi were called to Parma for a specialized medical consultation. The precise cure, however, became a point of controversy, for some surgeons, like Donati, judged the predicament easily solvable with a procedure we would today call a hymenectomy, while others, like Fabrici, preferred a less drastic solution, hoping that nature would cooperate in due time and fearing an unclear outcome—not a small fear at a time when antibiotics were not available and so many new mothers died of puerperal fever following even normal deliveries.[54] Margherita was a princess after all, and surgeons were notoriously unwilling to intervene on problematic female cases. Realdo Colombo, for example, had refused to enlarge the vagina and remove the rudimentary penis of a hermaphroditic female "Ethiopian" because surgery was too complicated.[55] Months went by after the first rush of consultations. Margherita, who in the meantime was allowed to enter Mantua and had quite charmed the Gonzaga court, was sent back to Parma—officially to be "cured," and privately for the Gonzaga to buy time in order to figure out what to do next. The quandary thus reached stage three and became exclusively political. For the Farnese, Margherita had to remain a wife, because family honor needed to be preserved and a "returned" wife amounted to damaged goods. For the Gonzaga, Margherita could not remain a wife, because her tenacious hymen was making her an investment gone sour. Rather than shining as an icon of honor for her family, Margherita's armored hymen had slowly become a sociopolitical battleground capable of provoking state anxieties; if the *hortus conclusus* of the unexplorable bride could have suggested to the theologically minded a virginal modesty, the entire medical apparatus of two courts was now busy documenting, categorizing, and certifying instead her pathology.[56] In Mantua an agitated Duke Guglielmo started soliciting theological opinions on the subject.[57] He also promptly stoked the pope's fear that the lack of a legitimate successor could open the doors of Italy to the "contagion" of Protestant reformation.[58] Thus even more agitated cardinals on both the Gonzaga and the Farnese side began maneuvering the pope's ears to their particular family cause.[59]

Fabrici would certainly have been able to intervene on a labial fusion or to open up a hymeneal ring if necessary, since he had already operated in instances of vaginal occlusion. In fact, he described the exact procedure in a case so similar to that of Margherita that one would be tempted to think he was speaking of her, had not the case been reported years later, or so he says. In the presence of a "vaginal orifice that was united . . . as happened to the wife of a certain man who wanting to be with her found the place shut, nor he could do it before the labia had been opened surgically,"[60] Fabrici recommended this pelvic procedure: the woman must lie down, her legs bent and then tied, apart, to the table, her elbows placed under her knees ("sotto alle ginocchia"). Then a *siringotomo* (an instrument used generally to operate on fistulae) with a cutting edge or a very long knife ("lunghissimo coltello") with a very long handle ("con un manico lunghissimo") cuts a slit "with one or two delicate incisions, slicing a line in the middle of the labia that had been previously marked with ink and had been probed and investigated on the outside with the index finger and on the inside with the knife."[61]

This line—or lack thereof—in Margherita's body was soon "probed and investigated" by the fingers of so many doctors and surgeons that hardly a province in Italy was left unrepresented.[62] With the well-respected, future saint Cardinal Carlo Borromeo refereeing the final outcome on behalf of the pope, who had him rush from Rome to Parma specifically for the purpose, the number of doctors called to the Farnese court for a last collaborative consult to scrutinize the intimate part of an adolescent—a most unusual occurrence at the time—is staggering: three doctors for the Farnese court, among them the Roman Andrea Marcolini da Fano (a student of Gabriele Falloppio) and a certain Balestra, as well as two doctors for the Gonzaga, Marcello Donati and Tiberio Delfino.[63] Then there were three medical practitioners accompanying the cardinal, that is, two from Milan, Giuseppe Canali and Diomede

Borro, and a surgeon named Voltolina from Pavia.[64] Rounding out the list in the consulting room were also the Bolognese Giulio Cesare Aranzi; the *protophysicus* Zaccaria Caimo, an expert on legal medicine in Milan; and a certain Cassoli—all testifying to the seriousness with which the medical consultation was undertaken on the part of the Farnese, the Gonzaga, and the pope's representatives. And then there were two gentlewomen from the court in Parma, Maria Teresa Langosca and Eufrosina Pallavicino; two Milanese ladies, Margherita Meravaglia and Teodora Panigarola; and a nun from the Ospedale Maggiore, Sister Vittoria.[65] To be sure, the witnesses to this anatomical lesson were fewer in number than the twenty-seven who had supervised in 1498 the sexual apparatus of Queen Jeanne de France, whom her husband, King Louis XII, had submitted to a humiliating scrutiny of her private parts because she was thought to be sterile and he wanted to marry Anne of Brittany.[66] Still, the Farnese's examination room must have been quite crowded.

For Margherita it was sheer mortification, even though on February 18, 1583, she willingly gave herself to the inspection. As the master of entertainment Cesare Cavriani had written a few months before to Duke Guglielmo, Margherita had declared herself ready even to be flayed alive (*scorticare*) as long as she could go back to live with her husband in his society.[67] But if the prospect of being touched, scrutinized, poked, scanned, studied, and labeled by so many peering eyes was nightmarish to her, it must also have been unsettling to the professorial body. As Fabrici, who did not intervene in this new cycle, wrote, "One should not be amazed that the ulcerated opening of the vagina conjoins easily, because women, particularly the most honest, show quite unwillingly their external parts to surgeons."[68] Earlier there had been visits by a number of midwives. One, Madonna Antonia, had left Margherita particularly elated, for she had expressed no doubt as to the feasibility and ultimate success of a surgical intervention. There was some skin covering almost the entirety of the bride's vaginal opening, she had found, which was easy to cut away. She had also marveled at why the doctors had not felt it themselves earlier.[69]

Upon arrival, the team of doctors had to postpone their physical examination because Margherita was having her period. In order not to lose time, Zaccaria Caimo thus proceeded with an interview that made the young princess blush as she proffered tentative answers. Caimo's questions were specific: Was Vincenzo capable of an erection? She answered yes. Was he able to insert his member? Little, she offered. Was he hurting her? Somewhat. Did she spread her seed (the question was pertinent since it was understood then that women's bodily reactions mimicked those of men)? She could not feel it. Was her menstrual blood red? It was. And so Caimo put forward his medical opinion: Margherita had a normal apparatus and, in his opinion, could be "cured."[70] The same day Donati wrote to Guglielmo in Mantua, telling him that most probably Margherita's sexual organ was going to be incised in a way that would take into account the size of Vincenzo's organ.[71] In preparation, bipartite pincers ("tenaglia bipartita") were inserted in her body to enlarge the vaginal opening and to allow the doctors to probe to their satisfaction.[72] The day before surgery, she was administered the usual purge, and priests in all city churches were told to pray for her. The ascetic cardinal Borromeo also began a diet of bread and water.[73]

For the sake of professional seriousness, it was agreed that everybody had also to be on the same page when speaking about the hymen, given the confusion about this body part at the time. The college of doctors thus added a sideshow of comparative anatomy: four certified virgins of a nearby convent in Parma were asked to have their pudenda examined, while their *pudore* (modesty) was compensated with a congruent dowry, in order to familiarize the consulting group with the look and feel of a hymen.[74] In a period in which mostly older women and midwives performed manual exams, Margherita's case, with the lineup of hymens that it required, was manna for scientific research. Still, ocular proof was apparently dispensable when expressing an opinion. Cesare Pendasio had never seen, let alone touched, Margherita, but had nevertheless offered his expert medical opinion two months earlier in a letter from Venice. In describing pathological cases, he surveyed the term "feminine enclosure" (*chiusura muliebre*) in all its plausible meanings—invoking both Greek and Latin culture.[75] He also described how to open these blockages. Some could be simply exposed by using one's hands followed by unguents and powders. Others required the scalpel more than once; the recommended technique was to make a cross-like cut, the way Celsus did, and to incise around and transversally, in the manner of the Arabs. Finally, some obstructions could be addressed by applying corrosive salves ("medicamenti corosivi") and add, if necessary, an ad hoc cut with the knife.[76] He praised the comparative use of virgins and felt sure that surgery could be successful, whether or not doctors such as Fabrici and Aranzi were to perform it themselves.[77]

In the end, surgery was never scheduled, even though, according to the pope's own doctor, Marcolini da Fano—who stormed out of the consulting room, enraged at the overt intrusion of politics into the bedroom—it was the correct thing to counsel. He even pledged his own head that he was right on the issue.[78] In a conversation that the ducal counselor Zibramonti had with Cardinal Borromeo, we learn how divided on the problem were the other physicians: Zaccaria Caimo was unsure as to what to recommend, but in the end he felt that surgery would not cause Margherita's death; the two surgeons from Milan and Pavia were in fact worried that she would die if surgery were performed; and the others believed that Margherita's impediment was natural and that the problem that had rendered her marriage unconsummated rested with Vincenzo, whose organ was deemed too large for Margherita's body to accommodate and also insufficiently geared for sexual performance.[79] The doctors from Milan and Pavia recommended that Margherita take baths to soften her internal tissues. They also suggested inserting dilating instruments or, more simply, fingers.[80]

The rhetoric of shame that early modern culture employed to control female sexuality had transformed at this point into a rhetoric of blame that pitted the Farnese and the Gonzaga families against each other, flanked by their family cardinals. God's omnipotent eye, which, according to Augustine, should guide the individual to internalize the need for chastity and bodily control, had somehow metamorphosed into the impudent and suspecting eye of counselors and secretaries instructed to redefine the concepts of "virtue" and "honor" in terms of realpolitik. Refusing heatedly at this point the surgical solution that their own court doctor, Donati, had advocated earlier, the Gonzaga shamefacedly put Donati in charge of backing their latest position, namely, that Margherita be considered malformed, a *mulier excisa* (a woman with problems in her uterus), rather than a *mulier occlusa* (a woman with an imperforate hymeneal tissue). By definition, a wife's *incapacitas coeundi* makes her *inutilis* to her husband—or, in the language of the time, impotent. The marriage tie could thus be rescinded—and Pope Gregory XIII annulled it on October 9, 1583—for canon law is adamant on the issue: a union is invalid if it has remained unconsummated for three years due to natural causes (*dissolutionem matrimonii ex naturali impedimento*).[81]

Cardinal Borromeo had one more compelling thing to do in the name of *ragion di stato* (reason of state) before leaving Parma: persuade Margherita, who had turned sixteen in the meantime, to seal the virginity given her by an unassailable genital lock with the chastity of the mind. At this point not only the Gonzaga but the Farnese themselves, including grandmother, father, and powerful uncle, had abandoned Margherita, counseling reclusion in a convent, as if her physical impediment was somehow shaming the entire procreative Farnese line.[82] She had earlier written to the pope for help when the pressure to become a nun had become unbearable, but now her long and brave resistance was coming to an end.[83] Being repeatedly warned that her desire for a surgical solution was aberrant, given the risk of death in attempting it, she sadly agreed to take her vows on October 30, 1583.[84] She knew that the Gonzaga would not have allowed her to remain single, and thus potentially available for a future marriage, because that would allow for the possibility of her conceiving from another union—and this would have complicated the already problematic line of succession to the Mantuan duchy. As for the Farnese clan at large, she had by now become an embarrassment and a disappointment, and her grandfather did not delay the restitution of jewels she had received during her marriage and the payment of the expenses the Gonzaga underwent to properly clothe her. Everybody wanted this sad chapter to be put to rest forever.[85] Working on allegories of virginity, Bishop Basilio Gradi was able to dedicate his *Treatise on Virginity* (*Trattato della verginità*) just one year later to the by now well-known case of the coerced Margherita, who had just assumed the new name of Sister Maura Lucenia. He freely acknowledged that he had written the book to help "specifically those who are unhappy about becoming a nun," for everybody knew that Margherita's hymen had had to be pledged to Christ in order for political feuds between two of the noblest and most powerful families in Italy to be settled.[86] With the doors of the cloister of San Paolo in Parma locked after her—and we know that she remained a virtual prisoner within it for the next sixty years—Margherita's physical virginity became, by contract (or in religious terms, by vow), behavioral chastity.

Not that Vincenzo's sexuality was left unchecked, for to rescind the troubled Gonzaga/Farnese ties, Cardinal Borromeo had to ascertain beyond a reasonable doubt that Vincenzo possessed no physical impediment that would mar sexual performance. Such were the requirements for annulling a marriage following Tridentine norms, and even a prince had to subject himself to them.[87] Quite naturally there was a thorough anticipation that the final outcome would tip toward the political rather than the physiological, if the physiological turned out to be too problematic. After all, the Farnese were loudly claiming through their emissaries that Vincenzo had plenty of problems on that score. In various courts there was a rumor that Vincenzo was unable to have sexual relations because he appeared to have syphilis (the telltale sign in this case was loss of hair, although he did not seem to sport what was called the *pellarella,* that is, circumscribed baldness resembling a priest's tonsure).[88] Others were arguing that Vincenzo was known for having paramours in both Mantua and Ferrara, thereby confirming that he was sexually active. In the world of gossip there was talk that Vincenzo had a genital malformation, which could have made the sexual congress difficult.

To inspect the aptness of the prince's sexual functions, the team of doctors from Milan and Pavia that Borromeo had brought with him to check Margherita's pudendum in Parma set up two meetings with Vincenzo. The first consultation, which took place in Ferrara, turned out to be mostly verbal; thus a second meeting was scheduled in Reggio on February 15, 1583. Doctors were asked to settle the issue of whether the prince's sexual organ was unequally proportioned vis-à-vis that of Margherita ("et sia troppo sproporzionato alla natura d'essa S.ra"). On this score the doctors all agreed: it was, given also the princess's immature age and genital malformation.[89] Since there was also talk of a perianal fistula addressed when Vincenzo was a child, a problem that at the time was thought to potentially impede potency and generation, a clinical exam was done on the anal laceration. The fear was that the procedure of searing ("bottone di fuoco") the fistula could "have offended some little nerve or something similar for which reason the genital organ may have remained somewhat weakened and lean while the head remained as usual large, so that it perhaps happens that it may not valiantly be able to hold out for the needed exertion."[90] But the doctors were unable to open it to check it properly (the ducal counselor, Zibramonti, argued that it had not impeded sexual relations in the past and therefore that it was useless to expose it now and cause the prince undue pain); thus no unassailable conclusion was drawn on this score.[91] The third and most important step was to check whether the prince's organ was able to perform its marital duty, and thus it was agreed that

Vincenzo would retire to a room and call in the team of assembled doctors when he was ready for the exam. However, when the group arrived, he was unable to show off properly his manhood because, as the Gonzaga counselor punctiliously wrote back to Duke Guglielmo, "either he had no occasion to get excited or it was not perfectly erected, as often happens to men."[92] In their report following the medical examination of Margherita, some doctors had argued that the marriage could have been consummated, even considering Margherita's small pudendum, if Vincenzo had been able to keep his erection sufficiently for a time and if his organ were smaller—laying the blame for the failed nuptials partially on the Gonzaga doorstep.[93] From Milan a gazette scribe argued that "tests were made to determine whether Vincenzo could support a reasonable weight with his erect member and if he could thrust sufficiently against the palm of a hand so as to be able to pass through a maiden. Moreover, a model was made in the shape of his sexual organ to see whether it was so deformed as to cause impotence. Everything seems to show that he is potent."[94]

Given how embarrassing were the sexual trials and prying verifications to his inner sense of self, it is easy to understand why Vincenzo then felt he needed to show off his virility left and right. Cardinal Cesi, also affected by what had now become a contagious *hysterica passio*, claimed in a letter that "the bishop of Casale swears aplenty that he knows for a fact that the prince [Vincenzo] has deflowered two virgins and one of them he made pregnant."[95] With Vincenzo unleashed, possessing a hymen in the duchy of Mantua suddenly became a liability. Defloration having become part of the prince's agenda, rape could be imagined now as constituting not a crime (even one, to be sure, impossible to prosecute) but a simple transgression—just to try things out. The wife's physical predicament had launched, in short, the husband's behavioral deviance, for the impenetrable princess Margherita had put in danger, through no fault of her own, the hymens of other female subjects in Mantua and nearby towns. As Cardinal Cesi wrote again, certifying that his information could be trusted because he had it from his own physician, the well-known Bolognese doctor Gabriele Beato, the prince's sexual performances now even caused hospitalization for one unfortunate young woman: "Vincenzo wanted to try it with a virgin a few months ago and he was so potent that she had problems and it was necessary to treat her."[96]

Conquering the Hymen, Officially

Our story of virgins' bodies used for political reasons does not end here. Margherita had hardly entered the convent when Vincenzo was asked to engage in a form of highly supervised sexual encounter with a certified virgin as a sine qua non condition for a second marriage. If the potency proof in front of a team of doctors, previously discussed, was indispensable for issuing a judgment on the validity of his union with the Farnese princess, the second trial with a woman he did not know was just grotesque—unending fodder for tabloid sleaze. With this well-recorded occurrence, Vincenzo's story moves from the pathetic and the expedient to the crass, with no stone left unturned in reporting it. Here is how the events unfolded: a new bride, Eleonora de' Medici, was made available to the newly single Vincenzo soon after the demise of his union with Margherita, but he could not marry her, her father, Francesco I, and her stepmother, Bianca Capello, insisted, until he could demonstrate once and for all—through a test that outside parties could verify with their eyes and certify with their pen—that the obstacle to the consummation of his first marriage could be ascribed exclusively to his former wife's defective genitalia and not to his inability to overcome a hymen. This was a claim, after all, that the Farnese were loudly making on the heels of the first marriage fiasco. The last thing Grand Duke Francesco would have wanted for himself, he explains to his brother, Ferdinando, was "to become the joke of Italy, as it was the case in Parma, which for me would be a double smack in the face."[97]

Since this request was, all considered, not too honorable for the Medici, who were offering their daughter to Vincenzo, it has been argued that Bianca had insisted on it to humiliate the Gonzaga for having publicly disparaged her in the past. Indeed, when shopping a few years earlier for a wife for his son, Guglielmo Gonzaga had entertained the idea of marrying him to Eleonora but had preferred the more significant alliance and larger dowry to be gained through a union with the Farnese line—a choice that the Medici were not likely to forget. At the time it was murmured that Guglielmo, who was looking for honorary titles (and indeed had just gotten the right to have his son addressed as "prince"), was finding it highly inappropriate for the Gonzaga to tie the knot with the newly stained Medici family, not only because Francesco had married the parvenu and untitled Bianca, whose first husband had been conveniently murdered in Florence when their relationship had become serious, but because it was widely believed that Bianca had been involved with the puzzling accident that just a few years earlier, in 1578, had killed Francesco's first wife and, as it turns out, Guglielmo's sister-in-law, Joanna of Austria.[98]

The reason behind a certifiable demonstration of Vincenzo's potency was explained by the Medici Grand Duke himself in a letter to the Duke of Este, Alfonso—and his words could scarcely hide a sadistic need to denigrate Vincenzo: "My purpose is to remain assured that the 'friend' can consummate the marriage with a virgin, and therefore let's do the test, and let's choose carefully a healthy maiden whom we know for sure is a virgin."[99] It did not matter that a month earlier, on December 11, 1583, a friend of Vincenzo, Cesare d'Este, had written a formal declaration ("fede") to the grand duke in which he said and affirmed ("dico e affermo") that he knew for sure that Vincenzo had engaged victoriously in amorous battles.[100] Nor did it matter that Cesare's father, Duke Alfonso himself, wrote to the grand duke to reiterate what his son had written.[101] A genuine test needed to take place.

Why Vincenzo agreed to this public assessment, which was scheduled to take place in the city of Ferrara, where his sister reigned as duchess, is unclear, since it is a given that people in position of power lose their authority when they allow their private fallibilities to be checked by outsiders. In fact, when Guglielmo heard of the request from Florence, he immediately recoiled and reminded his interlocutor that the gossip about his son's potency was coming from a very dubious source: the Farnese.[102] A more psychologically convincing explanation could be that Vincenzo, who had also balked at first, only to see court murmurs about his *impotentia* increase exponentially, felt that he could rely on his age and bravado nature. In any case, he was by now sufficiently traumatized by publicly verifiable sexual demonstrations that he refused to sign an initial agreement in which he had three hours to successfully prove himself in an encounter with one of the two virgins found for the try-out and departed suddenly from the Este duchy to the scorn of Francesco de' Medici, for whom "what cannot be done in a night cannot be done in two either."[103]

Soon a second choice was scheduled in a much more neutral territory, Venice. There by contract, Vincenzo consented to a certified sexual congress with a virgin chosen by the Medici, and the encounter had to be successfully concluded within twenty-four hours from the moment he arrived at her lodgings. He was allowed three tryouts and could leave the room in between. In a missive after the event, Francesco explained to Philip II—even the king of Spain needed to know—why he wanted to be sure that the goods were delivered: "There was a certain rumor from the Farnese side that the prince was impotent, [and] we did not want to sign a marriage contract without knowing for sure of his potency, and thus decided that a test would be undertaken in Venice, where we sent a woman with whom he was able to make us convinced and assured of the vanity of that hearsay."[104] The woman was Giulia, a Florentine with a certified maidenhead, who appropriately enough was never given a last name throughout the copious correspondence, for she had no other value than her commodified anatomical property. Giulia was promised a dowry so that she could be recycled into the marriage economy, since as a poor orphan from the Pietà she had almost no chance of marrying.[105] Then, closely guarded to assure that she would do nothing to imperil her hymen, a woman guardian was put at her heels "to instruct Giulia [and] advise her not to force some instrument on herself before she had sex with him."[106]

To put it crudely, Vincenzo was unable to triumph over Giulia's *signaculum virginitatis* at his first try. The culprit was given to abdominal problems that affected him after his friends fortified him with too many oysters before the meeting, but since we know from many sources that Vincenzo often suffered from abdominal abscesses, we may likely blame other undiagnosed medical conditions rather than oysters for the fiasco. Full of misgivings after such a blatant fumbling, Vincenzo immediately inquired back home whether he could marry elsewhere, for there had been talk of a union with a princess of Lorraine. His father cruelly scolded him. At this juncture no new marriage could be in the works for his son with such a cloud over his sexuality, Guglielmo wrote through his secretary. Better for Vincenzo "to ascertain first what His Highness can do" before entering into any agreement.[107] If he wanted to repeat the tryout, the father went on, it was capital for him to "self-examine his strengths, and when he felt that they are such that his weakness could well be attributed to stomach problems and not to impotence, then he should repeat the test."[108]

So a second meeting was arranged within a few days.[109] This time Vincenzo was able to demonstrate to the peering eye—and probing hand—of the Medici's envoy, Belisario Vinta, that a heterosexual congress was taking place and that his organ was correctly conjoined in the sexual act with that of the woman sharing the bed with him. Asked by Vincenzo as per previous agreement to enter the bedroom at the appropriate time to check things out, the scrupulous Vinta put his hand "between the two hairy parts, until I touched her pubes and slammed against the solid member that the young girl had in her body."[110] And so life imitated literature, for all over Italy the episode of Messer Nicia touching the sexual parts of the disguised Callimaco, who was making love to his wife under false pretenses in Niccolò Machiavelli's *La Mandragola*, had constituted for decades an endless occasion for jokes on cuckolded husbands.[111] The example may have made the Florentine envoy Vinta chuckle at the connection. On the other hand, what a fall from grace was he reporting: the allegedly legal right, the *droit de seigneur*, to take the virginity of a serf's maiden, about which Vincenzo may have fantasized in private, was here reduced to a secretary's account of whether a prince could be sufficiently dexterous to trounce a hymen. Vinta's letter to Grand Duke Francesco back in Florence was extensive, accurate, full of tidbits, and serious—a perfect chancery report. Soon other letters announcing the event, some sarcastic or at the very least vulgar in tone, began to circulate.[112]

Later, Vinta conducted an extensive exit interview with Giulia to certify himself one more time that a hymen had been obliterated as needed. I surmise that this would constitute the first historically recorded interrogation of an *ante litteram* sexologist zeroing in on what women "feel" during defloration and intercourse. Much later, in the middle 1950s in fact, Alfred Kinsey would study in depth similar psychosexual experiences (as Masters and Johnson would do soon after) and catalog them scientifically. (It pays to notice that Kinsey's wife, Clara MacMillen, had an unbreakable hymen that impeded the consummation of their marriage until it was surgically slit.)[113] Kinsey's particular interest was not in the physical reaction of women engaged in sex for the first time. But in a well-appointed Venetian bedroom, the conscientious functionary Vinta did just that: an official interrogation that allowed him to write a report card on what women rarely tell and often fake.[114] Giulia's responses to Vinta's detailed inquiry reveal more about what those of the era believed women should feel during the sexual act than what women actually feel—and these responses all played along the

Galenic and Hippocratic corpus' lines. Since it was thought, for example, that women's bodies react just like men's, Giulia was asked whether she felt her seed descend at the end of the sexual act ("se ella avesse buttato seme"). She said she believed it dribbled down her private parts the second time she had sex as well as the third time. The back of her shift was dirty indeed, but she did not know, she said, whether it was blood.[115] Since at the time it was unclear whether there was much difference between lubrication and female seed, Vinta was interested in seed not because it overlapped with female pleasure but because it replicated male semen, which in this particular case was essential for Vincenzo's performance to be successful.[116] It was understood at the time that women have pleasure both in pouring out their seed and in receiving in their womb male ejaculation, so Vinta asked whether she felt the male seed pouring out of her body once she got out of bed. Giulia obliged by answering that she felt so while sitting. Did she herself have an orgasm? She was unsure but was aware of something happening in her body twice, she offered ("se ella habbia sentito piacere nel buttare il seme—dise che alquanto le era parso di sentirne due volte"). The word "orgasm" was of course not used, but Vinta's interest in Giulia's uterine secretion had plenty to do with the view that women released seed during sex, a release that mimicked men's ejaculation, although being that a woman's body was inferior and less efficient vis-à-vis that of a man, the quality and amount of a woman's seed were inferior to those of man's *verum semen*.[117] Did she experience some discomfort? Yes, she admitted, and had asked Vincenzo on his third assault to stop. Did she cry out of pain or shame? Pain, she answered. Would she like to see the prince again? Yes, she would—and there is no need here to ask why: Giulia was an orphan with no prospects in life, but if she managed to become pregnant in the act, she could land a commensurate dowry to raise a child and get a convenient husband in the bargain. Having been callously used by those above her, Giulia knew that she now had a chance to scheme for a better future for herself.[118] She was then asked one more time whether she felt that she had lost her virginity that night—the reason for the experiment after all—but she demurred. She did not know much about this threshold, she said, and lowered her head onto her breast ("Domandata un'altra volta del parerle d'essere sverginata o no—disse che non se n'intendeva, et ficcava il capo in seno"). Seeing her visibly uncomfortable, the peering secretary thankfully ended the interview.

Vincenzo too was not left alone after the event. He had to show his sexual apparatus to a doctor appointed by the Medici family, Piero Galletti, who rushed to write about the examination directly to the grand duke. Galletti's task was officially to prove or disprove some notions that were circulating about Vincenzo's sexual apparatus, which had already influenced the physical examination that had taken place in Reggio exactly thirteen months earlier for the purpose of having his marriage to Margherita annulled. By now the queries had become even more ludicrous, and Galletti was asked to comment specifically not only on whether the prince's member was disproportioned but also on whether he was missing a testicle and whether his testicles were unbalanced because of his fistula.[119] Galletti was able to observe and manually check Vincenzo's sexual organ twice. The first time it was—in his word—"lowered" (*chinato*), and he could observe that "it was ordinary but well-proportioned, and the same was for the testicles; and having put my hand under the two testicles, I found no disease or hindrance whatsoever."[120] The second time, he was called into the bedroom by a surely amused Vincenzo himself, waiting for him in a state of erection. Here Galletti did "touch and carefully manipulate it [the organ] with my hand and also I handled the testicles and was quite satisfied, for the member's width and length were bulky, but not outside nature, and the forms of the maid that received it have not suffered any lesion."[121] For Galletti, and for those who paid for the bedroom checkup, what was important was not the size of the prince's member—in fact, its proportion, rather than being read as a sign of Vincenzo's virility, as would popularly be the case today, was judged problematic in the current medical literature, for it was understood that semen challenged with a long journey toward the womb could become colder and therefore nongenerative.[122] Of paramount importance instead were his testicles and his ability to have an erection, for what was at stake for the Medici in light of their daughter's promised wedding (and this statement assumes that there was some seriousness in the whole charade) was not so much Vincenzo's libido but his ability to produce and deliver semen in light of a dynastic marriage furthering the Gonzaga line.

All's well that ends well, and one month later, on April 29, 1584, Vincenzo married Eleonora, with whom he would have six children.[123] Not surprisingly, his problems with hypertrophic or just regular hymens continued to be the basis of salacious anecdotes throughout the years and even a voyeuristic movie, *Una vergine per il principe,* which came out to great fanfare in the 1960s.[124]

Threatening Anatomical Parts

To move away from the scandal that surrounded these events and return to the issue of female sexuality, I would like to examine briefly what our story teaches about women's bodies, because two schools of thought have had their say regarding the hymen: that of doctors and surgeons, who spoke of obstacles such as films, veils, lids, membranes, covers, plies, meninges, flaked skin, brittle textures, and bandages—the vocabulary used by Fabrici and Donati in the case of Margherita Farnese—and that of church fathers, who, just as euphemistically, referred to cloisters, hedges, seals, locks, shut doors, enclosed gardens, and sealed fountains—the vocabulary used by the papal envoy, Cardinal Borromeo. Both schools had one purpose: to tell women that their sexuality was not their own to administer because patriarchy and God were checking on it. But given the attention that the hymen was attracting in the medical arena at the time, one imagines that anatomists may have used this "flap" to start rethinking the Galenic homology that fully presided in those years over the understanding of the functions of the male and female body. According to Galen the female body, because of its humid and cold humors, was inferior to the male body, which was instead dry and hot. The sexual parts of either males or females were often represented in a similar fashion: outside for men, because heat would bring them out, and inside for women, for lack thereof. In this system, males and females were not absolutely different. Ovaries were called female testicles, and the vagina was described and even illustrated—as in Vesalius's figurations of the male and female genital anatomy, for example—as corresponding to the penis.[125]

So would the newly recuperated and thoroughly examined hymen, which was not present in the male body, confirm that the two sexes were not so physically similar after all? Let me move sideways briefly and point out that in those same years, another part of the female sexual apparatus, the clitoris, had just been fully described. The Hippocratics had correctly affirmed the existence of this "little hill" (*kleitoris*), and Peter of Abano had stated that "having the upper orifice near their pubis rubbed" can bring women to orgasm "for the pleasure that can be obtained from that part of the body is comparable to that obtained from the tip of the penis."[126] But in general medieval doctors confused the function of this organ or simply forgot about it—just as had happened with the hymen.[127] Now both organs, although correctly named, began to be conveniently deemed of no use and to be persistently described as minuscule and hidden. One was breakable and the other was "so small and hidden" (così esiguo e nascosto), as Falloppio put it—or, as Vesalius authoritatively claimed, "a new and useless part."[128] If the hymen had to wait for a man to bring about its hara-kiri, the function of the clitoris was predicated on the notion that it was superabundant, important for pleasure according to Realdo Colombo, who asserted he had discovered it (although Falloppio had also correctly identified it a bit earlier), but with no physiological purpose, unless of course "women hermaphrodites," as the Bolognese doctor Constanzo Varoli put it, used it to remove their sexual behavior from a heterosexual context.[129] It is indeed only the "monstrously" enlarged clitoris of the tribade that got the attention of illustrators in the period; the "normal" one remained a visual taboo.[130]

Here one can grasp the irony: the same organ that was described as minuscule and of no use was at the same time depicted by some doctors as too threatening—exactly like Margherita's tiny but inflexible hymen. Vesalius felt that the clitoris was some sort of sport of nature (*naturae lusum*), not an organ, and feared that because of the "incompetence" of some anatomists (he was chiding Falloppio in this instance), the clitoris could stand for "the rudiments of a tiny phallus."[131] Colombo too used words for the "sweetness of Venus" (*amor Veneris*) that seem to describe a peculiarly male body part: "if you touch it, you will find it rendered a little harder and oblong to such a degree that it shows itself as a sort of male member."[132] Thomas Bartholin called it "the female yard or prick." It resembles, he argued, "a man's yard in situation, substance, composition, repletion with spirits, and erection."[133] No wonder that at times surgeons thought that it should be removed. In his *De curtorum chirurgia per insitionem,* Gaspare Tagliacozzi explained, for example, that sometimes the clitoris grows so much that it needs to be removed because it causes "many problems or turpitude. Therefore the woman needs to lie down and one takes whatever is superfluous with a pincer and then cuts it out with a chisel."[134] Reading through the literature of the period, one cannot help but feel that the medical interest in removing an unproblematic clitoris was spurred by a precise libidinal and moral reason: to remove the issue of female lustfulness.

No matter how threatening it was when compared to the phallus, still the clitoris was—just like the hymen—hard to find for some dissectors. It is true that doctors at the time were seeing a smaller clitoris than the one women physiologically have, because the bodies available for anatomy lessons were usually those of old women whose muscle and erectile tissue had, as we would expect, shrunk or thinned with age, just as surgeons, unlike midwives, were unable to detect the presence of a hymen, because most of the female bodies they were allowed to dissect belonged to hanged prostitutes. Indeed, we have to wait for the anatomical waxes of Clemente Susini, who was reproducing the dissections of anatomist Francesco Antonio Boi in Florence in 1803–1805, to see clearly and for the first time the correct size of the clitoris, with all its constitutive parts: vessels, prepuce, glans, and *corpora spongiosa*. It turns out that this organ is much less "small and hidden" than the apprehensive Falloppio had judged to be the case.[135] But only in 1998 did photography finally make clear the clitoris's precise measurements, when Helen O'Connell, a urologist at the Royal Melbourne Hospital of Melbourne, with the help of John Hutson, a pediatric genital reconstruction specialist, correctly mapped out the dorsal and cavernosal nerves of the clitorises of ten women by capturing the 3-D structure of the member. In the process, O'Connell found it to be quite dissimilar from the lilliputian piece that anatomy books, such as the ubiquitous *Gray's Anatomy* textbook in America, have routinely described. In fact, it was double the size.[136]

That it took a long time to have a correct female anatomical reconstruction constitutes, of course, a story of its own; that it is perhaps just as well, for this organ's miniaturization saved many women from clitoridectomy and infibulation over the years, constitutes indeed food for thought. Whether the anatomy of another bodily feature that belonged only to men—the prostate—contributed to substantively differentiate men's and women's bodies in the mind of early modern doctors will necessarily need to be the subject of another study. The prostate was described first in 1536 by Niccolò Massa, another professor of anatomy and surgery in Padua, and illustrated by Vesalius in 1538. A detailed drawing of the prostate, which correctly shows it as one entity, was done, unsurprisingly, by the very doctor called to fix Margherita's problem first, Girolamo Fabrici.[137]

In any case, since both hymen and clitoris culturally signified much more than they did materially—as loci of anxiety about women's agency, representation, and power—the medical discovery or recovery of their existence meant little right away. But soon enough, as more female sexual parts were closely examined by doctors entering the field of gynecology alongside midwives and as the knowledge learned in hands-on dissections began to supplant commonplaces on how bodies were conceptualized, the supposedly somatic nondifferentiation between the male and the female body started to crumble.[138] Already by the end of the sixteenth century André Du Laurens could argue forcefully that "no similarity comes in between the vagina and the male penis; none between the uterus and the scrotum; neither in the structure, form and size of the testicles the same, nor in the distribution and insertion of the spermatic vessels."[139] Shortly after, in 1611, Caspar Bartholin declared the parallelism between the male and the female organ an inept one.[140]

As for Margherita, her militant "superfluous" was addressed both politically, by making a recorded spectacle of it and its owner in the examining room, and scientifically, by pretending that any such observation could be objective. For the doctors who recommended surgery, Margherita's virginity had to be violated in order to make her body pliable and normal—that is, acceptable physically and morally—and correctly owned, as in Freud's argument in "The Taboo of Virginity": "This experience [of defloration] creates a state of bondage in the woman which guarantees that possession of her shall continue undisturbed and makes her able to resist new impressions and enticements from outside."[141] For the doctors who did not recommend surgery, Margherita's virginity was instead a scandal, because in repudiating ownership, her no-longer-chaste body was exposing the fickle basis of patriarchal authority. Thus, once the hymen that was originally the guarantor for the Gonzaga of a chosen bride's biological and social appropriateness proved that chastity and virginity can be a masquerade, state and church moved in to contain the woman's resistance. Although it would be correct to presume that the use of that "very long knife" that makes "one or two delicate incisions" in the *vulvar ostium*, as Fabrici put it, could have corrected Margherita's physiological problem, the Gonzaga and the pope's representative not only forbade a solution but also required that her subjecthood be thoroughly expurgated from their society. Margherita had to become a nun, a nonentity—that is, a nonhistorical subject—and had to lose both her name and her status of princess by speedily cloistering herself. For this schema to work perfectly, reclusion for life had to be her choice rather than an outside imposition: she was thus invited by Cardinal Borromeo to stay for a while in a convent in Milan, where she was treated well and was able to enjoy musical soirées, in order to see that her willfulness in insisting on a surgical operation was narcissistic and thoroughly sinful. After all, if she were to die following the procedure she would go straight to hell, having committed suicide, and what Christian girl would risk such an outcome for the sake of presiding over an active life at court? In the end, as testimony to the disconcert created by an undecidable virginity, Margherita not only was rejected by everybody in power but was so tormented by her brother Ranuccio Farnese, the new Duke of Parma, that years later she had the courage to expose her harassment in a tearful letter to Pope Clement VIII. In it she begged him to have her transferred from Parma to a convent in Rome, so that she could be subjected to a more benign guardianship.[142] In "The Taboo of Virginity," Freud explains this hostility on the part of men as castration anxiety: "It cannot be disputed that a generalized dread of women is expressed in all these rules of avoidance. . . . The man is afraid of being weakened by the woman, infected with her femininity and of then showing himself incapable."[143] No wonder that to prove to himself that he was sexually "capable"—and to exorcise Margherita's puzzling clout—Ranuccio populated her convent with all of his bastard daughters.[144]

But that Vincenzo himself may have been perhaps unable to exorcise the memory of Margherita thirty years later is much more surprising. Yet we know that a few weeks after he lost his wife, Eleonora, Vincenzo started to reconsider marriage, ostensibly "in order not to live in sin," as the Mantuan gentleman Lucio Arrivabene communicated to Francesco Maria II Della Rovere, Duke of Urbino.[145] The new bride, according to Maria Bellonci, may have been Margherita herself. Between the end of 1611 and the beginning of 1612, Bellonci writes, Vincenzo instructed his secretary, Annibale Chieppio, to make inquiries with Federico Borromeo, the nephew of that other cardinal, Carlo, who had supervised the monachation of Margherita, to see whether the possibility of remarrying his long lost Farnese bride could be accepted at the Vatican.[146] Assuming such conversations actually took place (and how fascinating the idea would be!), Vincenzo's death in February put a swift end to it.

Margherita survived every member of the Gonzaga clan for two generations; she also survived the devastating plague brought to Italy by the German Habsburg troops marching south in 1629 to invade the Mantovano and besiege Mantua in order to oust the Gonzaga Nevers, the cadet branch of the family that claimed the duchy's succession once the Gonzaga line, which Vincenzo had thought he had assured with the sons he had generated in his second marriage, dried up a few years after his death.[147] This epochal catastrophic occurrence together with the sack of Mantua in 1630, from which the city never recovered, was so passionately evoked by Alessandro Manzoni in *I promessi sposi* (*The Betrothed*)—a novel that every Italian student has to read and criticize for weeks in high school—that it has rightly become, through the decades, an integral part of the national mythology. To think of it, the Gonzaga tragedy—and the subsequent destruction of the body politic that sealed it—was also, as fate wanted, the consequence of a lack of procreation, one that involved Vincenzo's sterile daughter-in-law Caterina de' Medici. Were not the event utterly heartrending, one would be tempted to read justice in it. Princess Margherita Farnese Gonzaga, who liked so much to sing and dance and even created an elaborate ballet of women warriors in the short time she resided at the Mantuan court with her husband, did indeed not like being Sister Maura Lucenia in a cloistered cell in Parma.[148]

2

The Aesthetic Cure

Skin Disease, Noses, and the Invention of Plastic Surgery

> Medicine sometimes snatches away health.
> Sometimes gives it.
>
> —Ovid, *Tristia*

> Better to hunt in fields, for health unbought,
> Than fee the doctor for a nauseous draught,
> The wise, for cure, on exercise depend;
> God never made his work for man to mend.
>
> —John Dryden, "Epistle to John Dryden of Chesterton"

SOMETIME IN THE YEAR 1595, Vincenzo Gonzaga I, fourth Duke of Mantua and Monferrato and munificent sponsor of art, music, and theater—a Renaissance prince in every sense of the word—realized that he had a physical difficulty that required some creative addressing. Historians are in agreement today that this particular ducal predicament was mostly political, like the one I follow in Chapter 3. Vincenzo's crusade against the Turks in Hungary—his first out of three—was at a standstill. Militarily speaking, the resourceful duke, who saw himself as a new-age warrior, loved hunting and firearms, and collected precious foreign armor and military gadgets to embellish his armory, had been able to engineer a victorious armed conquest at Visegrád.[1] This raid, as the letters sent home suggest, left him exhilarated. But the attack constituted all the success he could boast of on the battlefield. In the meantime, many, many soldiers within the large Christian encampment were becoming incapacitated by recurring attacks of dysentery. Vincenzo was indeed the prince who had rescued from prison the poet Torquato Tasso, whose epic romance, *Jerusalem Delivered,* detailing the heroic sorties of the Christian heroes Tancredi and Rinaldo during the first Crusade had filled his adolescent days; he was indeed the prince whose grandmother, Margherita Paleologo, a member of the family that had originally ruled Constantinople and the Eastern Roman Empire, could have motivated her eager descendant to entertain a crusade against the "infidels," but his dreams of glory were fading fast as his soldiers continued losing limbs and life.[2]

Alternatively it could be said that Vincenzo was enjoying glories other than military ones in Hungary, for he had become legendary for his munificence and for the splendor of the court he had brought along, which included a retinue of five musicians under the leadership of maestro composer Claudio Monteverdi, as well as cooks and even a bishop protecting a tabernacle with the relic of Christ's Most Precious Blood. He also brought doctors and apothecaries (supplementary medicine was often provided by his wife's uncle).[3] It was well known, for example, that when asked to surrender, the Turks insisted on doing so only to the "pasha of Mantua," an outcome that surely pleased Vincenzo's ego, although it did nothing to increase his martial reputation within the crusaders' camp. This military expedition was going nowhere, and Vincenzo had already spent 100,000 scudi. Then, suddenly and without communicating his decision to the other commandants, he decided to return home.[4]

There was at the time an official explanation for the duke's rushed departure from the battlefield, even though many did not believe it, and it was medical: Vincenzo had developed what doctors called a painful and disfiguring facial infection, an erysipelas. This streptococcus bacterial infection (*S. pyogenes* in modern medical terminology) manifests itself in immuno-deficient patients in reddish skin plaques and pustules, usually around the eyes, cheeks, and ears, and is accompanied by high fever. These plaques also migrate to other parts of the body, mostly to the lower extremities. The painful rash was the result, a counselor wrote, of the duke having spent three days fully armed and on horseback repealing constant Turkish attacks.[5] To find relief from his pain, Vincenzo first decided to move out of the field camp to Colmar, in

Possonia (lower Hungary). As an anonymous contemporary chronicler confirms, once lodged in a comfortable palace in Colmar, Vincenzo's erysipelas improved quickly ("pigliando essa molto miglioramento per conto di detta Crisipilla").[6] But then the duke developed a leg erysipelas ("colà lo prese una risipola alla gamba") so excruciating that in the end he was advised to forget returning to camp and move to Vienna. His health did not improve dramatically there either, and thus at the beginning of October 1595, Vincenzo left for Mantua, traveling partly by water and partly by carriage. He arrived home on November 29 and immediately asked for medical relief.[7]

In this chapter I connect Vincenzo's relentless search for a way to address his skin problems to the invention of reconstructive plastic surgery of the face as delineated in *De curtorum chirurgia per insitionem*—a magnificently illustrated book dedicated to him by Gaspare Tagliacozzi (1545–1599), one of the doctors involved in tackling the duke's aesthetic as well as physical disabilities once he returned home. Tagliacozzi was professor of surgery and chair of theoretical medicine at the University of Bologna and "the greatest anatomist of our time," according to the renowned scientist Ulisse Aldrovandi.[8] He was called to the Gonzaga court in February 1596, three months after Vincenzo's return from the battlefield, when, unsatisfied with the treatment he was receiving from his doctors or in too much pain to deliberately disregard his condition, Vincenzo had instructed his secretary, Tullio Petrozzani, to organize a larger consultation with well-known physicians and to invite the Bolognese doctor as an outside superconsultant. In a letter to the Mantuan philosopher Federico Pendasio, who was teaching at the time in Bologna, Petrozzani described Vincenzo as "having twice suffered from erysipelas of the face and about the entire head, and having certain other disorders."[9]

Surely pleased by the invitation of a duke "who seeks him and from him expects great benefit to his health, which may it please God to restore to him," Tagliacozzi rushed to Mantua to assess Vincenzo's "indispositione."[10] He had been asked to time his arrival with the first day of Lent, when the highly choreographed carnival festivities requiring the duke's presence would be over, and "when other Most Excellent Doctors will be here to consult and deliberate on the case of His Highness, who trusts greatly in the judgment and great prudence of the said Messer Tagliacozzo, and who will show himself a most grateful Prince."[11] The

Bolognese doctor did not stay long, for within two weeks he was back in Bologna.¹² We have no record of what decisions he and the medical team summoned to court took regarding Vincenzo's facial eruptions. A month later, in April, Tagliacozzi was again called to Mantua. Still no mention was made of the specific trouble affecting the duke, although we can assume that the problem had to do with his face. Whatever cure Tagliacozzi proffered this time must have been somewhat beneficial, for a rumor started to circulate following his visits to the Gonzaga court, a rumor soon reaching Rome, that Vincenzo liked Tagliacozzi so much that he was trying to lure him to Mantua by doubling the salary he was receiving in Bologna.¹³

Thankfully for us readers, not much later, on August 17, 1596, the duke himself—writing from Porto, a summer residence where he loved to retire—specified what part of his face was troubling him the most: the nose. In a letter to Francesco dall'Armi, a nobleman working for the Gonzaga in Bologna, Vincenzo asked to petition Tagliacozzi for the unguent the doctor had given to his relative, Cardinal Scipione Gonzaga (1542–1593), a few years earlier, in 1586: "Be good enough to say to Messer Doctor Tagliacozzo that I should like him to let me have a little of that so famous unguent to apply to my nose ['per ongermi il naso'] and with which it is said he cured that [i.e., the nose] of Messer Cardinal Gonzaga, may he now be in heaven."¹⁴ Tagliacozzi was unable to go himself to Mantua this time but sent a student, Giovanni Battista Solimei, with "a certain ointment for the nose of His Highness" (unto per il Naso di S. A.) and the recommendation on its use.¹⁵ He advised the duke to treat his nose with the thermal waters of Villa, one of the baths at Bagni di Lucca deemed to be highly beneficial for skin problems. As he wrote from Bologna on August 22, 1596, "My Very Serene Lord and Most Honored Patron, I am sending to Your Very Serene Highness the unguent about which Messer Francesco dall'Armi spoke to me in your name. You will anoint the excoriated parts of the nose with this at night, and in the morning will wash them with a little warm *acqua della villa.*"¹⁶ We do not know whether at this juncture Vincenzo's nose problem was aesthetic or pathological, that is, whether he was having an episode of acute skin rash with *vescicles* and *bullae* (perhaps a form of cutaneous tuberculosis) or was showing signs of developing, say, a saddle (syphilitic) nose.

Tagliacozzi returned to Mantua on March 23, 1597, but this time, rather than for a medical consultation, his journey was to promote the massive book on reconstructive surgery of the nose, lips, and ears he had just finished writing, *De curtorum chirurgia per insitionem,* the first book ever published on plastic surgery, which he dedicated to Vincenzo three days later (Fig. 7).[17] The duke was a military man, Tagliacozzi wrote in his acknowledgments, and therefore no patron could appreciate more his work on how to "re-make" men's parts:

> Thus I dedicate my firstborn offspring to your Highness, the Most Serene Duke, and entrust it to your protection, chiefly because of my unceasing respect for your house, which has always honored me.... The other and also very important motivation behind my wishing to publish this work embellished with your most distinguished name rather than that of any other is that the house of Gonzaga has always been known for its prowess with swords. Because camp followers and those who deal with arms often incur this type of injury, I thought it fitting to dedicate a book dealing with martial injuries to military men.[18]

Beyond reasons of patronage, then, Tagliacozzi chose Vincenzo because he was a man of arms, and military men needed to have their noses, lips, and ears reconstructed. Why? A logical explanation could be that these three body parts extruding from the face are often at risk in soldiers facing unforgiving encounters with swords and rapiers on a daily basis. Soldiers were also occasionally victimized after having been defeated, especially when engaged with Turkish squads, which may have wanted to inscribe a mark of infamy on their faces with a disfiguring but nonlethal cut. It did help, of course, that Vincenzo was known to be one of the first Renaissance rulers to abide by the politics of compassion, for in his military campaigns he had been praised for instituting ambulances and camp doctors for soldiers, and had the sick and wounded carried back to the army base to be assisted and cured.[19] Reconstruction of injured body members was exactly what Tagliacozzi addressed in his book.

Perhaps more to the point, military men were also in need of the clinical attention of a surgeon like Tagliacozzi because as a result of being away from home, sometimes for years, and of migrating from region to region, they were notoriously being infected by syphilis and thus had diseased, sunken, or missing body parts. Tagliacozzi's biographers, Jerome Pierce and Martha Teach Gnudi, imply that Vincenzo's

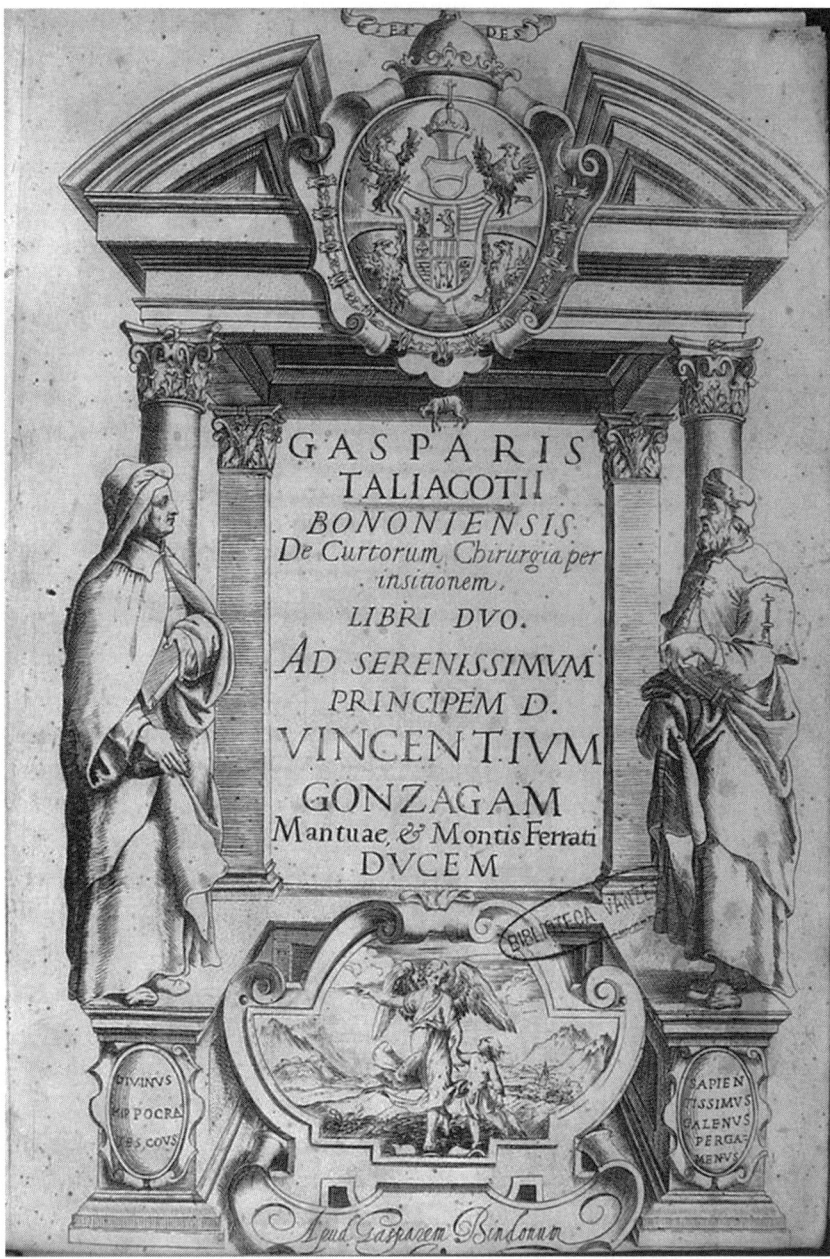

Fig. 7. Gaspare Tagliacozzi, frontispiece dedicated to Vincenzo Gonzaga, in *De curtorum chirurgia per insitionem* (Mantua: Bindoni, 1597). (Photo: Biblioteca Vincenzo Pinali, Sezione Antica, Università di Padova, Padua.)

request for the ointment used by Cardinal Gonzaga meant that he himself was syphilitic, but in a subsequent collaborative writing they choose to be vague on the issue and no longer identify Vincenzo's nasal problem.[20] Many contemporaries, in any case, have suggested that Vincenzo had developed syphilis, and indeed at least one of the cures he underwent through the years, the *cura del legno* (guaiacum), was the treatment of choice for syphilis. In a letter from Padua of April 20, 1602, for example, Giacomo Alvise Cornaro, having heard that Vincenzo was undergoing the *cura del legno,* complained that the duke should have sought better remedies for his problem. What this health problem was, however, Cornaro leaves unmentioned.[21] And as early as 1580, there was a rumor that Vincenzo was impotent due to syphilis because he was losing his hair. More recently, Adalberto Pazzini has argued that the presence of infected boils coming back with a certain frequency in Vincenzo's body would indeed point to syphilis.[22] One of the most common visual results of syphilis is a depressed nose, but none of Vincenzo's portraits save perhaps one shows what appears to be a saddle-nose deformity (Fig. 8).[23] To be sure, a court painter could have been asked to correct any facial feature that the duke—his employer—would have found unpleasant to register for posterity, but then saddle noses are also present in diseases such as scrofula (which probably corresponded to herpes zoster in Italy and is commonly referred to as St. Anthony's fire), lupus, leprosy, yaws, and erysipelas, to name a few, so a diagnosis of syphilis would not necessarily put the issue to rest. Many of these pathologies, in any case, point to tuberculosis as their originating factor. Scrofula, for example, is tuberculosis of the lymph glands of the neck and typically manifests itself with swollen nose and hands. Lupus is a form of cutaneous tuberculosis. The so-called *mal di formica* (ant disease), which spread arithmetically in Italy toward the end of the sixteenth and the beginning of the seventeenth centuries and no longer exists today, manifested itself with redness and itching (the patients felt as if insects were walking all over them) and produced face cancers with a lengthy but nonfatal development. We can think of it as a form of lupus. The guaiacum itself, being a mucolytic agent, was used to relieve not only skin problems associated with syphilis but also respiratory problems in patients affected by pulmonary tuberculosis. As Chapter 3 which more closely examines Vincenzo's co-pathologies, makes even

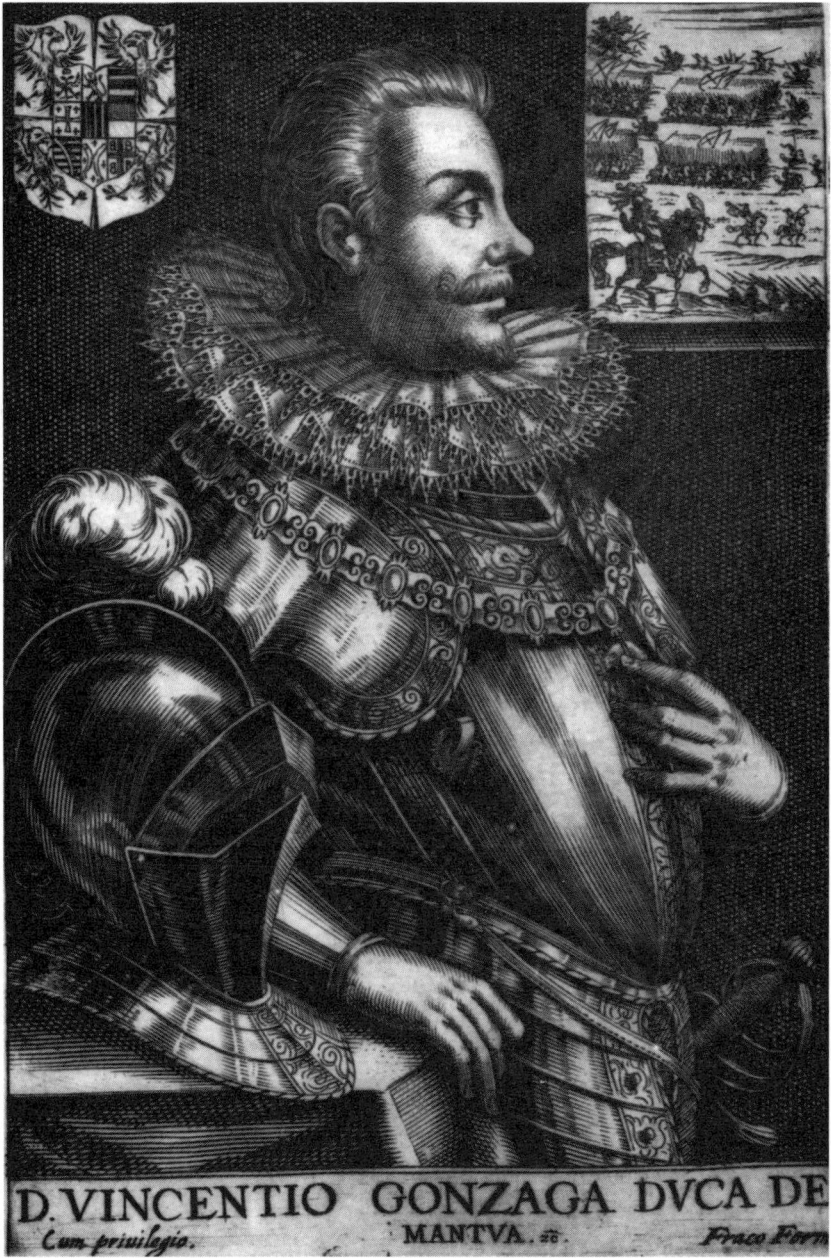

Fig. 8. Giacomo Franco, "Vincentio Gonzaga Duca de Mantua," Plate 23 in *Effigie naturali dei maggior principi et più valorosi capitani di questa età con l'arme loro* (Venice: Apud Iacobum Francum, 1596). (Photo: Biblioteca Nazionale Marciana, Venice.)

clearer, tuberculosis seems to have been Vincenzo's core health problem.

Vincenzo did not have Tagliacozzi perform any surgery on his face of the kind the Bolognese doctor punctiliously illustrated in his book. Even when one year later, on March 28, 1598, Tagliacozzi was again urgently called to Mantua to cure Vincenzo for unspecified problems, as testified by two letters—one by Tagliacozzi and the other by dall'Armi, both to Annibale Chieppio, the ducal secretary—we can assume that the cure was once more topical rather than surgical: that is, it was addressed with unguents, gelatins, and lotions and not with scissors, forceps, and retractors.[24] I would argue that Tagliacozzi saw Vincenzo as a natural choice to be the dedicatee of his scientific work not because the duke needed facial surgery himself, although he had facial problems, nor because he knew men who needed it, although skin pathologies like dermatitis and fungal infections were endemic at the time, but because toward the end of the sixteenth century he was firmly associated in courts all over Europe with aesthetic refinement and love of beauty, no matter how costly these hobbies were to the Mantuan treasury. In this reading, Tagliacozzi did not see his groundbreaking treatise as a how-to book on remodeling—as best as a surgeon could at the time—disfiguring facial features but as the pathbreaking way science could match the aesthetic canon that Renaissance artists were following en masse in their work and that so motivated Vincenzo's passion for collecting. As Giorgio Vasari famously stated, "The artist achieves the highest perfection of style or *maniera* by copying the most beautiful things in nature and combining the most perfect members, hands, head, torso, and legs, to produce the finest possible figure as a model for use in all his works."[25] If artists could imitate God in creating beauty by correcting imperfect body parts; if Neoplatonic philosophers such as Marsilio Ficino could persuasively argue in *De Amore* that beauty is the mirror of the human soul, and thus it is a benefit for man to be handsome and to look for beauty; if even politicians such as Baldesar Castiglione could argue in *The Book of the Courtier,* alongside Ficino, that there are moral advantages to being beautiful in that good-looking individuals have an interior moral goodness ("Li belli son buoni"), then why should surgeons not use their scalpel to remake man as a piece of art in a recombined pleasant order, fully aware of the importance of proportion and symmetry, as in God's handiwork?[26] Almost two centuries earlier, Petrarch had praised humans expressly for their capacity to correct bodily deficiencies, for a human being "learns to make wooden feet, iron hands, [and] wax noses, . . . erects failing health by medicines, excites weakened taste by flavor, and restores ailing sight by eyeglasses."[27] This was after all the claims that the anatomist Andreas Vesalius had made in his groundbreaking *De humani corporis fabrica* (1543). Indeed an interest in cosmetic surgery, together with a concern that a heavily scarred face should get back some of its natural beauty through surgery, was shared in the sixteenth century by a number of famous surgeons, such as Gabriele Falloppio, Girolamo Mercuriale, and Giovanni Tommaso Minadoi—all professors at the University of Padua.[28] Recently Mariagrazia Gadebush Bondio has identified the 1580s as the moment in which the patients' desire to correct their disfigured faces moved surgeons from somewhat philosophical disquisitions—on whether surgery with its accompanying pain and risk of infection and the use of prosthetics could be justifiable for aesthetic reasons—to practical analyses of case histories showing that ugliness (*turpitudine*) could be corrected through surgical interventions.[29]

There was no man in power at the time in Italy more interested in aesthetic refinement, no man more involved in pricey artistic collection and more obsessed with magnificence, from both a narcissistic and a sensual point of view, than Duke Vincenzo. He was a hedonist par excellence, known for believing that fundamental happiness was a state of mind. He was an aesthete of sensual materialism, deluding himself over and over into thinking that possession of beauty—women, objects, art, jewels, clothes—constituted his life-affirming right. Through the years Vincenzo had been the unofficial but de facto buyer and master of style not only for his court but also for the imperial court of Rudolf II of Habsburg. The emperor used to prod Vincenzo continuously with letters to both identify what was worth collecting and to find collectible items in Italy—from bric-a-brac to masters' paintings—to display at his refined court in Prague.[30] Vincenzo employed artists in Mantua who were repeatedly asked to go to Naples (as in the case of Frans Pourbus) or France and Spain (Peter Paul Rubens) to paint portraits of the most beautiful women in the world to put in his private *camerino*, so that he could enjoy looking at their fair, feminine proportions in his spare time.[31] Through the years Vincenzo sponsored the best writers of his time, from Torquato Tasso, whose epic romance he revered, to

Giovanni Battista Guarini, the refined "inventor" of the pastoral play. Vincenzo also employed the best singers and actors—Claudio Monteverdi's operas *Arianna* and *Orfeo* were composed at his court; the greatest opera singer of the time, Adriana Basile, was lured away from Naples to shine in Mantua; and the most famous commedia dell'arte company in Italy at the time, the Fedeli, was on his payroll. Through the years Vincenzo, who had been educated by a famous mathematician, Giuseppe Moleti, supported learning, recruited renowned professors for his children, invited Galileo to his court, fostered the literary and scientific production of the Mantuan press of Francesco Osanna, and authorized the first university in Mantua, run by Jesuits: the Peaceful University of Mantua.[32] Through the years Vincenzo maniacally collected not hundreds but thousands of expensive memorabilia, to the point that when the Gonzaga collection (that of Vincenzo, of his predecessors, and of his son Ferdinando) was put up for sale in 1626–1627 (that is, fifteen years after the duke's death), the list included 2,000 paintings and 20,000 precious objects. The sheer number of these artifacts made the collection one of the most coveted in Europe.[33] In *La celeste galeria di Minerva,* Adriano Valerini, an actor and poet who worked in Vincenzo's court, had indeed imagined a gallery of works of art that sported portraits of the most important patrons rather than the customary paintings and sculptures. Vincenzo's imagined place in this context was that of a colossus.[34] Even on his deathbed and well aware that the end was near, Vincenzo had a last request: that his beloved collected pieces be brought to him. He kept touching them, lovingly kissing them, and crying over them, we are told, as if they were too beautiful to be let go. Vincenzo was a high-end materialist who needed to surround himself with magnificence. Thus his worshiping of beauty could not only spur a science of rejuvenation in Mantua, as evident in his own avid creation of a botanical medical garden (*Orto botanico*), the third in Italy after those recently established in Pisa and Padua, but also justify, if not motivate, a radical experimentation with aesthetic surgery.[35] Tagliacozzi knew his man.

Rhinoplasty as Remedial Surgery

Plastic, as in "plastic surgery," has nothing to do with plastic as containing synthetic material. Rather, in the original Greek, *plastikos* meant to shape, to contour, to mold. Plastic surgery thus has the scope of restoring body parts that have been devastated: that are injured, misshapen, or missing. Its function is not merely cosmetic but corrective and reconstructive; in fact, only in the past fifty years has plastic surgery become mainly cosmetic. Gaspare Tagliacozzi was the first surgeon in Europe to claim plastic surgery as an important branch of medicine and to offer the distinction between beauty surgery, which he named *chirurgia decoratoria,* and remedial surgery, which he named *chirurgia curtorum.* In his book Tagliacozzi argued that the face was important to one's sense of self and well-being, and this was the reason why facial surgery was recommended, even though for some such an intervention was considered superfluous. The face indicates "character," he wrote; "it distinguishes one person from another; . . . contains the main essence of our appearance. The face reveals age and beauty and distinguishes between the sexes. It displays man's dignity; finally, it is a true image of our souls and exposes most full our hidden emotions."[36] Thus, facial lesions are prejudicial to one's dignity and beauty, he wrote; the medicine that cures beauty does not substitute unnatural attributes for the natural ones that an individual once had but gives integrity back to a man, and therefore reconstructive surgery has a right to be placed next to other medical branches.

Unfortunately, no matter how much a person disliked his or her nose, rhinoplasty in the sense that we today give to the term—a surgery that modifies the shape of the nose by intervening internally on its cartilage or bone—was not available in the early modern period. In fact, such was hardly the preoccupation of Tagliacozzi, for he made plain that he was interested only in plastic replacements of the nose and gave precise explanations, supported by detailed drawings, regarding the surgical interventions he could perform. Since the procedure Tagliacozzi used was also predicated on aesthetics—and he specifically stated that there is no point to taking a deformity away by adding another—one could argue that no nose surgery is purely reconstructive.[37] It also pays to notice that although today women, much more than men, constitute the gender that most seeks out plastic surgery, none of the Renaissance doctors refer to nasal interventions on women. In fact, I have come across only one case of plastic surgery on a woman's nose. It was done in 1592 in Lausanne by Jean Griffon, who had heard of Tagliacozzi's technique from a pilgrim returning from Italy.[38]

It turns out that the history of rhinoplasty preceding Tagliacozzi's intervention is also very much Italian. With the exception of Hippocrates, ancient Greek medicine did not mention repairs of nasal injuries.[39] The Roman encyclopedist Aulus Cornelius Celsus described the possibility of repairing a disfigured nose by using nearby facial parts.[40] But Galen was uninterested in the issue, although his humoral theory would be frequently used in later physiognomic theorizations, so much so that even in the late eighteenth century, Johann Caspar Lavater saw in the beautiful nose—one not too long and decisively not too curved—the sign of a beautiful character.[41] Some doctors in the Middle Ages, such as Lanfranco of Milan, Guy de Chauliac and his pupil Pietro d'Argellata, Rolando Capelluti, and Henri de Mondeville, broached the issue of nose repairs and even addressed concerns about aesthetic results, but no surgeon mentioned transplant.[42]

The first historically documented intervention on a noseless person made by taking the skin necessary for the reconstruction of the nasal pyramid from the forehead or cheek (*ex ore*) comes from Catania, Sicily, where the surgeon Gustavo Branca Minuti got a license from King Ferdinand I of Sicily in 1432 and opened a shop where he reconstructed noses, lips, and ears. It has been hypothesized that since a similar technique—the transplant of a skin flap from the cheek—was described in the *Sushruta Samhita*, the basic treatise of Hindi medicine, around the fifth century B.C., Branca Minuti may have learned of it through a journey made to Persia, where Hindi teaching was known, but this connection seems far-fetched.[43] In any case, given the obvious disfiguration that the method of forehead flap advancement involved, we may assume that a patient must have really wanted a new nose to risk permanently scarring other nearby facial features. Already Gustavo's son had felt the need to address the problem of nasal reconstruction along a more aesthetic line and had modified his father's surgery by taking the skin not from the face but from the patient's arm. This transplant required a more complicated intervention, in that arm and nose had to remain attached for a period of at least three weeks before skin separation and reshaping could begin.[44] It is at this point—when forehead rhinoplasty was abandoned because it was aesthetically unpleasing—that corrective surgery met, however awkwardly, beauty surgery, in that attention to correcting a physical deformity for aesthetic reasons resulted in no more scarring.

The Branca technique was sufficiently known outside Sicily to be illustrated in surgery manuals, such as that of 1527 by Alessandro Benedetti, a professor of anatomy and surgery at the University of Padua.[45] But the doctors most well known in the next century for their ability to reconstruct noses were the brothers Pietro and Paolo Vianeo, who had a shop in Tropea, in the southern region of Calabria. The Vianeo method was briefly described by Ambroise Paré, who had a patient, a scion of the Saint-Thaon family, in need of a new nose because he had had enough of his fake silver nose, and who therefore came all the way from France to visit the Vianeos in Italy. He was very pleased with the results.[46] A contemporary account of the brothers' work comes from the historian Camillo Porzio, who wrote of a man who had his nose sliced by a jealous husband and who thus went to Tropea to get a new one.[47] He too was satisfied with the procedure. Either the surgery must not have been too painful or the patient's love was beyond bounds, because when the husband died, Porzio writes, the patient ended up marrying the woman who had caused the injury, however unwillingly.

A full narrative of how the Vianeos used a pedicle flap graft to rebuild a nose would have to wait for the Bolognese doctor and charlatan Leonardo Fioravanti. Visiting Tropea incognito in 1549 to see how the famous brothers operated, Fioravanti feigned that he needed to duplicate their surgery in order to cure a rich and wretched patient of his, Cornelio Albergati, who had lost his nose in a fight. He was generously allowed to sit in for five surgeries, which he later described as successful, and thus was able to replicate the Vianeo technique in his own practice, especially in Bologna. This remained, however, not the only method Fioravanti used in his practice, for he also claims in his writings that he was able to reattach noses without the need for complicated surgical reconstructive rhinoplasty by simply using his secret balsam mixed with urine. The case in point was that of his patient Andrés Gutiero, whose nose had been severed in a duel. As he retells it, Fioravanti picked up the stump from the sand, urinated on it to disinfect it, reattached it pronto to the Spaniard's face, and finished the procedure with his curative balsam. Great was his surprise when upon uncovering the wound a few days later, he found not a much feared suppuration and necrosis but a nose perfectly reattached. He gave all due merit of course to the pap that he had formulated and that he was hoping to sell left and right.[48]

By Fioravanti's time, the question of how to fabricate a new nose and what to use when doing so was debated by a number of doctors. In *Chirurgia magna,* Andreas Vesalius—or rather the pseudo-Vesalius, for it appears that this text was actually the work of its editor, Prospero Borgarucci—had earlier been unconvinced of the advantages of surgical interventions on the nose. The procedure described in the book involved taking the biceps muscle, rather than skin, for the reconstruction of the septum—quite a painful process.[49] Following him, Gabriele Falloppio too felt that a superficial muscle was needed for surgery and, greatly exaggerating the time of recovery, wrote that it might take up to one year for the new nose to properly look like one. He also appropriately addressed the pain that the patient experienced at surgery and declared that he would have preferred to live without a nose rather than with a fake one acquired with so much difficulty.[50] Similarly Ambroise Paré thought that the new nose was not worth all it involved, given the length of the procedure to attach it and the suffering on the patient's part; moreover, the new nose could suddenly detach itself if one blew it too harshly, he argued, and its color, especially when the temperature outside was low, was not exactly fleshlike.[51] Girolamo Fabrici also criticized the method as being "very laborious, difficult and long," and so painful that "those who have submitted to it would not undergo it again if they should again have need of nose reparation."[52] Paolo Zacchia, who is today considered the founder of legal medicine, stated that a malefactor could legally have his nose redone through the Tagliacozzi's arm flap method because the pain that surgery would cause him was sufficient punishment for whatever crime he had committed.[53]

Still, the well-known Paduan doctor Girolamo Mercuriale, whose consult had often been solicited in Mantua by Duke Guglielmo, had nothing against nose surgery. It is indeed in a letter to him in 1587, "De reficiendo naso," that Tagliacozzi first explained his surgical method and hinted that his hefty book on the surgery of mutilation (*curtorum chirurgia*), delayed because the accompanying figures were not quite ready, would soon be sent to press. Tagliacozzi's procedure required not a muscle from the hand but skin grafts from above the elbow and thus, at least theoretically, his method was not unduly painful. Tagliacozzi in fact rebuked both Vesalius and Paré for arguing that nasal surgery meant excavating a hole in the arm, which surely would have made the operation unjustifiably agonizing. Instead he argued that the surgeon needed only to graft skin, and "the patients find the procedure so bearable that even apart from the work itself [i.e., the result] it wins universal admiration. Moreover there are other operations in surgery much more painful and difficult."[54] Tagliacozzi also introduced Mercuriale to two patients on whom he had performed surgery, and although their new noses did not appear totally natural, they seemed functional to Mercuriale, who hoped that this method would slowly progress to perfection. Tagliacozzi also mentioned by name a few patients whom he had treated surgically, noting that they were so satisfied with their new noses, they liked them more than the ones they had been born with.[55]

Ten years after the letter to Mercuriale on rhinoplastic procedures revealed the details of Tagliacozzi's daringly novel approach, the book *De curtorum chirurgia per insitionem* came out—illustrated in punctilious details—to divulge the method to future doctors. Here Tagliacozzi did not acknowledge his debt to the Vianeo brothers or to Fioravanti, who operated at the time in the same city, Bologna, and whose medical writings were a recommended reading for university students, no matter how controversial was the man's reputation. More damningly, Tagliacozzi did not acknowledge the pioneer work of his own teacher, the anatomist Giulio Cesare Aranzi, who repaired noses successfully in Bologna during his academic career and who in fact used the new technique of grafting from the skin rather than from the muscle, according to a Polish student of his, Wojcieck Ocsko, who studied in Bologna in 1565 and wrote on the Aranzi method upon his return to Poland a few years later.[56] Since Aranzi had died by the time *De curtorum chirurgia per insitionem* came out, Tagliacozzi was conveniently able to claim that he got the inspiration for his technique simply by examining nature.[57] By that time the Bolognese doctor was well known, and his consults on face and nose, like the one to which he was invited by Duke Vincenzo, were greatly sought after.

The Tagliacozzi method required an incision on the patient's arm over the biceps for the purpose of forming two parallel lines. Subsequently the doctor would loosen the skin and put linen dressing under it to promote separation. Four days later he would dress the wound and encourage scar formation by treating the skin regularly for fourteen days. At this point he would cut the flap at one end, leaving the other end securely attached to the man's arm in order to avoid necrosis. Then, two weeks later, he would graft the connected flap onto the nasal stump and keep the patient's arm attached to the nose by means of a strong halter. After another twenty days he would cut the flap from the arm. Two weeks needed to go by before the surgeon could finally start shaping the nose and attach it to the upper lip. This last procedure required a number of subsequent steps, but if the patient had survived sepsis—and that at the time was a big "if"—the goal was at least at hand (Figs. 9–12). Tagliacozzi also indicated the best time to perform the surgery and addressed at length the issue of pain and the difference in color and sensibility of the nostrils.[58] This technique of tissue transplantation became known as the "Italian method."[59]

Tagliacozzi insisted that he was creating not virtual noses but healthy ones. His repaired noses were lifelike, he wrote, although of a lighter skin color, and they were more responsive to cold temperatures. All other problems connected to them were mostly of a cosmetic nature and easily addressed, he added, such as the issue of hair growth on the nose. The kind of sedation he used on his subjects during surgery is not stated, but there were a number of techniques that a doctor could follow on the operating table at the time. Since ether was introduced only in 1842, offering the patient alcohol; imbibing him with various herbals, such as mandragora and belladonna; compressing his carotid artery to induce unconsciousness; or using a soporific sponge impregnated with henbane, water of nightshade, or other sleep-inducing components to produce narcosis were the surgeons' methods of choice.[60] Most important was the doctor's swiftness in using the knife. Patients were generally bled profusely before surgery to make them numb to pain; they were also routinely tied to a chair or to a bed, or held down by assistants to impede movement. Before the invention of the antibiotic and the anesthetic, opting for unnecessary surgery was a deadly business at least 50 percent of the time due to either infection or shock following surgery; records exist of patients literally fleeing the operating table.[61] Wanting a new nose must have thus seemed a sine qua non to individuals willing to undergo what, all considered, was an unnecessary operation. Still, Tagliacozzi insisted that his surgical method was not unduly painful:

> The surgeon uses a very small blade to cut the skin, which is held with a forceps [Fig. 13]. The incision can be completed very quickly, often

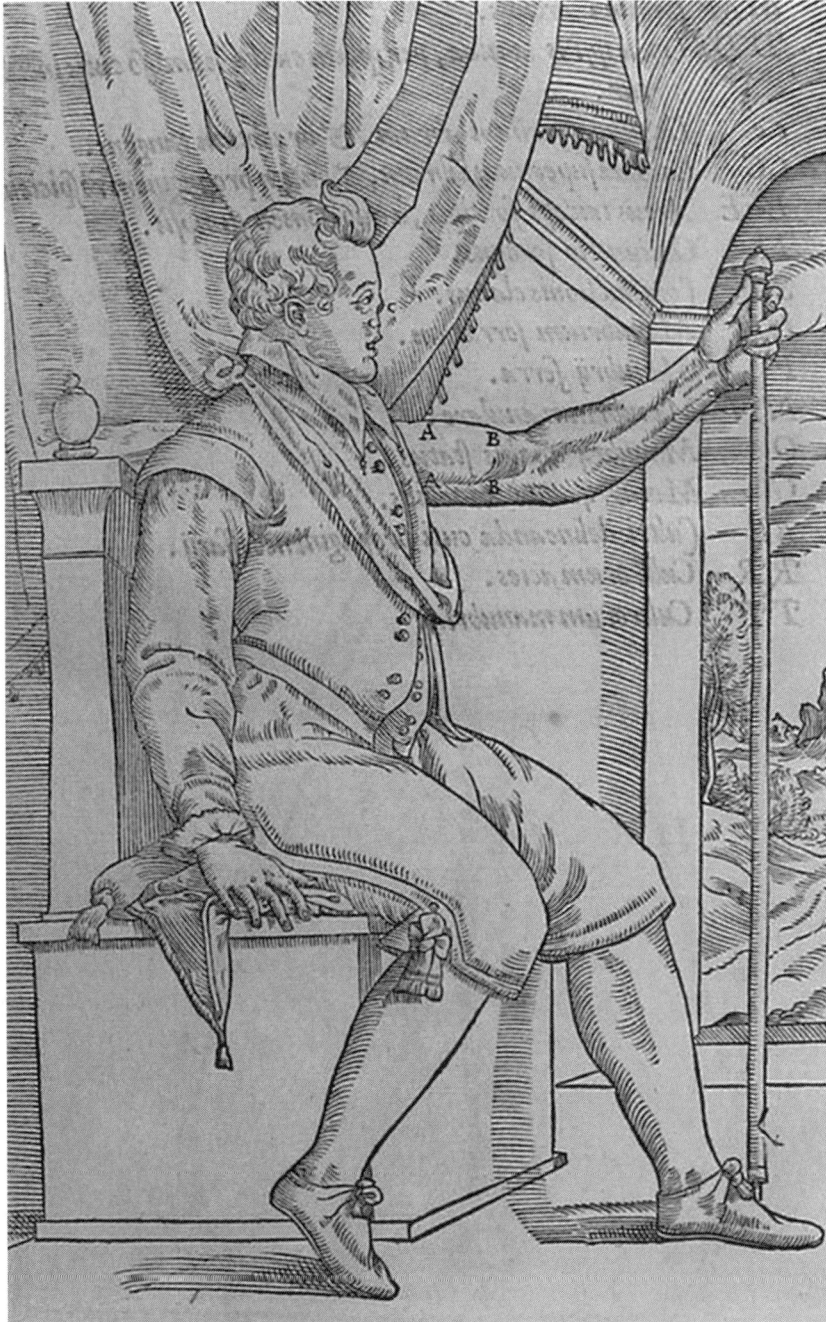

Fig. 9. Gaspare Tagliacozzi, "Icon Tertia," in *De curtorum chirurgia per insitionem* (Mantua: Bindoni, 1597). (Photo: Biblioteca Vincenzo Pinali, Sezione antica, Università di Padova, Padua.)

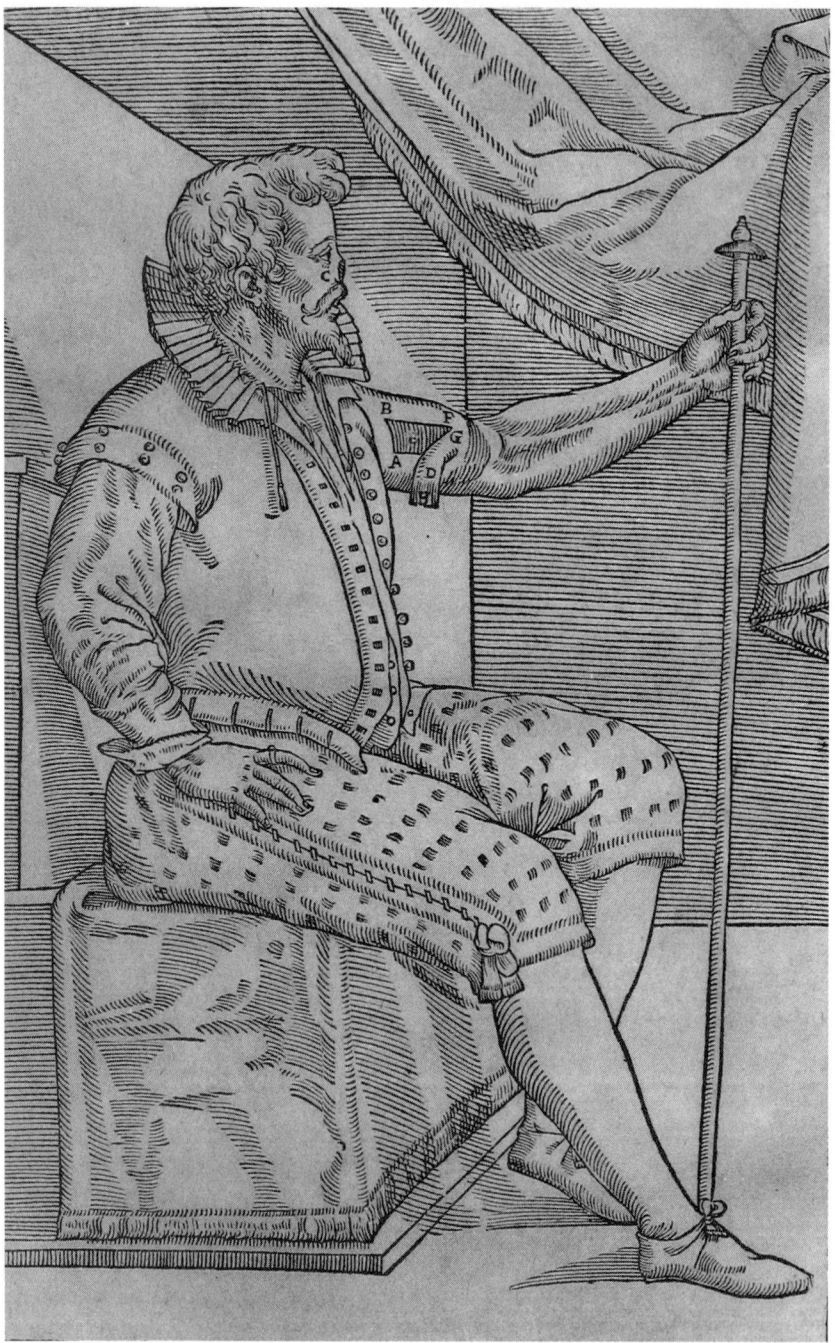

Fig. 10. Gaspare Tagliacozzi, "Icon Quinta," in *De curtorum chirurgia per insitionem* (Mantua: Bindoni, 1597). (Photo: Biblioteca Vincenzo Pinali, Sezione antica, Università di Padova, Padua.)

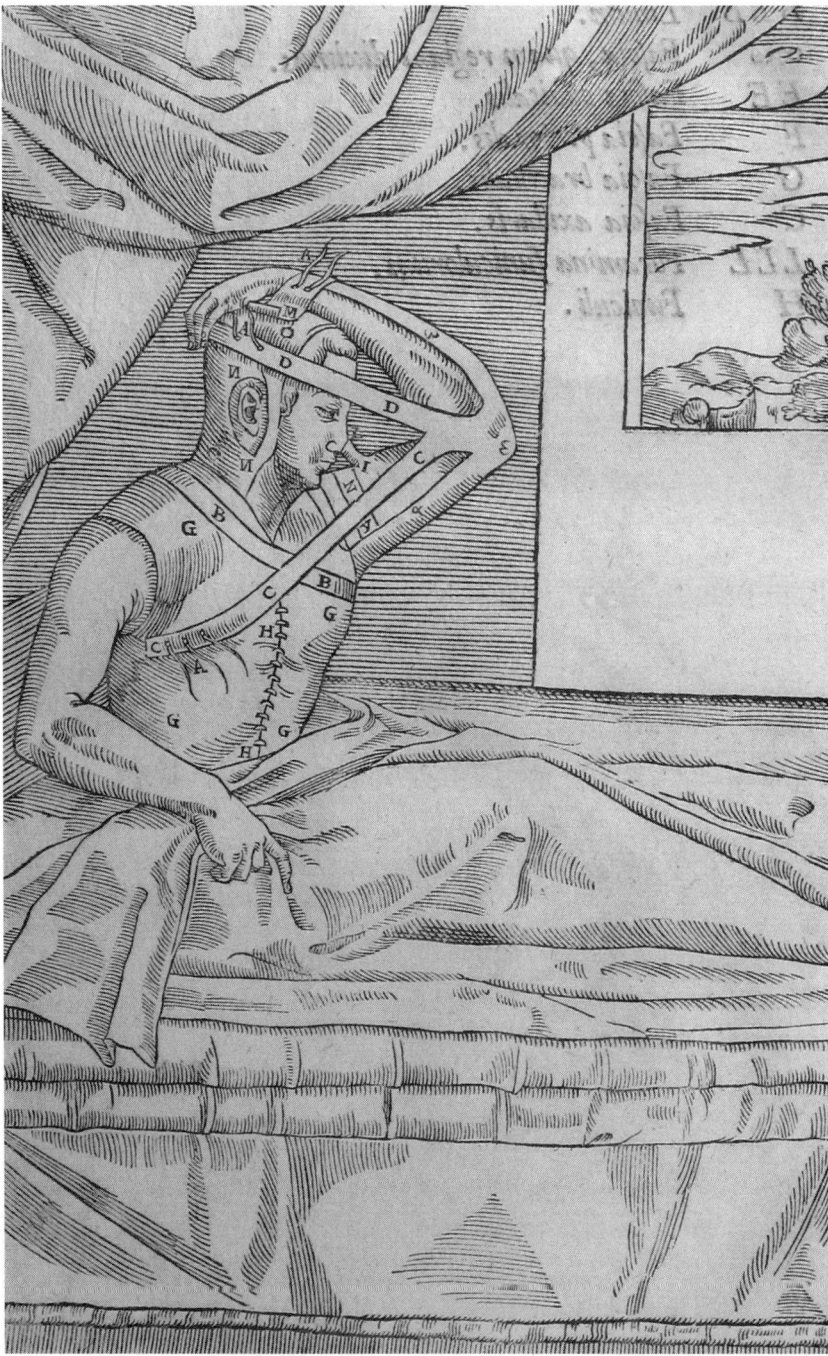

Fig. 11. Gaspare Tagliacozzi, "Icon Octava," in *De curtorum chirurgia per insitionem* (Mantua: Bindoni, 1597). (Photo: Biblioteca Vincenzo Pinali, Sezione antica, Università di Padova, Padua.)

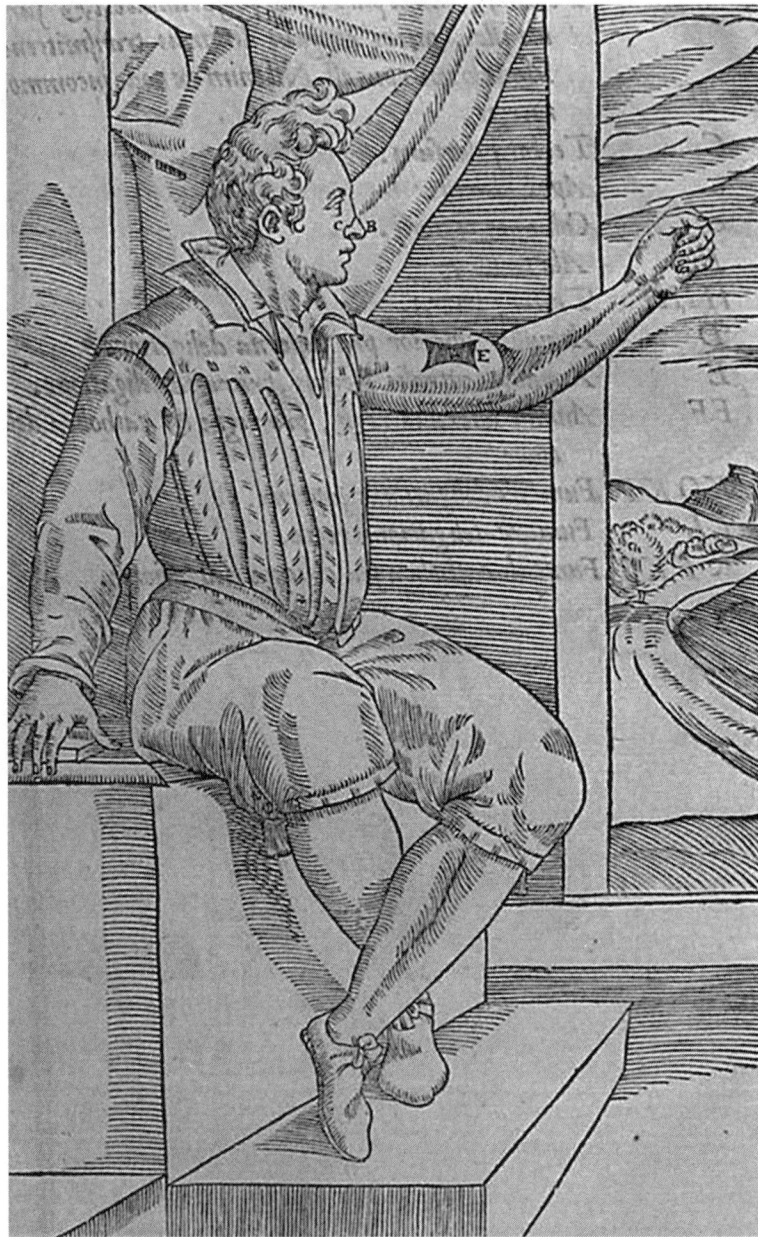

Fig. 12. Gaspare Tagliacozzi, "Icon Decimaquinta," in *De curtorum chirurgia per insitionem* (Mantua: Bindoni, 1597). (Photo: Biblioteca Vincenzo Pinali, Sezione antica, Università di Padova, Padua.)

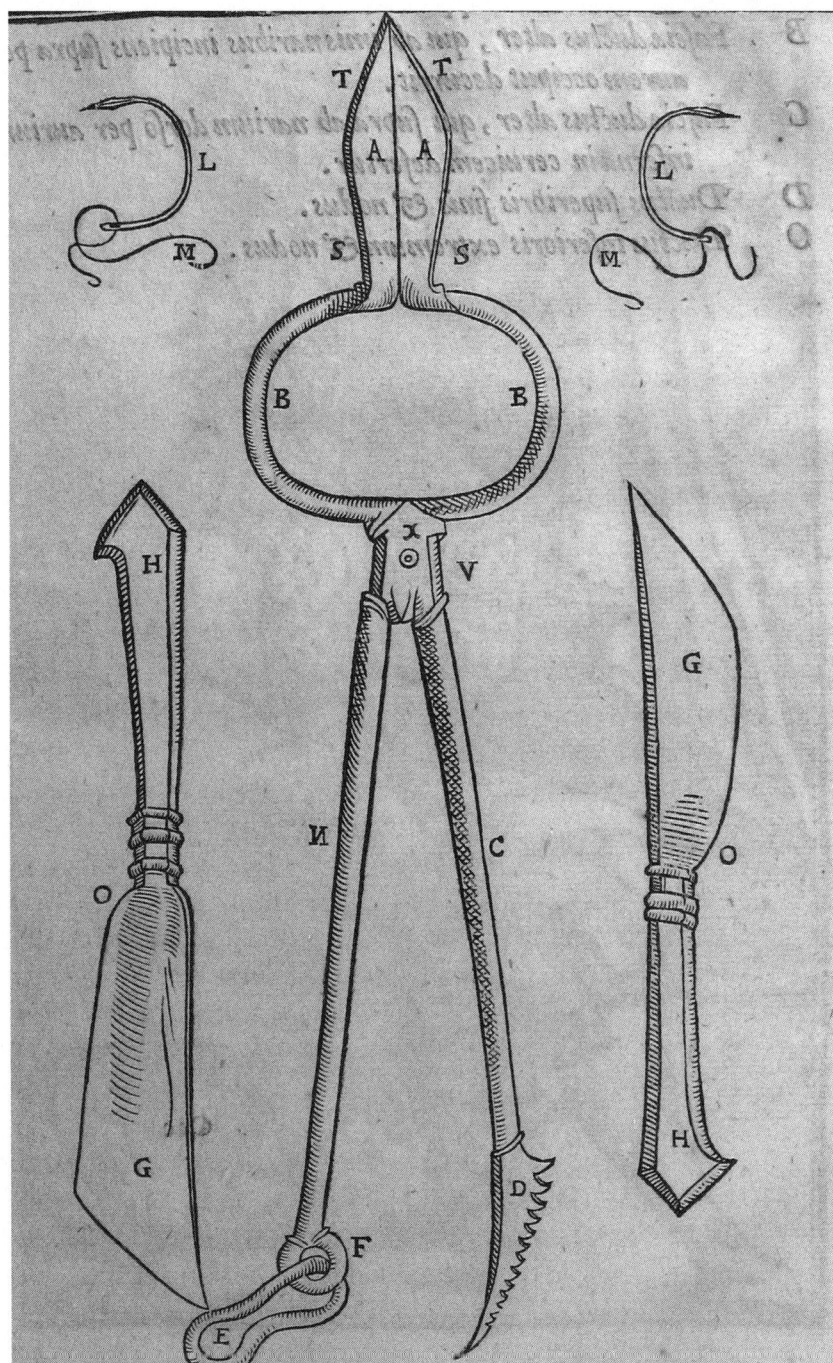

Fig. 13. Gaspare Tagliacozzi, Surgical Instruments, in *De curtorum chirurgia per insitionem* (Mantua: Bindoni, 1597). (Photo: Biblioteca Vincenzo Pinali, Sezione antica, Università di Padova, Padua.)

before the senses perceive it. This is hardly difficult to believe if one realizes that the constriction of the forceps dulls the skin's senses and, therefore, the perceived impact of the knife. This stage, then, is painless and swift. . . . The removal of the graft from the arm is equally swift and almost as painless. The only difference between this stage and the taking up of the graft is the lack of forceps; in the latter procedure, the skin is numbed by constriction, and in the former, the skin has regained a moderate capacity for feeling pain. The small size of the incision is, nevertheless, a mitigating factor. Although the shaping of the nose is a slow and long-lasting process, it is not violent or painful, because the recently grafted skin has not yet attained the proper balance needed in order to acquire sensitivity. The grafting of the skin to the base of the nose cannot, however, be carried out without pain. After all, parts that are endowed with acute sensitivity must be excoriated, incised, and pierced with needles. None of these activities can be accomplished quickly, and none provides pleasure to the patient. . . . It should by now be clear that my procedure causes little or no harm to the patient and is notable for the speed with which it is performed. Moreover, the operation is quite safe, because we stretch, cut, and shape only skin and avoid the large blood vessels completely.[62]

In remaking a nose, Tagliacozzi was realistic: the new nose would meet no beauty standard, he wrote, although he kept aesthetics on his mind as he trimmed and shaped, patient permitting, the stub that he had manufactured in the place where a nose once was. Renaissance ideals of beauty vis-à-vis the nose, of which he and his patients were obviously well aware, were in any case spelled out in numberless pamphlets, in collections of cosmetic recipes, and even in advice books written in Italian rather than Latin (and thus more accessible to the middle class to which they were addressed) by qualified medical practitioners. For the Venetian doctor Giovanni Marinello, for example, writing in 1574 *Gli ornamenti delle donne*—a book centered on female beauty and beautification techniques—the perfect nose is small, thin, and turns up slightly. No aquiline noses for women, he argued, for the ideal nose proportion from the base to the tip should be the length of a finger's knuckle. The nose should also be of the same color of the ears or less reddish. Curly noses ruin a profile, he stated.[63]

In the art of the period it appears that slightly longish noses were good attributes for both men and women. Titian's idealized beauties—La Bella, Salomé, Flora, the Venus of Urbino, and the Venus with the Mirror—all sport longish noses. Indeed, even when he painted a real woman, Eleonora Gonzaga della Rovere, Titian chose to lengthen her nose, as recently demonstrated by forensic pathologists studying the Uffizi portrait of Eleonora and a three-dimensional scan of the skull believed to belong to the duchess.[64] Michelangelo, another artist whose long life span and lengthy accomplishments cast a shadow throughout the sixteenth century, famously sported a flattened nose, which he broke during a brawl in youth and which became very much part of his legend. I mention him here, however, because he flatly refused to shorten David's nose, showing thus that nose sizes have complicated psychological connotations, even when artists are drawing from a live model.[65]

Unlike artists, poets avoided talking about noses, especially female noses, altogether. In the Petrarchan canon, which informed all manner of literary inquiry at the time, there were only two facial features—the nose and the ears—that were never mentioned in the catalog of Laura's attributes, as if they were two traits on the idealized face of the beloved object so improper that they could not even be alluded to. The others, however—the eyebrows, the eyes, the cheeks, the mouth, the lips, and the teeth down to the neck—were all lovingly surveyed and appreciatively compared to stars, pearls, marble, and corals. In his footsteps, Renaissance Petrarchists never made the nose part of any narrative. In poetically portraying the incomparable beauties of Alcina in *Orlando furioso*, for example, Ludovico Ariosto went as far as mentioning the nose but did not describe it.[66] Noses were mentioned in satirical writings, as we would expect given the lower nature of that genre, but they mostly belonged to men.[67]

Noses in Culture

Today surgery on one's nose is meant to beautify a given facial feature or to hide racial attributes, for there are no individuals walking in the streets without noses. At the most fundamental level, having a nose is in fact the sine qua non for an identity, for a person without a nose cannot be easily identified as belonging to either gender, male or female. Even the church required in the past that men have noses if they wanted to become priests, just as it required priests to lack no part of their genital apparatuses, thus excluding castrati and eunuchs from holy orders. As Thomas Aquinas wrote, "Si sit talis defectus qui maculam natabilem inferat, per quem obscuretur personae claritas, ut abcissio nasi."[68] This prohibition was already present in Leviticus 21:18, where it is written that men with *charum*, that is, men with flat noses, cannot become priests in the temple. In canon law the loss of a nose could plausibly mean the termination of a marriage. Would a new nose reinstate one, the rhinoplast Otto Hildebrand mused a few centuries later?[69] Clearly lack of a nose in men meant lack of masculinity.

It also meant lack of power, for cutting off one's nose was often the penalty for subordinates, for women, and for criminals. Slaves were occasionally punished this way, as illustrated by the 1561 reprisal against two runaway Turkish slaves, whom Cosimo de' Medici condemned to have their ears and noses cut off but not their eyes taken out, for they were still needed for labor.[70] In Byzantine law, rapists were punished with *denasatio* (de-nosing). In Rome in the 1580s, Pope Sixtus V ordered that thieves be disciplined no longer with a mark of infamy but by cutting off their noses, although we do not know whether this bull was actually applied. Even missionaries were implicated in cutting off the noses of unredeemable pagans, and some kings lost their noses for losing a war. At other times it was sufficient to cut off the tip of one's nose to signify punishment and retaliation and to brand that person for life.[71] This was occasionally done, for example, to ambassadors or captured soldiers. The famous skinning and quartering of the Venetian commander Marcantonio Bragadin in Famagusta, Cyprus, in 1571, by the Ottoman general Mustafa Pasha was preceded, for example, by the cutting off of his nose and ears, an event traumatic enough for the Venetian republic to be continuously reenacted in tragedies performed in the succeeding years.[72]

Lack of a nose meant specifically sexual profligacy. Not for nothing a silver nose and a stench of sulfur give Satan away in one of Italo Calvino's contemporary fables.[73] Adulterous women or women who prostituted their daughters were sentenced to have their noses cut off by the Normans, who dominated Sicily in the late eleventh and most of the twelfth centuries—and let us remember that the first nose surgeons were from Sicily.[74] In the baroque plays of Margherita Costa, women with long or missing noses are associated with sin and prostitution.[75] This sort of gendered punishment is easy to categorize, for women were typically thought of as valuable as long as they were attractive. But men too risked their noses when they strayed sexually onto other men's property, as in Virgil's *Aeneid*, in which Deiphobus was punished with *denasatio* for having committed adultery with Helen.[76] Under Venetian law, occasionally the passive partner in a homosexual relationship was condemned to have his nose cut off, whereas the active partner's punishment was to be publicly executed—a reflection, Guido Ruggiero suggests, of the fact that the passive member of the couple was perceived as feminized and easily led astray and thus deserved a punishment that would mark him as womanly.[77] And indeed nuns who wanted to avoid being raped when marauding soldiers raided their convents sometimes chose to cut off their noses to appear repulsive, and thus preserve the virginity of their body and their marital tie to Christ. Self-disfigurement "as an extreme measure of virginal defense" is documented in a number of medieval convents.[78] Tagliacozzi too registers the case of England's Saint Ebb, who cut off her nose and persuaded her fellow nuns to do the same in order to "ward off the calamitous sexual desires of the invading Danes."[79] Even more startling, cutting off noses after rape was the punishment inflicted on women at times of sack, plunder, and war, thus marking them for life as abjects and rejects of their own society.

Lack of a nose or a sunken nose also meant disease, for syphilitics had inscribed their inner decay for all to see in their noses—and there were plenty of such instances in the sixteenth century. In cases of congenital syphilis, the parents' "sin" also condemned the offspring to become objects of pity and horror, as can most famously be seen in the missing nose of Erik, Gaston Leroux's phantom in *The Phantom of the Opera*. In his unpublished treatise, "Del Disonore," Tagliacozzi's friend and known anatomist, Giulio Mancini, distinguished between a scarred body, which meant valor and courage, and a mutilated body, which meant that the individual had undergone punishment, such as, he wrote, the severing of his nose or ear. Tellingly, the diseased body of the syphilitic registered for him the transformation of the noble, honorable body into the debauched remains of the sexual profligate. To avoid such a corporal disintegration, Mancini suggested that young men keep before their eyes the painted portrait of a syphilitic gentleman with a rotting nose—that, he thought, constituted a sufficient deterrent to randy desires.[80] Girolamo Fracastoro, the first doctor to assign the name "syphilis" to the disease ravaging the times, was quite specific in describing the ways by which syphilis literally obliterated body parts, at least in its tertiary stage: "In those in whom the disease [syphilis] attacks the upper parts, foul drippings appear, which in some eat away the palate, in some the uvula, in some the fauces, and in some the tonsils—in some the lips are consumed, in some the nose, in some the eyes, and in some the whole pudenda."[81] Shakespeare's curse in *Timon* well illustrates how a putrefying nose spelled general decay:

> ... Consumptions sow
> In hollow bones of man; strike their sharp shins,
> And mar men's spurring.
> Crack the lawyer's voice,
> That he may never more false title plead,
> Nor sound his quillets shrilly: hoar the flamen,
> That scolds against the quality of flesh,
> And not believes himself: down with the nose,
> Down with it flat; take the bridge quite away
> Of him that, his particular to foresee,
> Smells from the general weal.[82]

A major motivation for the preoccupation with nose reconstruction at this specific period in time may have thus originated from the widespread course of syphilis, which affected all social strata. It is true that by the end of the sixteenth century, syphilis was no longer the thoroughly disfiguring and revolting disease it had been during its endemic years in the late fifteenth century; however, no specific interest in operating techniques could have surfaced when the disease first presented itself, because surgical procedures became more common only with time.[83] This also explains the repeated recommendations in manuals on how to correct a smelly nose, the result of the widespread circulation of people affected by tertiary syphilis.[84] As evidenced in paintings and drawings from *alba amicorum* (books of friendship) illustrating life in Italy of the period, the era saw the first use of the handkerchief. In addition, how to keep a nose clean and what to do with a handkerchief after it was used was appropriately discussed in manuals. In his *Galateo*, Giovanni della Casa offers the most suitable behavior for gentlemen on the subject.[85]

Finally, lack of a nose meant defeat. Among the litigious, vendetta-bent, and banditry-plagued early modern society, amputating the defeated enemy's nose in a duel was a sign of spite—leaving a man alive but marked, for all to see his failings and weaknesses. The astronomer and alchemist Tycho Brahe, for example, lost his nose at twenty to the rapier of a fellow nobleman in a brawl in 1566 over an argument about who was a better mathematician. For the rest of his life Brahe sported an artificial nose made of silver and gold, which, he wrote, he kept attached with an ad hoc adhesive balm. However, when Brahe's tomb was opened in 1901, his nasal bridge showed that the prosthetics were actually made of a lighter and therefore more wearable material, copper.[86] Loss of a nose was sufficient to start even a fratricide war, as in the case of the Corsi and the Donati, or so recounts Dino Compagni in his Florentine chronicles of the thirteenth century, when Ricoverini de Cerchi's nose was slashed during a spring dance by an unnamed Donati clan member.[87] Hence it is possible to argue that a man's honor resides in his nose, and Annibal Caro easily appropriated the metaphor in *La nasea:* "The nose is the seat of majesty and honor in man, in consequence the bigger one's nose, the greater one's honor . . . to be without a nose is one of the greatest dishonors that can befall a man. Today Sicilians say that if one loses one's nose, one loses one's honor."[88]

Following up on the issue of honor from decidedly another angle, Giambattista della Porta argued in those very years that the nose corresponds to the penis and the nostrils to the testicles, since there is proportion between the face and all body parts. Those with large noses are more masculine, he offered, and from this "comes the saying: from the largeness of the nose you will know of that other largeness."[89] Yet Carlo Borromeo, a most famous ascetic canonized in 1610 (he had negotiated the end of Vincenzo's first marriage), was known for having a very large nose, so much so that in a letter by Caterina Gonzaga, Vincenzo's daughter-in-law, to her brother Cosimo II in Florence, St. Carlo's nose is indicated as precisely a horrible model to follow when painting a face, and she begs the painter Bronzino to stay clear of it: "I wish that these [Mantuan] artists learn how to make noses, since the one that they are painting of mine is three times that of St. Carlo."[90] It could be argued that Borromeo sublimated his sexual urge into religious inflexibility were it not that this assertion had little evidential support, as doctor Laurent Joubert argues, "Do all men have the same size or caliber, in every dimension? It is certain that they do not, even though one may say: *Ad formam nasi cognoscitur at te levavi.* And this is because the proportion of members is not observed in all men. Several who have a stunning trunk of a nose are flattened elsewhere, and several who have flat noses are well endowed in the principal member."[91]

The association does not come as a surprise, for the Venetian doctor Giovanni Andrea Della Croce (Joannes Andreas Cruce) had argued that one of the reasons why a new nose could not be attached was that the nose is a "spermatic part."[92] Indeed, according to Alfonso Corradi, after Tagliacozzi's death, many nose surgeries were done no longer by surgeons but appropriately by Norcini castrators, who were customarily employed to cut off the "spermatic" parts of prepubescent boys' sexual organs when the craze for castrati took over the musical establishment.[93] The association between nose and genitalia was made most forcefully as recently as last century in a series of letters exchanged between Wilhelm Fliess and Sigmund Freud. As the correspondence shows, women, and not men, were the most involved in nose issues for the two doctors, for in their noses was the seat of emotion and sexual passion: the gastric spot, according to Fliess—a Berlin otorhinolaryngologist, who assiduously wrote on "the therapy of the neurasthenic nasal neurosis" and operated on the noses of at least 156 patients to correct their sexual dysfunction. Of these, only a dozen were men.[94] Sander Gilman has since argued that the reason for Fliess's and Freud's concentration on women is that Jewish men, no matter their long noses, were already "othered" as lacking, following their ritual circumcision. Thus, now women too participated to the "cut around."[95]

The Afterlife of the Tagliacozzi Method

We do not know how many reconstructive nasal surgeries Tagliacozzi performed during his lifetime, how many total columella, septum, and nasal tips he fixed, but when he died, just two years after the publication of his book in 1597, his technique was well known in Italy among surgeons. Sadly Tagliacozzi did not leave a school behind, and his method died off during the course of the seventeenth century. In 1788 the University of Paris went so far as to forbid any nasal surgical procedure, and the entire method of nose transplantation practically had to be discovered *ex novo* in the nineteenth century, not as an Italian but as a Hindi technique. This was thanks to British colonial exchanges, for in 1816 the English surgeon J. C. Carpue described a method of nasal surgery employed on two patients that used a forehead flap, a technique coming from Indian procedures dating back to Sushruta.[96] Soon after, the German doctor Carl Ferdinand von Graefe, who invented the term "rhinoplasty," put Tagliacozzi back into the picture when in his book on plastic surgery—the first to come out following Tagliacozzi's 1597 opus—he described three kinds of surgery that he performed on the nose: the first was using skin from the face, following the Indian method (although von Graefe was unaware of it, this was actually the original Italian method of the Sicilian Branca team); the second was grafting it from the arm, following the Tagliacozzi method; and the third was modifying the arm flap, which came to be called the German method.[97] In the end it was another surgeon, Johann Friedrich Dieffenbach, who provided the most influential technique for nose reconstruction. His preference was to use the forehead skin, including the hair-bearing portion, rather than the arm, because it offered skin of better quality. He also lengthened the incision so that there was less twisting of the pedicle and better blood circulation, and illustrated the technique in a series of plates that document how aesthetically pleasing the new noses could eventually become.[98] In those years the French doctor Philippe Blandin, who also preferred long incisions from the forehead to the nose, suggested a new term, "autoplasty," for procedures involving skin grafted for aesthetic surgeries, but Dieffenbach preferred Tagliacozzi's term, "beauty surgery," to describe reconstructive surgery.[99] Then, in 1837, an American surgeon, Jonathan Mason Warren, returned to the Tagliacozzi technique, although he used the forearm rather than the biceps, because the patient was too muscular.[100] It would take World War I—when the number of badly injured soldiers coming back from the trenches made the issue of reconstructive surgical treatment timely as well as necessary for reintroducing horribly wounded men into society—for plastic surgery to be again practiced on a large scale. In the meantime, by the middle of the nineteenth century, the introduction of skin grafting had made interventions on the nose aesthetically pleasing.

Tragically, by the eighteenth century Tagliacozzi's name—and, more to the point, his teachings—had turned into a subject of ridicule. Here is what happened: less than two months after the famous surgeon's death and burial in the convent of San Giovanni Battista in Bologna, where two of his daughters were cloistered, some nuns claimed to have heard a voice proclaiming that Tagliacozzi was a damned man. They thus rushed to unearth the anatomist's corpse and carried it away from the burial ground to the convent's walls, from which they threw it.[101]

Following this superstitious exhumation, the Inquisition intervened to investigate the charges while Tagliacozzi was temporarily reburied in unconsecrated land. Unfortunately neither the church nor the convent—along with the tomb where the surgeon was originally buried—exist today, for under Napoleonic law they were dismantled and became military barracks. The documents relative to the trial, once kept in the Archivi del Foro Archiepiscopale and the Tribunale dell'Inquisizione in Bologna, have also been lost, but we have a note written in the second half of the seventeenth century by Gerolamo Sbaraglia, a professor of medicine and anatomy. This note was inserted into a copy of Tagliacozzi's *De curtorum chirurgia,* which was owned by a fellow doctor at the University of Bologna.[102] Here it is stated that the body of Tagliacozzi, who was accused of magic by jealous people, was fully absolved of heresy on July 15, 1600, and that the accusers were condemned.[103] Tagliacozzi was subsequently reburied in a newly constructed monumental tomb, situated in the convent where he was originally inhumed and where his son was also buried a few years later. These tombs as well no longer exist.

The academic establishment at the time, however, read the news of Tagliacozzi's untimely exhumation in a much different light. Here we move from the original accusation of unorthodox and magical practices on the part of cloistered nuns into the area of class and money. Since rhinoplasty was thought to be a lengthy and excruciatingly painful enterprise, could it be possible, it was argued most famously by nondoctors, that a new nose could be fashioned not by grafting skin from one's arm but by paying for somebody else's body part, say, that of a slave? In chapter 18 of his book, Tagliacozzi had made clear that such a grafting procedure was not impossible, technically speaking, but was thoroughly unreliable, because it would have been very difficult to keep two people immobilized for the considerable amount of time it would take for the pedicle to attach. He chose not to elaborate on whether such a surgery could have even been successful.[104] No matter: the issue had less to do with the possibility of having an outstanding outcome than with the argument of what happens to a nose transplanted onto another's face when the original owner dies. This constitutes the theory of the sympathetic nose, and it is tied not to a medical but to a philosophical and religious issue: that of one's soul. Let's hear the explanation of the problem that the philosopher and theologian Tommaso

Campanella—Tagliacozzi's contemporary who refers not to Tagliacozzi but to the Tropea brothers—proffered:

> A friend asks me: "Of whose soul was the [re-made] part of the nose living, of the slave, or of the master? If of the master, why did it die when the slave died? If of the slave, why did it continue to live away from him, since any members cut off perish? Furthermore, why does the grafted scion not die when the tree dies from which it was cut? And why does the son not die when the father dies, whose seed he is?" I reply that, according to the soul given of God, yesterday the soul was living which was in the whole, which is vilified in its subject. For the [re-made] part of the nose is not separate like a worm in the belly, but united to the whole.[105]

Campanella's assertions are illogical, but many like him believed in the unity of the soul and argued passionately about it. It did not take long for Tagliacozzi to be satirized for taking the nose needed for the master not from an inferior's arm but from an inferior's buttocks, as in Samuel Butler's *Hudibras*:

> So learned Taliacotius from
> The brawny part of Porter's bum,
> Cut supplemental Noses, which
> Would last as long as Parent breech:
> But when the Date of Nock was out,
> Off dropt the Sympathetik Snout.[106]

The comments then reappeared in Voltaire's *Candide,* in which the syphilitic doctor Pangloss indeed sported no nose. In his usual mocking vein, Voltaire saw a kind of reparatory reunification at the donor's death when the flesh used for the nose was buried next to his derrière.[107]

When all is said and done, the association of the nose with racism has remained for a long time attached to the issue of plastic surgery. For until fifty years ago, when corrective surgery gave way to cosmetic surgery and doctors increasingly started to be asked to rework the osseous nasal skeleton from within rather than to transplant new noses, the category of patients that had sought rhinoplasty until then were almost exclusively of Jewish descent. As Sander Gilman has argued in a series of pathbreaking studies, by diminishing a nose's size and reshaping its form, Jewish men and women could pass for Aryans and unobtrusively belong to the society in which they had come to live in America. It was only after World War II that new noses were increasingly sought by

Jews and non-Jews alike, and only in the 1990s that plastic surgery, having become thoroughly entwined with the notion of beauty as socially and economically important, crossed gender lines and became the surgery of choice for women.[108] Yet the racial aspects of rhinoplasty have not died. One has only to read the tabloids and gossip magazines to see that the overwhelming preoccupation with, say, Michael Jackson's nose exposes other anxieties. For in seeking not only a feminine nose a la Elizabeth Taylor but a slender nose like that of an Aryan, Michael Jackson proved, as Jews in the past could testify to, that "passing" is difficult. In Jackson's collapsed and discolored proboscis, America read not the wunderkind's personal desire, even if extreme, for a virtual white, racially unmarked self, but the confirmation that no matter how much you "wash the Aethiop white," as the saying goes, he remains black at the core. For Jackson's disappearing nose has been satirized both for giving his face a monkey-like look—and note the animalistic connotation of this remark—and for testifying to his ever-diminished masculinity and "sinful" sexual desires, if not practices.

And this brings me back to our story. At a time when surgery was gradually becoming a profession rivaling that of medical practitioners in prestige and revenue, a brilliant surgeon like Tagliacozzi thought the moment was ripe to assist moneyed patients who desired to correct debased facial features in becoming social "men" again, just like God had made them. His problem was that the medicine available at the time was inadequate to cure the majority of the health problems that were presented to him. Tagliacozzi could remake noses, but infection could easily take the life of half of his subjects. At this moment in history, he was also unable to cure Duke Vincenzo. Whatever pomade he gave him for his face and nose provided the duke only some temporary respite. Whether Vincenzo had gonorrhea, syphilis, erysipelas, or tuberculosis is beyond the point here. None of these illnesses could be properly addressed at the time, for they could not be eradicated until the development of sulfonamide drugs and antibiotics. In fact, Vincenzo lived many years in their company.

In another sense, however, Tagliacozzi the visionary surgeon and Vincenzo the curious aesthete were pursuing identical goals. The modernity of Tagliacozzi's conception—his daring technique of restoring aesthetic appearance through intervention on facial deformities, despite the pain—does indeed match the longings of a duke committed to live under the sign of the beautiful, the striking, and the splendid, no matter the political and economic consequences that these choices could generate vis-à-vis his Mantuan subjects. Vincenzo's enthusiasm for artistic sophistication was so contagious, we are told by historians, that even those who criticized him often ended up falling under his spell, thus proving again and again that hyper-aesthetics is a transmittable, even eagerly sought after, syndrome.

3

The Comfort Cure

Managing Pain and Catarrh at the Spa

> The old get old and the young get stronger . . .
> Your ballroom days are over, baby.
> Night is drawing near.
> Shadows of the evening crawl across the years.
>
> —Jim Morrison, "Five to One"

Sometime in the year 1601, Vincenzo Gonzaga I, fourth Duke of Mantua and Monferrato and munificent sponsor of art, music, and theater—a Renaissance prince in every sense of the word—realized that he had a difficulty that required some creative addressing. Historians are in agreement today that this particular ducal predicament was, like the one I followed in Chapter 2, political: Vincenzo's crusade against the Turks in Hungary—his third and last—was eerily looking like his first or second, and again it was not going well.[1] Four months into his war east, Vincenzo was contemplating a camp decimated by disease (half of his army had died) and recurrent floods. In one of the first registered instances of chemical war, he had even ordered that poisonous gasses, prepared back home by his apothecaries, be hurled into the besieged city of Canissa (Nagykanizsa or Grosskirchen) in order to hasten at least one victory, but this gimmick too had proven unsuccessful.[2] Disagreements over tactics with the new imperial commander, Colonel Hermann Roswurn, who privately judged the Gonzaga commander militarily inept—he, the great-grandchild of the condottiere Francesco Gonzaga—were making his life miserable.[3] A radical resolution only could keep somewhat intact his leadership and political ambitions, no matter how ego crushing the compromise was at present. Thus Vincenzo resolved to push aside his dream of martial glory and, with haste, left the encampment, its contents, and the wounded soldiers behind to return to Mantua.[4] He arrived home on December 19, five months after his departure.[5]

There was at the time an official medical explanation for the duke's rushed return home, even though many did not believe it: a rheumatism or catarrh of the knee. From the correspondence of those days we know that Vincenzo's long-standing knee and leg pain had become excruciating during his stay abroad, and no relief suggested by the doctors in his retinue had provided more than a palliative alleviation of symptoms. Not long after his arrival to Canissa, for example, in a letter of September 6, 1601, to his sister Anna, Archduchess of Innsbruck, Vincenzo had complained that his intermittent fevers (he referred to them as a *quartana*) had now become a daily occurrence and that he was suffering from his usual swollen knee ("solita enfiaggine al ginocchio").[6] Later that month, writing on September 29, 1601, the ducal counselor Alessandro Striggio informed Eleonora de' Medici back home that the duke had to remain in his pavilion in Canissa to rest because of continuous issues with his knee.[7] Indeed, following his return from Hungary, Vincenzo spent a few years trying to address some pervasive bodily pain, a long-standing problem that had recently become unmanageable. This required all sorts of topical cures, unguents, elixirs, tinctures, tonics, and brews, most of which did little to relieve his aches, so that in the end the customary comfort treatment of his days, a visit to the spa, offered the most viable alternative.

Vincenzo's pilgrimage to spas all over Italy as well as throughout northern Europe turned into an almost yearly event after that painful episode in Canissa; when he lacked time, he kept his water-for-health routine alive as much as he could back home. He loved, for example, to dip into pools and water sources, even though swimming was not considered beneficial to one's health at the time.[8] He also devotedly followed alternative water therapies, such as bathing in salt water or drinking bottled mineral water imported for his use from curative fountains as far away as Spa in the Catholic Flanders. In this chapter, taking my cue from Vincenzo's cyclical water cures, I am interested in reconstructing the spa culture of the early modern period and examining what exactly spas were thought to address and treat in a historical period that was not in any way identified with baths. The dictates of Galenic medicine at the time—which recommended keeping one's pores closed to avoid contracting infectious diseases—together with more sweeping hygienic requirements increasingly enacted by local governments to contain the spread of syphilis, were meant to make some watering spots obsolete.[9]

Whether people believed in the miraculous power of mineral mud baths and the rejuvenating properties of hot springs or whether they used a sojourn to a watering place more prosaically to escape the pressures and the duties of court and city life was usually beside the point. A spa resort, even a primitive one, provided patients with a measure of comfort that the medicine of the time was unable to deliver. For the people with the means to afford a trip to a watering establishment as well as for the local poor who crowded these places, seeking a water cure was a hands-on choice meant to reduce distress and minimize disability, given the array of identifiable diseases (some of them nonexistent today, which makes their identification both difficult and dubious) for which no long-lasting relief was in sight. They did not mind, while there, to submit themselves to a variety of invasive therapies and rehabilitative routines in order to address their afflictions, as many of them had already undergone mind-boggling, aggressive treatments at home. I am not talking here of simply resorting to emetics, suppositories, and leeches to expel the bad humors thought at the time to cause illness, but of the long list of toxic recipes that the homey pharmacopoeia was extensively producing, such as, to give just an example, viper meat or viper-infused wine (*vino viperino*) to fight scabies, elephantiasis, syphilis, ulcers, scrofula, and a range of other disfiguring syndromes.[10]

At the same time spas offered plenty of entertainment and relaxation. Musicians with bagpipes and other string instruments often entertained their sick patrons while sitting in the pools with them; waiters floated luscious food and wine on trays so that the stomach had its recompense too; and masseurs hired for muscle relief waited for customers on tents built for the occasion next to the pools. Last, but definitely not least, tempting youthful male and female companions were on call for those in need of letting loose otherwise, and they were so ubiquitous that even Dante lamented the promiscuity and immorality they brought to Bagni di Viterbo, a place typically frequented by popes and the Roman curia.[11] In the evening, nearby gambling facilities provided plenty of amusement and frisson; moreover, the presence of people from similar social classes fostered unconventional, often unanticipated, economic and political deals or cemented marriage alliances.

The Duke's "Indispositions"

Vincenzo's bodily afflictions—or, as he called them, "indispositions"—were many, though not by any means unusual for people of his life and times, an age that, unlike ours, had none of the benefits of immunization, antibiotics, and sulfa drugs. Thus, before I present a chronology of Vincenzo's spa stays, I would like to attempt a diagnosis of the duke's health problems at this stage in his life, based on contemporary documents, for "the language of pain," to use a quote from Roy Porter, "—was it moral, physical, emotional, localized, behavioral?—reveals much about perceptions of selfhood and the hieratic organology of mind, body, heart, soul, nerves; and also about the meaning of maladies."[12] Medical nomenclature has obviously changed in the intervening centuries, and diagnoses have to be accordingly readjusted. Moreover, since Vincenzo's remains have not yet been found, we lack the support of diagnoses by forensic pathologists in coming up with a comprehensive identification of his health problems; thus any conclusion is subject to revision. There seems to be agreement, however, that Vincenzo suffered from chronic rheumatism of the knee, as in the instance that motivated the end of his Hungarian campaign. His complaints of localized swelling, stiffness, inflammation, weakness, and pain in the cartilage of his knee seem to be the result of an autoimmune disease: rheumatoid arthritis—that is, a chronic and inflammatory type of arthritis. Of course it is possible that the pain was a bursitis of the knee, coming, say, from long journeys on horseback with knees bent, although bursitis may not have caused the significant pain that by all accounts afflicted Vincenzo.[13] The pain could have also been the outcome of a traumatic condition, a meniscus injury following a fall from a horse or a wound in a joust.[14] More likely, however, the duke's crippling arthritis can be read as another manifestation of that double medical pathology that for generations coursed through the Gonzaga dynastic line—male as well as female, sometimes alone and at times together—and that was never fully understood by contemporary medicine: rickets and tuberculosis.

Skeletal disorders among the Gonzaga point to rickets. Medically speaking, when rickets affects the bone tissues of the spine, it produces a vertebral disease, such as a hunchback deformity (the case with many members of the Gonzaga family from previous generations, beginning with Paola Malatesta and followed by her son, Ludovico Gonzaga, and immediately after by Ludovico's son, Federico). The celebrated family mural by Andrea Mantegna of the Gonzaga and retinue in the Camera degli Sposi in the Ducal Palace in Mantua shows that this disease was so common in the family that it could be realistically accommodated even when an artist was engaged in celebratory depictions. When rickets affects the articulations, it produces a degenerative disease such as arthritis, as with Vincenzo.[15] In his case, the disorder seems to have gone undiagnosed, probably because he bore no visual marker of it, unlike his father, whose pathological spinal curve spelled the presence of rickets.

But Guglielmo's hunched back could have just as well alerted to the presence of Pott's disease (tuberculous spondylitis), a tuberculous arthritis that causes softening or collapse of the vertebrae. And indeed a series of recorded illnesses that Vincenzo suffered through the years would lead us toward a diagnosis of tuberculosis, which in Vincenzo's case affected not the spine, like his father, but the knee and other body parts, often the skin. Signs of arthritis in the knee quite early in life could mean that Vincenzo had developed osteoarticular tuberculosis of the knee, a most common location of non-vertebral, extrapulmonary tuberculosis.[16] Localized germs coming to the knee as a result of wounds or circulated from other parts of the body by blood would have infected the joint, which felt warm, tender to the touch, and swollen. This form of arthritis, often involving just one joint, was very common at the time and usually presented itself during infancy or before adulthood. It was accompanied by low-grade fever, muscle spasms, and tiredness. As tuberculosis destroyed the cartilage in the joint and the bone, it provoked abscesses, which were then called cold abscesses, because there was neither redness nor heat in the affected area, just swelling without inflammation. The abscess produced a yellow-green liquid that filled the joints. If the abscess opened, and this could happen in a different location in the body, it produced a fistula (or, as we know it today, a psoas abscess, which was often confused with a fistula) that usually spread through the perianal region via lymph channels, bringing with it anal pain, fever, and cough.[17] Often it did not heal. We know that Vincenzo had a fistula localized to the left of his anus, for which he underwent surgery before puberty—and it was later examined more than once to evaluate whether it constituted an impediment to the *copula carnalis* with his first wife, Margherita.[18] Also Vincenzo's erysipelas—an acute streptococcus infection of the skin, for which he sought Gaspare Tagliacozzi's intervention in 1595—could be another manifestation of tuberculosis, affecting the skin this time, although in the past there were no established connections between the two ailments. (In the third military campaign of 1601, Vincenzo had erysipelas affecting his lower extremities.)

We also know from letters that Vincenzo obsessively communicated with apothecaries and charlatans, looking to find a way to address pain, fever, or simply the acute discomfort caused by his chronic headaches through compounds of animal and mineral products. Most notoriously, he was interested in the transmutation of metals through fire and in creating potable gold (*aurum potabile*)—an alchemical elixir made of very small particles of pure gold in permanent solution that were thought to be digestible. Until recently, colloidal gold was used to address tuberculosis, rickets, and several kinds of arthritis, and these indeed were Vincenzo's pathologies.[19] For example, the alchemist Giacomo Alvise Cornaro, a frequent correspondent of the Gonzaga court and friend of Galileo in Padua, wrote to Vincenzo in 1607 that he felt it was possible to "reduce [gold] into a most healthy medication."[20] Gold was also used in popular medicine as an antibacterial agent, a preventive in skin diseases such as erysipelas and dermatitis, and was given to syphilitic patients as an alternative to mercury, as for example in the case of Vincenzo's great-grandfather, Francesco, the husband of Isabella d'Este.[21] I mentioned in previous chapters that some documents suggest that Vincenzo could have been afflicted by another infectious disease—perhaps syphilis or gonorrhea, given a sexual career marked by indiscriminate access to multiple partners, and it is easy to confuse arthritic and syphilitic or gonococcal pain of the joints. Last, Vincenzo used tobacco pills, which at the time were recommended to cure intestinal colics, of which he had many, perhaps another form of intestinal tuberculosis; as well as abscesses, wounds, gout, and syphilis.[22] He also used jalap, which was mostly indicated as a purgative for children but was employed against syphilis and to relieve water retention; in fact, Vincenzo's own counselor and personal doctor, Marcello Donati, had written a treatise on it, *De radice purgante*.[23]

Other documents, such as a letter by Donati, refer to the duke suffering and immobile as a result of a gout attack.[24] In the past, the word *gout* was used interchangeably with *arthrytys* and *podagra* (though the latter term was not necessarily applied when excruciating pain affected the toe)—that is, it was described as the painful inflammation of one or more joints. We know that gout is a metabolic disorder caused by excessive uric acid in the blood: urate crystals deposit in the tissue of joints, and in time their surface is destroyed with consequent chronic pain. The disease is associated with the upper and affluent merchant classes because of the food rich in red meat and proteins that they could afford to eat. Guglielmo was gout stricken, and we know that gout has a hereditary component. Moreover, gout as well as syphilis, which afflicted Vincenzo's grandfather and great-grandfather, can alter the distribution of minerals in the body, giving rickets to the next generation.[25] On the other hand, gout usually develops after the age of forty and is sometimes accompanied by a fever, whereas the letter by Donati referring to this medical condition was sent when Vincenzo was twenty-seven and includes no mention of a fever relegating the duke to his bedchamber. It is possible that Vincenzo was also a gout sufferer, but it is more probable that this diagnosis was used in a general sense. For example, Petrarch identified his leg problems following a bad fall from a horse as "gouty," but he had most probably caught an infection. Similarly, the pain of Galeazzo Visconti, the ruler of Milan, about which Petrarch wrote profusely to deride a famous doctor who presumed to start curing it with fresh eggs, was most probably not gout but rheumatoid arthritis, as with Vincenzo.[26] Most recently, Christopher Columbus's death, routinely attributed to gout, has been revised as being the outcome of reactive arthritis, a form of arthritis that follows infection and is marked by influenza, fevers, and painful gout-like attacks.[27] Thomas Sydenham made the first clinical distinction between rheumatism and gout in 1666. His specific diagnosis does indeed support the case of Vincenzo as suffering from acute rheumatism:

> It begins with shivering and shaking, and presently heat, restlessness and thirst; and other symptoms which accompany Fever. After a day or two, and sometimes sooner, the patient is troubled with a violent Pain,

sometimes in this, sometimes in that Joint; in the Wrist and Shoulders, but most commonly in the Knees; it now and then changes places, and seizes elsewhere, leaving some redness and swelling in the Part it last possessed.... When this Disease is not accompanied with a fever it is often taken for Gout though it differs essentially from that, as plainly appears to anyone that well considers both Diseases.[28]

For the specialists who diagnosed the duke's illness, Vincenzo's pathology of the knee joint and his chronic form of "gout"—manifested with joint stiffness, tender skin, sores, and pus—may explain why doctors often talked of catarrh in referring to the duke's swollen knee. Catarrh is an acute laryngeal infection, and indeed many private documents seem to imply that Vincenzo was suffering from some form of chronic catarrhal bronchitis. But in the early modern period, and in fact until sometime in the twentieth century, the word *catarrh* had many more applications than would seem pertinent today and was used for all parts of the body in which there was retention of fluids. Thus, for example, one could talk of a catarrh of the knee as well as of a catarrh of the stomach. Letters that mention the duke's problems with catarrh seem to make no distinctions between a bronchial affliction and an acute form of osteoarthritis presenting "water in the knee." In May 17, 1602, for example, a few months after his return from the third crusade, Vincenzo wrote to his wife's uncle, Ferdinando I de' Medici, that he was going to the baths in Spa to cure his catarrh (here he was referring to his knee) because there were no suitable medicines to address it otherwise ("appropriate medicines to remedy the indispositions caused by this catarrh of mine").[29] A catarrh in his knee motivated him in 1607 to take sea baths in Sampierdarena, a resort three miles outside Genoa, as publicized by an anonymous contemporary report: "The Duke of Mantua, Vincenzo Gonzaga, has come here to the sea to take some baths for a knee that has offended him with catarrh."[30] An unspecified form of catarrh, perhaps bronchial this time, was very much what four years later made Vincenzo vow to go on pilgrimage to the most famous holy site in Italy in the early seventeenth century, Loreto, together with his wife, as we learn from a letter by Giovanni Pietro Tornatore from Milan to the ducal counselor, Annibale Iberti, of March 16, 1611: "Since His Excellence is oppressed by catarrh, it is being said that he has made a vow to go to the Holy House of Loreto together with the duchess, his wife."[31] An unremitting attack of catarrh, seemingly bronchial, was also observed and lamented during Vincenzo's final days in February 1612, when he lay prostrate with intermittent fevers and pneumonia.[32]

Catarrh, also referred to in the past as rheum or rheumatism, was thought to be caused by a displacement of humors in the body, since it had an exudative character. Technically, catarrh was a flowing down of humors from the head (from *kata*, meaning "down," and *rheum*, meaning "I flow"), but the Hippocratics used the term to describe all sorts of fluxes. Shigehisa Kuriyama brilliantly summarizes the problem in reviewing past anxieties about catarrh:

> The distillation could flow down and out of the nose, in which case, the catarrh would be given the more specific name of *koryza*. Or it might run down the throat, causing the inflammation and hoarseness known as *branchos*. Descending lower still, into the lung, it could induce coughing and fever, or worse, slowly consume the lungs in that fatal malady called *ptisis*. And this was just the start of terrors. The defluxion might pour into the heart and provoke spasms and palpitations, or into the stomach and intestines, wreaking havoc with the digestion, provoking vomiting or diarrhea; or into the womb, and cause the menses to turn white. Accumulating in the kidneys or the bladder, catarrh formed stones and blocked the passage of urine; collecting in the joints, they provoked the swelling and ache that we still call rheumatic. When acid fluxes stagnated in the back muscles, they became the sharp, piercing pain of sciatica; when they gathered in the toes, they induced the gnawing agony of gout.[33]

The varied impediments caused by a catarrh coming from the fluid of the blood are based on an understanding of the body as an excremental machine, following Galenic medicine. People mostly believed that when the humors were not in perfect harmony, they had to be excreted so that proper function could be reestablished. Ambroise Paré and Marcello Donati were of the opinion that catarrh was flatulent matter caused by imbalances of phlegm or bile. Not so, claimed Giovanni Tommaso Minadoi, a professor of medicine at the University of Padua, in his treatise on arthritis, *De arthritide*, published in 1602—the very year of Vincenzo's most serious first bout with the disease. For Minadoi, the cause of arthritis was a flux of excremental matter in the articulations caused not by a specific humor but by any humor. He pointedly excluded meteorological causes (*intemperies*) for the disease and argued that besides hereditary factors, patients suffering from rheum were not only, as we could guess, old men and sedentary persons but also the most active ones, especially the most sexually active—a category that fit the swaggering Vincenzo to the hilt. A doctor, Minadoi wrote, needed to address arthritis with medicines that made it difficult for the flux to go toward the joints. He also advised ways of strengthening the body and recommended that patients avoid "cold" food, such as milk, beans, and ice. Finally, he suggested that sufferers shun external cold and move to a hot and dry climate.[34] In the first medical treatise fully dedicated to the subject, *De catarrhis* (1672), Richard Lower offered a precise ad hoc therapy to address the disease. Initially the patient had to drink very little, he ordered, in order to dry up the source of the supply, and had to follow a restrictive diet. Phase two, if needed, required drawing blood. Phase three involved administering cathartics as well as diuretics. If there were still no tangible results, fluid had to be eliminated "by opening small fontanels in the neck, arms or thighs, or by applying vesicants to these places."[35] It was also recommended that the patient sweat abundantly once or twice a day, thus "eliminating the fluid and moisture through all the pores to make the body properly dry."[36] It was indeed a tenet of Galenic medicine that disease could enter the body through the pores, and much has been written on the subsequent dislike of early modern men for cleanliness and bathing.

Thermal Healing

Although we identify a culture of bathhouses and thermo-mineral springs with the Roman Empire (Romans often built bathhouses close to mineral springs), medical baths had come back into fashion during the Middle Ages, no matter how much a full opposition from the clergy had tried to suppress it. Indeed, a number of baths that at the end of the Roman Empire had been used simply for speeding the maceration of linen flax or, more domestically, to dip just-killed animals in order to flay or pluck them were somewhat reconditioned to serve a sick clientele. It was specifically from the middle of the fourteenth century that the benefits of a thermal sojourn started to attract the attention of medical writers, so that, as Katharine Park argues, "though early fourteenth-century medical authors such as Pietro da Tossignano or Gentile da Foligno knew of relatively few such sites—Porretta, near Bologna, and Abano, near Padua, were the most famous northern Italian examples—early fifteenth-century writers on mineral springs, such as Ugolino da

Montecatini or Michele Savonarola, were familiar with hundreds of individual springs."[37] The culture of baths was not necessarily associated with the middle to upper classes, for in the Roman Empire as well as in the medieval and early modern periods, baths were accessible to the poor, who may have resorted to open-air pools, unlike the leisure class, but still sought relief to pain in mineral drinking and bathing. Technological balneotherapies with hot and cold springs were many, and patients therefore felt they could choose them more or less accurately, following the advice of their doctors or friends and according to the area of the body that needed to be addressed.

The claims of doctors did not necessarily help people decide what was best for them, as the lawyer Nicia, who was looking for a sojourn in a Tuscan bath to address his wife's supposed infertility in Niccolò Machiavelli's *Mandragola* (*The Mandrake*), complains: "I spoke last night to several doctors. One said that I ought to go to San Filippo, another to Porretta, a third to Villa, and they all seemed to me a bunch of birdbrains. To tell you the truth, these doctors of medicine don't know what they're talking about."[38] There were sulfurous springs good for gout, rheumatism, secondary syphilis, and chronic skin diseases—especially scrofula and psoriasis—and within this category patients were recommended to choose hot spring waters for rheumatism, gout, and syphilis, and cold spring waters for pulmonary and catarrhal problems. There were ferruginous waters for anemic, gouty, and catarrhal patients, but given that these waters turned reddish for the presence in them of iron, they were recommended for all sorts of female disorders, such as stopped menses, inability to conceive, and prolapsed uteruses. Then there were bituminous springs for internal problems; purgative springs for constipation, sluggish liver, abdominal ailments, and obesity; and acidulous springs for nervous, circulatory, and chronic diseases (they were thought to be good to address kidney stones but had to be avoided in the presence of active inflammation). There were also aluminous springs for skin diseases; calcic springs for kidney stones; and alkaline springs for gout, rheumatism, urinary calculi, and dermatitis. Seawater could be curative as well, and was recommended for rickets, for dermatological afflictions such as scrofula and chronic skin eruptions, and for sturdy joint problems. The different qualities of these waters had been known and described since antiquity by Pliny the Elder and Vitruvius, among others. Soranus of Ephesus had recommended baths to relieve mental stress. In his treatise on the property of the baths of Caldiero, outside Verona, Ventura Minardo listed seventy-eight ailments—from nausea to urinary problems, from vertigo to hemorrhoids, from scabs to swelling of the matrix, from gout to cramps, from ulcers to palsy, from fistula to melancholia—that could be successfully addressed by drinking the mineral waters there.[39]

A patient usually visited a spa in the summer, ideally in July and August, not only because the temperature was warm then, with less humidity, but because in other seasons an abundance of precipitation could compromise the ideal heat of the therm. Almost all Vincenzo's spa stays were in the summer, apart from the sojourn in Pozzuoli in southern Italy, which took place a bit earlier, in April. Renaissance spas hardly resembled the elaborate and often sumptuous Roman bath constructions dedicated to the well-being of the empire's citizens. Still, they were more than watering holes. In the fifteenth century, we know from Antonio Filarete's treatise on architecture that baths often sported "a loggia where one could stand to watch the bathers, and there were places to eat. In addition to this loggia there were rooms where one could go to rest after coming out of the bath. Up above there were similar rooms and halls and very beautiful places where one could stay most comfortably."[40] Baths were often left unroofed. Usually they were segregated according to sex; at times they also had a separate section for lepers. In vapor pools men wore linen trunks and a hat; women wore a camisole open at the side, although in some illustrations they are naked, as well as a turban or an elaborate head covering and jewels. Finally there were establishments with pools for animals needing cures for, say, chronic inflammations; horses especially were brought in to heal their hoofs. These pools were often situated close to those used by patients. Filarete listed a number of thermal baths well frequented at the time, such as Bagni di Petriolo, Bagni di Acqua (now known as Bagni di Casciana), and Bagni di Lucca.

As the letters regarding Duke Vincenzo show, patients drank the mineral water and took baths or submitted to mud baths early in the morning. Rich patients did not necessarily go to the thermal springs themselves but had the water or mud carried to their palace of residence, where they could be cured in private. The water therapy was followed by a light diet, for it was necessary to help the body's forthcoming healing process by generating good humors (and better blood) ahead of expelling the bad ones. Lampridio Anguillara recommended a diet that could modify the blood by using absinthe, "saracen truffle," gold, and pearls.[41] Doctors also advised patients to abstain from sexual intercourse, although the recommendation was often discarded; they were not to take a nap in the afternoon but could read books, listen to poetry, and play cards. The quantity of water recommended varied, and at times patients drank too much, on the understanding that if a small amount is good for one's health, a larger amount may prove better. During his sojourn in Caldiero, for example, Federico Gonzaga, Vincenzo's grandfather, went to the springs at dawn every morning, weather permitting, accompanied by his own musicians (in some illustrations of the period, musicians are shown sitting inside the pool); drank from eight to eleven eight-ounces glasses of water per day, paying attention to how much water was later expelled, whether through urination or vomit; did not eat for four hours after drinking the last glass; consumed a light lunch; did not take a nap in the afternoon but read, walked leisurely, rested, or played cards; and went horseback riding after dinner before retiring early. At times he returned to the springs later in the day to see who was there.[42]

Doctors were attentive to everything connected to the cure, since some patients responded badly to it and became sick or developed a fever. To facilitate evacuation, some patients were submitted to bowel-irritating enemas or had their skin oiled with "spirited" paps; as would be expected, these practices did not help in keeping the ailing serene. "Heroic" fasts, which were strongly recommended, together with attempts to stop sudoration with cold sponge baths and iced footbaths, could make the sick residents unresponsive or aggressive. At other times, for the sake of encouraging a contrary response from the body through excessive perspiration with heated sheets, patients were made to sit near burning braziers or to undergo long fumigations, which left some so depleted that they passed out. A challenging astrological or lunar combination could temporarily stop the therapy (a new moon, for example, meant that Federico Gonzaga did not take the water that day).[43] During Vincenzo's stay at Spa, at least one member of his retinue died. It was clear to both doctors and sufferers that mineral waters were not for everyone.

Doctors often recommended increasing the benefit of water therapy through bloodletting, so that humors causing the patients' problems could be expelled. Venesection was done directly in the pools, which as a result often turned red by the end of the day; enemas also took place there. Vaginal and rectal irrigations were performed on women to encourage elimination of whatever was obstructing their uteruses. Barbers and surgeons performed leeching and other minor surgeries within the pools or nearby. Cupping was frequently done on both men and women.[44] To encourage sweating through steam, bowls were placed on hot stones. At times the water contained herbs, such as mint, rosemary, oregano, and sage, to provide some feel-good aromatherapy; to increase circulation, patients were recommended to rhythmically beat their skin with bunches of leaves. Given the often incredible length of time spent immersing in the mineral pools, patients would often have food brought to them while they were leisurely talking with their friends (the "Bagni de Abano" etching displays a floating tray most probably used to deliver food) (Fig. 14).

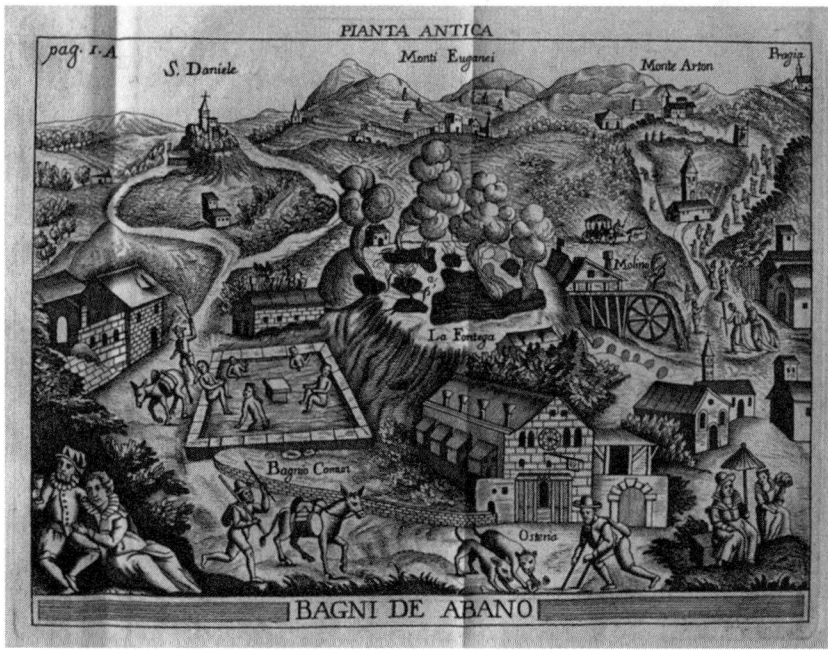

Fig. 14. Domenico Vandelli, "Bagni de Abano," in *Tractatus de thermis agri patavini* (Padua: Conzatti, 1761). (Photo: Biblioteca Vincenzo Pinali, Sezione antica, Università di Padova, Padua.)

References to Vincenzo's sojourns at spas occur in many documents throughout the years. Vincenzo broke rank, however, with his relatives, who had preferred stays in Tuscany or in nearby Caldiero in the province of Verona, as well as in Abano and Montegrotto near Padua (the case of Federico Gonzaga and of his son, Guglielmo Gonzaga). The thermal spa associated most with the Gonzaga through the decades has been Petriolo in Tuscany, which was recommended especially for arthritis. Paola Malatesta, the first woman in the family with a pronounced hunchback, more than once visited Petriolo in the summer to get relief for the pain in her joints from its hot, sulfurous waters. In 1461, for example, she went with her father Malatesta and stayed more than six months.[45] Likewise, Ludovico III Gonzaga sojourned in Petriolo in 1460 and 1475. His long stays were made easier, we gather from letters, by his habit of playing chess in the evening and of relaxing with the works of Augustine and Lucan.[46] Another favorite Gonzaga watering spot was Bagni di Lucca, also in Tuscany, where Vincenzo's mother, Leonora, underwent the cure in 1561. The hot springs of Bagni di Lucca (once known as Bagni a Corsena) were indeed highly recommended by the Paduan doctor Gabriele Falloppio, who had found them perfect for his hearing problems, as he explained in his treatise on healing waters, "De medicatis aquis atque de fossilibus," in 1566.[47] Michel de Montaigne too stopped at Bagni di Lucca in 1581 to address his kidney stones and stayed at Villa.[48] The "acqua di Villa" was recommended, among other things, for dermatological problems; as I mentioned in Chapter 2, Vincenzo had been urged by Gaspare Tagliacozzi to bathe daily his face and nose affected by erysipelas with "acqua di Villa," imported, bottled, for this purpose. Earlier, another doctor had given this same recommendation to his great-grandfather, Francesco, who needed to address facial skin complications most likely caused by syphilis.[49]

Going to the Spa

Unlike his relatives who preferred mostly Tuscan therms, Vincenzo sought relief to his acute pain in watering places as far north as Spa in Belgium, where he traveled more than once, and as far south as Pozzuoli in the Kingdom of Naples. Closer to home, he went to Lake Iseo in Lombardy for the air or perhaps for the mineral waters of Terme di Boario, and west to the shores of Sampierdarena, near Genoa, to see whether the marine air or salty seawater could provide the respite he sought for his aches. The duke's visits to spas started quite early, although the most extended stays followed the flare-up of the chronic knee pain he registered so effusively at the time of the 1601 crusade. Prior to 1591 he had found relief to unspecified problems by traveling west to Acqui Terme in the Piedmont region, a place well known since the Middle Ages for hydrotherapy, mud baths, and douches. Following this visit Vincenzo asked a doctor named Salamonio to prepare a report on the benefits of the town's bubbling spring water (the place still has a main pavilion called "la Bollente" for its hot water).[50]

We have abundant documentation regarding Vincenzo's journey to Spa in Flanders in 1599, a trip necessary to assure "a singular remedy to my indisposition," as the duke put it in a letter of May 7, 1599, to his wife's uncle, Ferdinando de' Medici, in Florence. Vincenzo had already planned a sojourn in Spa the year before, he explained, but was unable to make it; lately, he added, his doctors had urged him to be proactive.[51] Indeed, in June Vincenzo was already in Innsbruck (a regular stop on all his trips north in order to visit his sister), and then he proceeded toward Basel and Nancy. Later he visited the Brussels court and stayed in Liège and Antwerp. We know that hydrotherapy helped him, or so his wife, Eleonora, reported on August 20, 1599, to Belisario Vinta in Florence, who was going to inform her uncle.[52] Upon his return to Mantua, Vincenzo himself wrote on October 22, 1599, two separate letters, one to Ferdinando and one to the grand duke's wife, Christine de Lorraine, assuring them that he had returned in much better health and that the "indispositione" that caused him to use the waters of Spa had much improved.[53] Counselors and friends in Vincenzo's retinue too noticed progress in the duke's complexion within a few days of following the spa routine. As Ferrante (Ferdinando) Persia wrote from Spa to Annibale Chieppio in Mantua, on July 26, 1599, "His Highness has taken the waters for five days, and now he drinks 100 ounces every morning, sweats aplenty, and also passes the water out through urine. We all hope for a good outcome, God willing."[54] Vincenzo was still in Spa on August 5.[55]

By the sixteenth century, Spa had become a well-known watering place in the Ardennes mountains for aristocrats and merchants alike. Mentioned and praised in antiquity by Pliny the Elder, Spa had been "rediscovered," so to speak, by knights and noblemen in 1326. Henry

VIII Tudor took the waters to cure his rheumatism (or perhaps syphilis), and there were so many English tourists in Spa in the sixteenth century that the name has since become eponymous with thermalism. Henri's III of Valois's therapeutic vacation there in 1585 put this watering place on the map for French citizens.[56] As for the Gonzaga, in 1590 Ferrante II Gonzaga, who belonged to a cadet branch of the family, the Guastalla, had found much relief for an unspecified pathology following a twenty-day water therapy in Spa.[57] Later, Vincenzo's third son, Vincenzo II, visited Spa regularly to relieve his headache or to address the array of health issues procured by his syphilis.[58]

At the time of Vincenzo's visit, there was already a guidebook that illustrated the benefits of a hydrotherapy treatment in Spa. The booklet must have been quite inexpensive, since Persia, who was in the duke's retinue in 1599, was able to send a print in French to the ducal secretary, Chieppio, in Mantua, so that he could get a sense of what specifically was cured in the place.[59] In his letter to Chieppio, Persia gives a lengthy explanation of what Spa looked like at the time: the watering spot was in a valley surrounded by hills, he wrote, with houses built in the rustic style and a fountain in the middle of a square that spouted clear and cold water, which tasted like ink. The water was known to preserve its benefits for more than three years, he added, and this was why it was transported in great quantity all over the world ("portata in in grandissima quantità in diversi parti del mondo, come chi conserve la sua totale virtù et qualità per lo spatio di tre anni e più"). What was more interesting for Persia, however, was that two miles outside of town there was another fountain with better-tasting water. Early in the morning, a good number of gentlemen and ladies—especially women with irregular periods or people affected by the French disease—drank this water, he added, and happily cured themselves ("bevendo quest'acqua con i debiti ingredienti si curano con piena soddisfationi").[60] Not everybody got the same benefits from the cure, Persia continued. As for himself, he had tasted the water, and that was as far as he was going to go on the matter. On another point Persia felt compelled to comment: the fact that there were a great many women in the area taking the cure, although none at the moment appeared so beautiful as to make the men around them forget their "chastity." The ladies, he wrote, seemed to be quite delicate and always had their face covered. Besides, and here he switched to Latin, there was not much talk (*si soliquis minimi*).[61] Still,

Vincenzo found time to fall in love during this curative trip, and his secret visit to a woman's home in Brussels was judged to be damaging to his reputation.[62]

Vincenzo's visit to Spa in 1602 produced at first decent results. He left on June 8, following a day of conviviality and entertainment with his extended family and the performance of a comedy.[63] In a letter to Ferdinando de' Medici announcing his forthcoming journey, Vincenzo stated that he would leave his wife ("la Duchessa mia") in charge in the duchy's government.[64] And indeed soon after, Eleonora was engaged in making political and economic decisions in Mantua on her husband's behalf.[65] This sojourn in Spa was insufficient, unfortunately, to fully take care of Vincenzo's "indispositioni" that year. Early in the fall, after what was described as a long illness, the duke went to Lake Iseo, north of Brescia, in the hope that breathing more oxygenated air would improve his health. Writing to her uncle back in Florence on October 4, 1602, Eleonora expressed her hope that "the perfect air of those places could give him [Vincenzo] back his pristine health."[66] Vincenzo may have followed his physicians' counsel to relieve his emphysema or some other infection in an appropriately receptive environment, since it was a doctor's duty, as Bernardino Ramazzini was to write in his *La salute dei principi*, "to understand the nature of the air the prince was breathing and also harmonize it to his temperament and procure a just transpiration according to whether the prince's body was robust or frail."[67] But Vincenzo could have also taken the occasion to drink the waters of the mineral Terme di Boario, which were known since the 1400s and were recommended for the respiratory and urinary apparatuses.[68] At Boario it was also possible to undergo inhalation aerosol therapy to address chronic bronchitis or reduce edema of the mucous membrane.

The stay in Lake Iseo did not help Vincenzo much either, for in the spring of the next year, 1603, the duke decided to go south to the baths of Pozzuoli, and specifically to Agnano, where he underwent a different spa therapy—fumigations—in addition to aerosol inhalations. Pozzuoli was well known at the time for curing cutaneous diseases, and Vincenzo may have gone there to address his skin rash or fungal infection. He arrived in Pozzuoli on April 25 with a richly decorated ducal galley and was opulently feted by the local authorities and the viceroy. To be sure, in courts all over Italy the trip was treated as political, since it was well known that Vincenzo was trying to be named generalissimo of the Mediterranean by the viceroy of Naples, now that his post-Canissa desire to secure the title of governor of Flanders and Portugal from the king of Spain (he had sent Peter Paul Rubens to Spain to secure it with gifts) had not been satisfied.[69] Vincenzo chose to reside in Naples, but for a number of days and until Pentecost he took the cure directly in nearby Pozzuoli and Agnano.[70]

Together with Lucrino, Lake Avernus (which in the *Aeneas* Virgil made the entrance to the underworld), and Cumae (the official residence of the mythological Cumaean Sybil), the volcanic and continuously erupting areas of Pozzuoli and Agnano constitute the so-called Campi Flegrei (meaning, etymologically, "burning fields"). The area had been subjected to bradyseismic phenomena through the centuries, so that part of this smoky region, following some rising and sinking of the ground, had already disappeared under water by the tenth century or been reshaped with new hills created by earthquakes.[71] A few decades before Vincenzo's visit, a huge eruption of volcanic matter had radically changed the topography of the place, creating a new hill: Monte Nuovo, Europe's youngest mountain. The region constituted the best known and most elite resort of the Roman Empire—especially the town of Baiae, with its elaborate and luxurious mineral spring complex, which has now disappeared under water.[72] Pozzuoli (in Latin, Puteoli, "little wells") was a bathing establishment known for its sulfur caves, steam vents, bubbling sands, and four mineral springs that sported varied temperatures—all used to address not only arthritis and rheumatism but also sterility and obesity.[73] Today we have a stunning medieval illustration of what kind of balneotherapy went on in the area, thanks to a set of eighteen miniatures assembled in *De Balneis Puteolanis* by Peter of Eboli (1211–1220). From the images in this collection—produced in the third quarter of the thirteenth century to accompany Peter's poems—we can see how men and women bathed (in separate pools) or went to sweat in grottoes, what they ate, and how they dressed or undressed. The bath chambers offered different structures: some were round and domed; others were rectangular with flat ceilings. In the illustrations, some bathers seemed to be enjoying themselves with dance and games, whereas others were more attentive to the medical reason for their stay. There is also the illustration of an enema. The miniature of a man with a bellows fanning a flame to boost sulfur fumes seems to represent a common activity of bath helpers of the area; in another, a group of seven naked women bathe together while a man peeps through a window; and in still another, an old man with a walking stick is helped by a servant to descend the stairs leading to the bath. Another illustration is divided into two sections: one to undress and the other to bathe. According to Peter of Eboli, the Balneum Sulphatara in Pozzuoli "not only calms the nerves, but also cures scabies, produces fertility in the sterile, relieves pain in the head and stomach, removes tears from the eyes and restores keen sight. Furthermore it prevents vomiting, dissolves phlegm in the body and cures fevers."[74] Peter's manuscript was extremely popular (although he was not yet recognized as its author), and Vincenzo may have seen a copy, since this guidebook to the thermal spa has come to us in a variety of manuscript and printed versions. Vincenzo also went to the springs in Agnano, which contain sulfur and iron and resemble those of Vichy and Aix-la-Chapelle in France. An anonymous chronicler reported that the duke visited the "fumaroles," where "he sweated aplenty and we can hope that in due time this can help him."[75] Indeed, the area features pools of boiling mud called fumaroles, thermal mud-packing, and steam caves continuously spouting steam and mud, which were popular with patients suffering from gout, osteoarthritis, other muscle-bone traumas, and chronic cutaneous lesions—like Vincenzo. The local mineral water was used for both bathing and drinking.

But therapy was not the only reason one went to the Pozzuoli area, as Boccaccio hinted at when he called Pozzuoli the birthplace of Venus.[76] Cicero and Seneca had lamented the "vice" that coursed through Baiae; as Martial wrote, "In Baiae a woman comes as a Penelope and goes away like a Helen." Indeed, such seems to have been the case for the married noblewoman whose name is lost to history with whom Vincenzo fathered a child during his visit to Naples and Pozzuoli. This son, baptized with the name Francesco and raised in Naples, became a cleric and later bishop of Cariati and Nola.[77] Vincenzo also took the trip as an occasion to collect works of art, especially portraits of beautiful Neapolitan women, which he solicited for his private gallery in Mantua. Already by September 1603, seven portraits of Neapolitan gentlewomen had been sent to him; in 1607, Frans Pourbus, a Flemish painter at his court, was sent to Naples with the specific task of collecting more works of art and of painting portraits of the most beautiful local women.[78]

Still looking for ways to address his pain at a spa, in May 1607 Vincenzo went to an unspecified location on Lake Garda, halfway between Venice and Milan, but did not "get much relief from his knee pain."[79] Vincenzo may have gone to Lake Garda for the good air or simply for vacation. Given the season, he could have also briefly visited a nearby thermal spa, such as Sirmione, on the south shore of the lake, already made famous by the Latin poet Catullus. Even today, Sirmione's mud and sulfurous waters are used for rheumatism, respiratory ailments, and dermatological disorders. Vincenzo could have also stopped in Caldiero, the favorite health spot of his grandfather, Federico, who chose this location in the summer of 1524 before moving to the baths in Abano to undergo douche therapy—all to cure his unremitting urinary retention with "purgative waters." Vincenzo had an array of pathologies to address—including pounding headaches, which convinced him as early as 1592 to enter into a bargain with a holy woman in Mantua named Altea: she would take on herself the duke's headaches in exchange for him paying 15 scudi per month to honor the dead. When he failed to post the alms one month his pain returned, or so the story goes.[80]

In June 1607 Vincenzo wanted to go back to Spa and left Mantua for that purpose, stopping first in the duchy's western possession of Casale in the Monferrato region. Preemptively he had ordered his military commander general to move toward Corsica to clear the area of corsairs, since he wanted to travel north by sea.[81] But then he changed his mind. Still unwilling to let go of the benefits of water therapy, he ordered that mineral water be brought to him from Spa, a custom of which Henri III of Valois had already availed himself a few years earlier.[82] This water—transported for short distances in hollow containers such as pumpkins (*zucche*) to keep it warm, and in wooden tubs carried by mules or on barges—arrived three weeks later, on August 1, 1607.[83] Vincenzo had been thoroughly assured that "bottled" mineral water would not lose its benefits when transported, and in fact prior to his visit to Spa in 1602, he had been told by one of his most trusted alchemists, Giacomo Alvise Cornaro, that bottled mineral water from Spa was as good as water collected straight at the fount, provided that it could be warmed in a covered silver vessel in order to not let out any vapors. Therefore, the chemist suggested, there was no real need for a person of the duke's stature to make a journey to Spa.[84]

In the meantime Vincenzo had moved to Sampierdarena along the Genoa coast, where he arrived on July 8, magnificently received by the local authorities.[85] Already by July 14, the ducal counselor Annibale Iberti reported back to Mantua that the duke was in good health and was taking care of his leg pain with baths of seawater that he was having transported to his palace.[86] This palace, the Villa Grimaldi la Fortezza, sat along the shore of the Mar Ligure in the suburb of Sampierdarena and, like other Genoese palaces built at the time, sported luxurious private *stufe* (sweating baths), which although not technically thermal were judged "excellent for health" by contemporary doctors, thus fostering a lively bathing culture.[87] In a letter to Ferdinando de' Medici, Vincenzo wrote that the reason for his sojourn in Sampierdarena was to take certain baths, leaving unspecified whether he was bathing in the sea, having the seawater transported to his palace in wooden tubs, or simply using the *stufa* in La Fortezza.[88] In any case, we know that he underwent all three therapies, besides drinking the water transported from Spa, since an entry of July 6, 1607, in an anonymous Genoese diary mentions that "the duke was going to the beach to bathe (alla marina) in order to cure a knee full of catarrh."[89] Still, other health problems continued to afflict Vincenzo while he was curing himself: first stomach fits and then small kidney stones (*arenella*), "which caused some pains, but not too significant."[90] On August 24, 1607—a month and a half after his arrival—Vincenzo left for home, still afflicted by leg pain and swelling.[91]

As with his visit south to Pozzuoli and Agnano, Vincenzo did not let his health problems curtail some anticipated entertainment. This time he had brought along the tenor Francesco Rasi, who may have sang arias from *Orfeo*, which had been recently performed at court.[92] In the mornings Vincenzo went to the beach, bringing along his musicians; in the afternoons he played cards for two or three hours (games called Picchetto and Primiera, although the first day of his stay he played a much more dangerous card game for the pocket, called Los Buettos, and won 1,000 gold scudi); and in the evenings he hosted private banquets, listened to poetry and music with beautiful women (*belle ninfe*) in attendance, had comedies performed, or took strolls along the Riviera, where many gentlewomen flocked "to see and be seen."[93] At times Vincenzo would take along his friend Nicolò Pallavicino and a page and play the tourist. He thus visited the new Church of the Gesù and a number of nearby villas. One day the Genoese doge decided to surprise the Gonzaga by bringing a suite of eight galleys (*barcheggio*) filled with local senators and gentlemen along the shore fronting his palace. The visitors kept throwing all sorts of fruit—peaches, pears, and melons—as well as sweets and salami to the ladies on the shore until Vincenzo took off his hat, acknowledging with grace the doge and his retinue in the galleys.[94] Vincenzo spent so much money in Sampierdarena, that as Benedetto Moro wrote on September 6, 1607, from Verona to the Venetian Senate, "The duke was expected last night in Mantua, but his relatives and subjects were not too pleased, since in this trip to Genoa, which he has made simply because he liked to do so, he has spent almost 100,000 scudi that could have been put to better use for the needs of his house, which are not a few."[95]

Vincenzo went back to Spa in June 1608, following his son's lavish spring marriage in Mantua.[96] Already in February of that year, health issues had driven the duke to ask for the pills for a long life (*di lunga vita*) that a surgeon he had encountered at the time of his first marriage, Girolamo Fabrici, was giving to patients such as Galileo Galilei.[97] This time Vincenzo went to Belgium by land through France. In Nancy he stopped to see his cousin, Carlo Gonzaga-Nevers. He also spent some time in Paris with King Henri IV of Navarre, the husband of his sister-in-law, Maria de' Medici, and was entertained with banquets and ballets.[98] Once again the sojourn at a spa did not help much, and the pain continued to the point that the following summer Vincenzo had to postpone even such an easy commuting trip as the one from Mantua to his villa in Maderno for a few days, as we learn from a letter of July 6, 1609, because his leg would not cooperate.[99] In March 1611 Vincenzo again made a vow to go to the holy sanctuary of Loreto to get relief from catarrh ("His Excellence has been oppressed by catarrh") while also arranging to go to Sesto, presumably for another round of seawater baths and *stufe* treatments in the palace of Benedetto Pieno.[100] By now the health of his wife, Eleonora, had taken a downward turn. She died in September of that year, to be followed a few months later by Vincenzo himself.

The different hydrotherapy and balneology resorts that Vincenzo Gonzaga patronized both in Italy and abroad in the span of two decades have much in common: all were supposed to help with a variety of health issues, such as respiratory problems, digestive disorders, skin disfigurations, and diseases of the joints. Although the healing springs addressed some of Vincenzo's painful pathologies, they did not cure him. We must remember, however, that in past centuries, patients did not necessarily believe in the interventionist mandate of medicine and sought instead alternative ways to control pain and strengthen the body. Those who made the choice to go to the baths subscribed to the Roman dictum of living well—*balnea, vina, venus*—because it was understood that no cure would work without its accompanying entertainment agenda—women, cards, wine, betting. They were the sine qua non, then as now, of a day at the spa.

In the end perhaps Vincenzo, as many men of his time, may have entertained the wishful belief that mineral waters constituted a fountain of youth. After all, as recently as the late 1970s, the spa establishment of Baden-Baden turned up in the news for the elixir Gerovital, launched as a true "fountain of youth." Fountains of youth in which old men and women went in wrinkled and old and came out younger, refreshed, and even muscular were often depicted in contemporary illustrations, as in Lucas Cranach the Elder's famous panel of 1546, now in Berlin (Fig. 15). Let us not forget that in 1513 Ponce de León had fa-

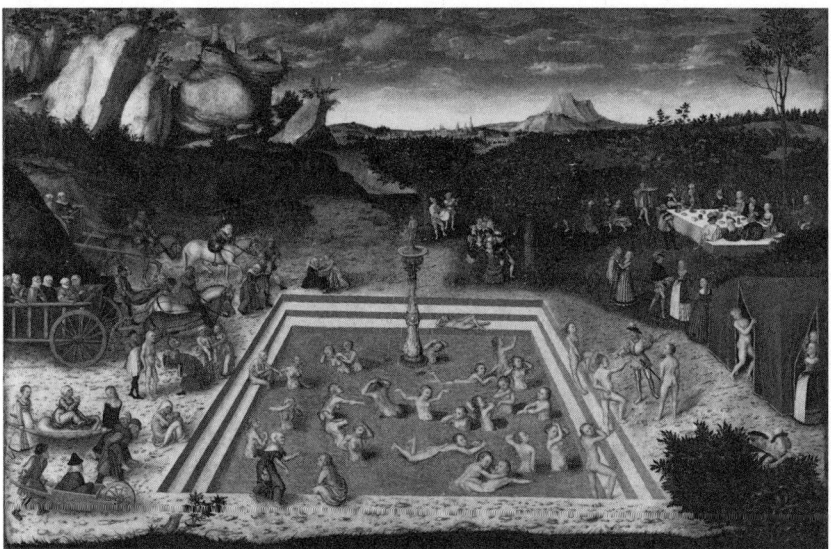

Fig. 15. Lucas Cranach the Elder, *Fountain of Youth*, 1546. (Staatiche Museen, Berlin. Photo: Art Resource.)

mously looked for a fountain of eternal youth in the mythical land of Bimini (Beniny) in the Bahamas (or Florida) to cure his impotence. Or so wrote Gonzalo Fernández de Oviedo in his *Historia General y Natural de las Indias,* an event confirmed by Antonio de Herrera in the very years that saw Vincenzo looking for solutions to his own health issues. The Ponce de León fountain increased longevity and sexual strength, he wrote, so that old men became strong anew, married, and engendered more children.[101]

Flush with money, endowed with a vivid imagination, and determined to provide a scientific reasoning for his desire, in his late forties Vincenzo too will turn to the New World for an ad hoc fountain of youth meant to rejuvenate the same particular body part that necessitated the vitality-restoring waters sought by Ponce de León almost a century earlier. His resolute, although undoubtedly anxious, search for a new, custom-made sexual elixir constitutes the subject of Chapter 4.

4

The Sexual Cure

Searching for a Viagra in the New World

> What shall I do with this absurdity—
> O heart, O troubled heart—this caricature,
> Decrepit age that has been tied to me
> As to a dog's tail?
> Never had I more
> Excited, passionate, fantastical
> Imagination, nor an ear and eye
> That more expected the impossible—
>
> —William Butler Yeats, "The Tower"

SOMETIME IN THE YEAR 1608, Vincenzo Gonzaga I, fourth Duke of Mantua and Monferrato and munificent sponsor of art, music, and theater—a Renaissance prince in every sense of the word—realized that he had a physical difficulty that required secrecy or, alternatively, a creative and perhaps radical solution. Historians are in agreement today that this particular ducal predicament was minor, although it hardly seemed so at the time to Vincenzo. He was approaching forty-seven, the very age that Dante had declared as delimiting the onset of senility.[1] This chapter looks at the events surrounding Vincenzo's search for a remedy to his predicament, which eventually led him to send an unknown apothecary, Evangelista Marcobruno, on a secret two-year journey by coach, boat, galleon, mule, llamas, and foot from Mantua to Genoa, then on to Barcelona, Madrid, Segovia, Seville, and Cádiz in Spain, and later to numberless stops in the New World, including Cartagena, Portobelo,

Panama, and Manta in Ecuador; Callao, Lima, and Cuzco in Peru; and Potosí and Chuquiabo (La Paz) in Bolivia, to say nothing about the return trip—to find a Viagra-like remedy (yes, so significant was this difficulty to Duke Vincenzo!) in that expanse of lands where all marvels were contained at the time.[2]

There was at the time no official smoke screen for the duke's willingness to pay for added pleasure by approving the travel of one of his provincial subjects, for it was well known in the court's inner circle that the sybaritic Vincenzo had recently been looking for some sort of medical remedy to enhance his fun in the bedroom. Already on June 22, 1608, for example, the correspondent Iacopo Spini was writing to Vincenzo from Florence that the knight Emanuel Cimenes (Ximenes), a Spaniard to judge from his name, had found an interesting libido enhancer, for he had "that worm [*quel verme*] about which I talked to Your Highness and besides I believe he also has many secrets with him."[3] Ximenes himself wrote on the subject on September 24, 1608, directly to Vincenzo from Antwerp:

> Most Serene Highness, following the order that Your Highness gave me, I did some research and found that in the Island of Carga, which is thirty leagues away from the city of Ozmus [Hormuz, now in Iran] on the mouth of the Euphrates there is a kind of frog [?] that the Portuguese call "Carangolo de Carga," which when kept [felt?] in one's hand achieves the effect which Your Highness mentioned to me. But this must be quite rare since another Portuguese who has served there as a soldier tells me that he never saw one, only heard about it. Being uncertain, I would rather exhort Your Most Serene Highness to make the essence or oil of pearl for a few months, for it is not dangerous and in a few months it procures a noticeable effect. Also the extract of satyrion, of which Your Highness deigned to get a little jar here, has a similar bountiful effect.[4]

Ximenes knew that shaved pearls were used to improve performance in bed because they came from oysters, whose aphrodisiac power is still recognized today; as for the power of satyrion to awaken the senses, this wild orchid—dried, powered, and drunk with wine—was so well known as a restorer of a man's sexual arsenal that already by the Middle Ages it could no longer be found locally, since the Greeks and Romans had used it to the point of extinction. As for the little blockbuster animal of which he writes—well, either it was living in myth or it was necessary to embark on a more dogged search in order to find it.

Vincenzo's discreet fantasy of resurrecting the flesh, anchored in male anxiety, narcissistic excess, and a peculiar dream of domination, occupies hardly a footnote within the multinational project of mercantile imperialism that marked the discovery of the natural beauties of the New World. Given the historical moment in which this personal drama played out, however, the panacean cure of which this aging conquistador of the bedchamber dreamed can serve as an instructive parable, allowing us to reconfigure what appears to be a trivial colonialist enterprise into an erotic of knowledge. By focusing on an unlikely protagonist—Marcobruno was by all means a provincial apothecary with limited scientific knowledge—I aim to provide in this chapter a lens with which to view early modern experimentations with pharmacology as well as to convey the curiosity, adventurousness, and methodical eagerness that at the beginning of the seventeenth century began to define how research was to be conducted by the natural philosophers: *ex vivo*, although not yet *in vitro*.

It is fair to assume, given the amount of information we have on the topic, that the early seventeenth century saw the dawn of an era marked by a thirst for wondering, wandering, and collecting. Medically speaking, the yearning to know through analysis, to explore the unknown through travel, and to understand the strange or plainly exotic through collection was matched by a commercial desire to deploy this novel knowledge, since an eager and flourishing middle-class, to say nothing of the moneyed nobility, was looking beyond God and current holistic approaches to address the everyday miseries that sickness and aging were inflicting on bodies. It is in this context that I situate at the frontiers of the unknown an Italian druggist whose aim was to match empiric fact with human imagination while faithfully serving his impatient patron back home.

By his society's acknowledgment, Duke Vincenzo could boast plenty of achievements by 1608. For starters, he had three campaigns against the Turks in Hungary under his belt. He had also most recently been an acknowledged power broker in the Italian peninsula, negotiating between the papacy and the Republic of Venice after the Serenissima's interdict.[5] In his official and almost identical portraits of those years, all made by Frans Pourbus the Younger, a Flemish artist in residence at his court, Vincenzo proudly wears the collar of the newly founded Order of the Redeemer (Fig. 16). His upright figure set against billowing

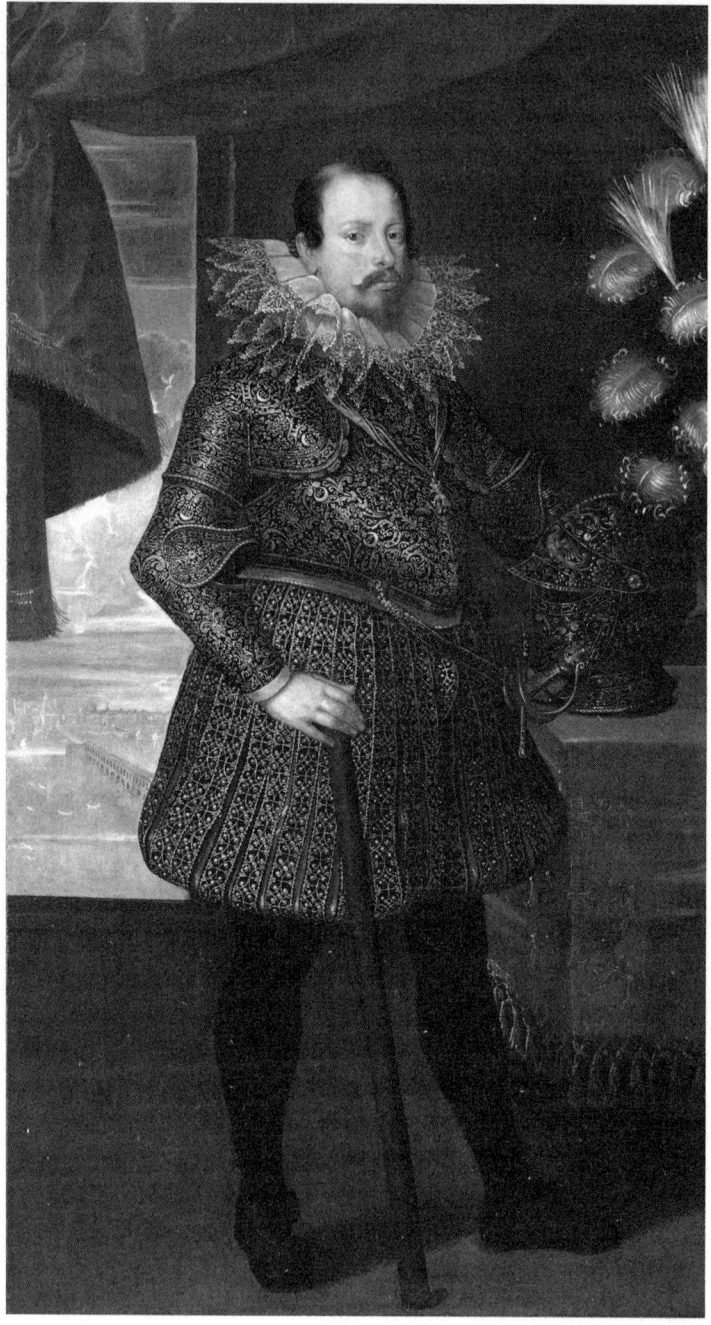

Fig. 16. Frans Pourbus the Younger, *Vincenzo Gonzaga,* ca. 1605. (Tatton Park, Cheshire, UK. Photo: Bridgeman Art Library.)

red curtains and accompanied by an array of phallic symbols—a sword, a ruler's baton, some flourishing featherwork on the helmet, and a well-padded codpiece—seemed to advertise time and again the self-image of a duke in charge or, as Patricia Simons would put it, of a ruler both alert and erect.[6]

Yet Vincenzo did "not seem to be at 46 in good health, in fact he was often troubled by a number of ailments," the Venetian ambassador Francesco Morosini perceptively reported to the Serenissima's Senate in the same year, June 21, 1608, perhaps because Vincenzo had "little discipline in life and continuous appetite for the things that give him pleasure." Still, Morosini added, the duke lived fully and ostensibly had no intention of slowing down.[7] Morosini knew his subject, for Vincenzo was famously known in courts all over Italy, as well as in France, Spain, Austria, Belgium, and Poland, for his unquenchable hunger for anything connected to beauty, collection, and entertainment. But by "living fully," people in the know had in mind not so much Vincenzo's refined aesthetic sensibility as his legendary promiscuity and excess, for the duke was notorious for his libidinous recklessness and extramarital liaisons, just like, to give a famous example, the libertine Pietro Aretino, who would ostentatiously boast in writing about his ability to inhabit his carnal landscape "forty times a month," no matter his age.[8] In his spare time that very year, for example, Vincenzo had a somewhat lengthy affair with a married woman named Elena, who wrote him a letter decrying his absence—she loved him as much as her own soul—while she was stuck at home with her husband.[9] As the Duke of Mantua in Giuseppe Verdi's *Rigoletto* sings, "This woman or that—they are all the same to me. . . . Constancy, that tyrant of the heart, I hate as if it were a cruel disease."[10] Vincenzo's appetites were enormous—and his ability to satisfy them seemed evident to many outsiders.

Thus at forty-six, the duke—for whom fidelity in sexual matters was like a disease—must have found it particularly punitive to acknowledge that he was having problems being constant even in pleasure. Or perhaps it was simply the other way around, and his problem was not age-related erectile dysfunction but priapic libertinism. Having tried everything in the bedroom, the resourceful duke might have longed to experiment with a different biostimulator to cure his legendary restlessness, for committed sensualists stop at nothing. That very spring, for the well-choreographed tournament that accompanied his son Francesco's wedding to Margherita of Savoy, Vincenzo had surprisingly chosen to march as Cupid's Petrarchan slave in the *Trionfo dell'amore* carriage. Taking what would have been rightfully Francesco's place, Vincenzo had made it clear that he thought of himself as a youthful prisoner of love, even as he was approaching senior amatory difficulties.

In Chapter 3 I hypothesized that Vincenzo's main medical problem was tuberculosis, perhaps accompanied by syphilis (or gonorrhea). It is well known that these two pathologies spur at times such trends as hypersexuality, satyriasis, sexual compulsivity, increased libido, even irritability and narcissism. Affected patients show little inhibition, and this could throw light, for example, on Vincenzo's almost pathological gambling; they also show a tendency toward euphoria and impulsivity, which may explain Vincenzo's reckless spending for everything that was, looked like, or felt luxurious, from expensive armor to expensive paintings. It is in this context that the duke's search for a remedy to indulge his high-flying style—money being no object—acquired urgency.

What Vincenzo sought to counter his andropause and revitalize his exhausted flesh had a simple name: *gusano*. It was not an Italian word, although the Mantuan dialect had the expression *gusar*, meaning "to enjoy, to experience pleasure." *Gusano* was a Spanish word with the widest meaning: worm, vermin, earthworm, spider worm, caterpillar, vermiform larva of beetles and flies (that is, grubs and maggots).[11] Where was this worm to be found? Maria Bellonci has suggested that the word *gusano* refers to the Spanish fly, that is, the cantharis, a species of the blister beetle (*Lytta vesicatoria* or *Cantharis vesicatoria*).[12] During the early modern period, the cantharis, dried in plaster form, was indeed used as a love stimulant in a number of electuaries, even though some doctors felt it could have lethal effects when taken unchecked.[13] However, using it directly as a penile ointment required courage or desperation, because although chemicals in the fly did increase blood flow to the genitals, they also tended to cause inflammation and blisters. In any case, the problem with this identification is that the cantharis is common in Italy, as well as in Spain, the Mediterranean basin, and even Britain. The duke may very well have tried the Spanish variant, but he was longing for something drastically new, whose aphrodisiac or topical powers he could validate personally more than once. His search knew no boundaries.

Enter the apothecary Evangelista Marcobruno, son of Giuseppe Marcobruno of the Pharmacy of the Coral and the Pharmacy of the King.[14] The seemingly conspiratorial communication between Duke Vincenzo and this mysterious pharmacist is today preserved in a rich array of letters, all dated from 1609 to 1613. It is clear from Marcobruno's correspondence—he presumably started his trip in May 1609, and the first letter is dated June 10, 1609, upon arrival in Barcelona—and from the ducal correspondence with the Gonzaga ambassador in Spain, Celliero Bonatti, that it was not in Spain per se but in the Indies and there alone that this fabulous *gusano* was to be found. It took some time to determine whether the *gusano* resided in the East or the West Indies, although Marcobruno, our indefatigable scientific investigator, was willing to travel to either place.[15] In fact, his desire was so great, he wrote Vincenzo on June 11 that he felt "it was taking a thousand years to get there and I pray God to preserve my health, so that I can happily satisfy your desire."[16] Still, the duke was not totally sure that his libido enhancers were in the West Indies, although Emanuel Cimenes in his letter of 1608 had hinted at that possibility. The importing firm of Carlo Hellman and heirs was making a similar bet, and in June 27, 1609, their correspondent, Gioan de Barlaymonte, had actually notified the ducal counselor, Annibale Chieppio, that a man working for the company in Goa, the East Indies—Giovan Battista Chiut—was not the right person to search for items for the duke, since the animals he was looking for could be found only in "Perù, which is a province of the West Indies, and therefore our man cannot be used for this purpose, since he goes to India." De Barlaymonte offered that if the duke really wanted these "animaletti," letters could be sent to the firm's correspondents in "Mexico, city of America" (Mexico Città di America), even though it would take two years for the fleet to come back.[17]

By this time Marcobruno had the upper hand, not only because he had already left Mantua but also because on July 14 he was able to confirm to Vincenzo that he had assembled indisputable proof from a missionary priest returning from the West Indies: the right *gusano,* he wrote from Madrid, was indeed in that part of the world. Thankfully for us modern readers, Marcobruno also revealed, without mincing words, what he was looking for:

> Signor, I searched so much in this court that finally an Indian priest was found with knowledge of the little animal for the erection of the

> penis [*dell'animaletto ad erectione virge*]. He says that it is no longer than a finger's nail, is hairy, is variously colored, has a head like that of a large fly, and when smeared over the member works marvelously, or put in oil for twenty-four hours grants the same result. It is to be found in Peru, in the valley of Chuquiabo. I also heard from him that there are some stones and gums of most great power there. I am feverishly waiting to go, if there is a passage to the West Indies, and Signor Bonatti has written to get the license. As soon as this is done, I will expedite myself there, forgetting all sorts of hardship in order to fulfill the order of Your Most Serene Highness.[18]

What Marcobruno was searching for in the immense continent of America was extremely tiny, but this detail seemed to present no insurmountable problem. After all, just a few days later that very year, Galileo Galilei was demonstrating to the Venetian Senate that there was a whole new world of minuscule beings visible through his newly invented telescope, which was waiting for man's mastering stare and appropriation.[19] Curiosity was the era's watchword.

Marcobruno wrote again on August 29, this time from Segovia, with more precise information on the form in which the *gusano* could be obtained and on the seemingly toxic effects accruing to its use without adequate preparation:

> Among the many Indians at court, I found a Franciscan priest who assured me that this *gusano* can be found in the mountains of the Andes, and the Indians bring them dried to the cities of Chuquiabo and Potosí. This worm is slightly shorter than a finger, variously velvety in color, and just by touching the member with it, this becomes so fearlessly erect that if there is no woman nearby one feels such a sharp pain to almost die of it. I have been unable to ascertain whether there is a male and a female species. This is what I heard from this priest, who was a guardian in that city and preached to his parishioners to abstain from using it. They are to be found in Peru, 400 leagues inside, and the convoy from Seville leaves this November for Peru.[20]

In a subsequent letter of October 20, 1609, Marcobruno confirmed that it was necessary to have close by an antidote when trying out such a stimulating pomade. As confirmed by a new Franciscan missionary from Genoa, who had been in Peru for twenty-eight years, men need to anoint the organ with a *gusano* kept in oil, and then for the antidote "they have the *contra hierva;* otherwise they would die. I could not know much about this, but it is to be found there."[21] In the same letter

Marcobruno reveals that an African slave had apprised him of another *gusano* with the same effect, called *dandastica*, to be found in New Spain, and if the intelligence were to be correct, he would have no problem in going there as well. For the moment, he was eagerly awaiting his departure with a fleet heading west because he knew where to go and what he must do, no matter the perils.[22] He was at work constructing his own poetics of colonialism. In his diary, Marcobruno mentions hardship and danger occasionally, but he mostly focuses on a comprehensive project of acquiring local knowledge, annotating it, and explaining it in familiar terms ("I will write on everything that will come upon me during the journey," he assured the ducal counselor), while making sure to get the goods and to return home safely to tell all.[23]

Arranging for the expedition had its own difficulties. First, it was brought to a halt by the fact that in August some *gusanos* imported from the New World had been found in the Sevillian market and subsequently sent to Mantua for the duke to test.[24] The experiment must have had only a palliative effect, for soon afterwards came the order to move forward with the journey. However, for an Italian not engaged in missionary work to be given passage on a Spanish galleon required special permission from the Spanish crown, which legendarily kept non-Spaniards out of the overseas colonies for fear of illegal trade or espionage. Thus, efforts were made to secure the king's imprimatur. On November 17, 1609, Philip III finally gave his approval, for the "Most Illustrious Duke of Mantua, my most dear cousin" had asked for it, and guaranteed the privacy of this matter in the New World. Evangelista Marcobruno was described in the license as a man twenty-eight years old, of medium height, white, and of large face and body. "Although he was a foreigner," no questions were to be asked of him. He was also exempt from paying the customary dues.[25]

Marcobruno, our bioprospector, left for the New World at the beginning of February 1610. The journey would deliver more adventures than he had conceivably bargained for, but he was willing to take them in stride. He belonged to a world that still believed that almost anything found in nature could heal. Thus, like any amateur Galenist, our pharmacist dreamed of combing Peru without respect to localities as long as the medicinal commodities he could find conformed to the humoral system of a deeply embedded Western medical tradition. Even more rewarding to him, he could experience personally, "as if I were a Christopher

Columbus," the adventure that the greatest Italian natural scientist of the sixteenth century, Ulisse Aldrovandi, had only dreamed of when he envisioned an expedition with writers, painters, and humanists to catalog the New World's nature. In the end, Aldrovandi was unable to get either funding or permission to travel from the Spanish king.[26] Marcobruno must have deeply felt the importance of his Atlantic adventure, because he was not shy about praising his stamina while casting his journey in the usual colonial metaphors of male penetration of an obscure and threatening interior. "If I were to narrate your highness the hardships I went through in the land of Peru," he wrote more than eighteen months later, on October 25, 1611, "for in six months I walked 673 leagues, so depopulated [is this land] that one has no memory of a similar journey, for fifteen days I passed through many precipices between mountains, and there are immense rivers to cross all year long."[27] However, as he would soon find out, this was not the most difficult part of his journey.

Peddling Potency

Let me pause at this point to delineate in bold strokes what the European pharmacopoeia of the time was offering to restore or enhance the sexual vigor of an aging prince. Food to stimulate the pleasures of Venus existed for all social classes and walks of life, even at hand in one's backyard. According to the Galenic theory of signatures, food that resembled the sexual organ worked to its advantage, so vegetables such as eggplants, broad beans, and similarly shaped comestibles were consumed to improve the odds of a successful sexual congress. Pigeons, cocks, pigs, and all animals known for their lasciviousness were also advocated; similarly, seafood such as oysters and shrimp were consumed to boost the libido. Flatulent vegetables, by contrast, were recommended only to men whose ardor had to be reduced, as in the case of ascetics and hermits, who were to eat lettuce or the aptly named agnus castus (chaste tree). When decrepit Nicomaco in Niccolò Machiavelli's play *Clizia* realized that he might have difficulties in bed with the young Clizia, he knew that he could rely on satyrion, which "as far as it regards that business, would rejuvenate a man ninety rather than seventy years old, like me."[28] To further improve his chances for success, he also planned to eat a dinner of pigeon roasted rare, fava beans, and onions, all cooked with various spices.

Most aphrodisiac recipes mixed plant and animal substances. Homemade poultices involved various vegetable oils or the fat of geese or donkeys, often blended with pepper to enhance the production of semen, honey to lubricate the organ, and basil to slightly irritate it. A simple formula suggested a diet of twenty eggs cooked with myrrh, cinnamon, and pepper, all eaten in the span of five to seven days. On the eighth day, a sexual feast was in the cards.[29] Then, depending on the money one wanted to spend, there were more exotic offerings coming from the East and dutifully sold by Venetian and Genoese merchants in local markets: ginger was supposed to have a congestive effect and thus was good for increasing the emission of sperm, aloe would strengthen the organ, vanilla and cinnamon would stimulate it, and so on. For everyday help in fostering one's sexual drive, carrying a talisman such as the mandrake root could give *in loco* results or make pleasure last longer.[30] More energetic methods fostered by professors of physics also proved popular, notwithstanding the extreme discomfort that some would cause. To be sure, one did not need to follow Pliny the Elder's suggestion that inserting the canine tooth of a crocodile into the anus would produce a speedier arousal, for a much easier recipe recommended massaging the sexual organ with ground gray clay mixed with the urine of a young bull, or putting the skin of a vulture over the member to render it robust. The marrow of a deer likewise guaranteed the same results.[31]

The expert advice of practitioners, herbalists, and distillers was so much in demand that the fees they charged for their decoctions, oils, powders, plasters, syrups, broths, philters, unguents, creams, gelatins, cataplasms, elixirs, paps, lozenges, philters, pomades, and infusions reflected their supposed expertise in the area. Often their instructions called for animals with phallic shapes or with a phallic lore in their history. Thus, many penises of bulls and cocks were sacrificed in the cauldrons of creative druggists. Giovanni Marinello recommended, for example, the powdered testicles of a cock drunk with wine before entering the bedchamber.[32] However, Caterina Sforza, a woman specializing in the secrets of love, preferred the dried penis of a donkey (*virgam asini exiccatam*) to marvelously magnify, as she put it, the sexual organ.[33] For Giambattista della Porta, a sure way to have strength in coitus was to consume the roasted and sliced penis of a wolf.[34]

Products from Cyprus were especially recommended, for Cyprus was famously the island of Venus; likewise, Friday was a key day for preparing decoctions and revitalizing broths. Take some drops of your own blood one Friday in the spring, another recipe recommended; dilute it with fresh sperm; and dry it next to a fireplace. Then put it in a pot containing two testicles of a hare and the liver of a female pigeon. After the compote turns into a fine powder, add some powder of hibiscus flower and dried leaves of endive. This therapeutic morsel is all that is needed to strengthen one's virility. Taken for three consecutive days, it can almost cause priapism.[35] Signora Isabella Cortese, an unconventional "professor of secrets," recommended, among other things, testicles of quails, large winged ants, moss, and amber to *far drizzar il membro*.[36] Relying as usual on the audience's understanding of Galenic medicine, Castore Durante observed that animals' testicles "afford excellent Nourishment to the Body, multiplying the Seed and increasing Copulation . . . and are good in cold weather for all ages and complexion, except decrepit and flegmatick men."[37]

Sometimes a single ingredient was needed to correct flaccidity, and this was especially true for remedies difficult to find in one's own country. The famous herbalist Pietro Andrea Mattioli was very much taken by

> a most marvelous herb to excite the venereal appetites that an Indian had brought, and by not just eating but simply touching this herb, men are incited so much to copulation that this herb made them potent to exercise sex whenever they wanted. It was said that those who had used it had made love twelve times, and some had heard the Indian, who was old and fat, say that he had done it seventy times using no more than a few drops of seed each time.[38]

Contrariwise, a tree in the New World was feared by locals as being able to make them impotent, and thus they would rather "get themselves killed than go under its shade."[39] Leo Africanus hailed the root of the African "surnag" in the western part of the Atlas Mountains, for it "has the virtue of comforting man's member and multiplying coitus to whoever eats it."[40] In short, the miraculous Viagra cure could be found anywhere east, west, and south in the known world, although not in the notoriously cold Northern Hemisphere, for "hot" was the operative word in the business of erotica.

It was toward the end of the sixteenth century, as the Paracelsian mineral-based chemical approach motivated countless apothecaries, chemists, and druggists to macerate and distill "mixts," that the early folksy pharmacopoeia of herbs and animals—a sort of personal *hortus sanitatis*—and the more expensive preparations from places farther away gave way to esoteric recipes that required alchemical preparations—the use of metals, such as gold, silver, and mercury, and the addition of pulverized precious stones, such as emeralds, pearls, and corals. As the new baroque yearning for the eccentric and the exotic met the same old desire for an effective cure to the scourges of the time—from plague to syphilis, from malaria to tuberculosis, from malnutrition to scabies— some of the new recipes ended up mixing more than fifty ingredients.[41] One could doubt that a humble southern Italian cook, Nicola, was the first ever importer of a New World medicament in Italy—cocoa butter, which he used to heal a wound on the foot of the great historian of New Spain, Gonzalo Fernández de Oviedo—but there was an army of Italian doctors, botanists, zoologists, historians, and impostors seeking passage in those decades to the New World to study its products or simply to check its allure.[42] Europe started to suffer from a pharmacological delirium as the number of named plants in herbals skyrocketed from 500 in Dioscorides—his text appeared in 1568 in a beautiful edition by the herbalist Mattioli—to over 6,000 in the work of the botanist Caspar Bauhin in 1623.[43] As tons of new phytotherapies and animal-based remedies—all enticing with their difficult-to-pronounce names— were shipped to European ports, often with no consideration given to the right season in which to harvest them, the most effective dosages in which to administer them, or the ideal climatic conditions in which they were to be kept, time and again they benefited only enterprising tradesmen. Historically speaking, and no matter the particular interests of merchants and the various experimentations of doctors and apothecaries, in the end the New World therapeutics did not have much of an impact on the official pharmacopoeia, which kept its fairly traditional approach well into the eighteenth century. Had people followed the recommendations or even the custom of local "American" healers regarding the medicinal use of their specimens, perhaps their introduction in Europe would have been more effective, but the dictates of Galenic humoral therapies were too imbued in patients' minds for doctors to ignore them for the sake of innovation.[44]

As the new century began, the interest in exotic and chemical compounds and in pharmaceutical experimentation was so strong that, concurrent with the steady increase in the number of named herbs, courts all over Italy began to create and staff their own botanical gardens and give the study of the new varieties to recently appointed university professors. In Mantua Vincenzo hired the famous Zenobio Bocchi. Requests to send specimens of his botanical garden abroad came from a number of courts. In the 1590s, the Habsburg, for example, asked for "jasmine from Catalonia, prickly pears, aloe vera, and other flowers from Italy" to be sent to Jacob Kurtz, who was furnishing his own garden.[45] The Gonzaga court also teemed with alchemists paid to supervise such preparations as tincture of coral, oil of iron, potable gold, and *menstruum* of mercury. Mantuan agents throughout Italy would either notify Vincenzo about finding the secret for the multiplication of gold[46] or complain that the process of extracting gold from silver was delayed by, say, the interruption of work due to the Easter holidays.[47]

As the use of poisons became more politically effective and the need for antipoisons was demanded both by Galenic medicine, which was predicated on freeing the body of poisonous humors in order to cure it, and by the vagaries of everyday life in a world where the water supply was never secure, laboratories of major cities started to provide "chemical" supplies to a concerned citizenship. Vincenzo was proud of his *nobile medicamento*, an antipoison medicine, which he was able to produce in such a large quantity that he could offer it for free to the poor "oppressed by the poison."[48] Even Romeo, in Shakespeare's *Romeo and Juliet*, knew that it was possible to find good poisons that killed quickly in Mantua. The universal antidote, the theriaca—a medicament considered so noble that it could only be prepared once a year, in public, and under official supervision—required a large amount of vipers' poison. Sometimes these animals were sold at such a prohibitive cost that the city of Bologna had to emit a *Bando sopra le vipere,* charging a fine of 25 lire to anyone who wanted to buy a viper, dead or alive.[49] No wonder that when Francesco, Vincenzo's son, became duke, one of his first acts was to fire all the alchemists on the Gonzaga payroll to save money—a gesture that unfortunately turned out to be rather ineffective.[50]

Cabinets of curiosities—the *Wunderkammern* of scientists such as Ulisse Aldrovandi in Bologna, often organized around the categories of *naturalia* and *artificialia* and sporting both botanical and animal artifacts from the Old as well as the New World—became magnets for sharing knowledge and were soon part of the must-see places frequented by ingenious new scientists and traveling university students. The Mantuan apothecary Filippo Costa owned a *studiolino,* whose incredible curiosities constituted "indeed a genteel theater of the rarest simples that our age has discovered."[51] The Wunderkammern of the Ducal Palace, decorated by Vincenzo with scenes of Ovid's metamorphoses, displayed ethnographic specimens, exotic real and fake natural history curiosities, deformed fetuses, and even a mummified cadaver.[52] The Gonzaga archives offer a keen sense of the fascination that *exotica,* grouped in typological inventories, had at court, as questions of cost steadily gave way to the pleasure of possessing a menagerie of unique artifacts.[53] Imports from America of wild flora and fauna and of raw minerals and precious or semiprecious stones were the most expensive. America was the land of desire, as Columbus had imperialistically claimed from the start ("This is a land to desire, and seen, is never to be left"), a place well worth the hunt, the fatigue of travel, and all related expenses.[54] It is within this context that Evangelista Marcobruno's search in faraway lands needs to be placed. For an apothecary with an enterprising mind and a sensualist with a megalomaniacal ego, the trip to the miracles of the West Indies made sound sense, both scientifically and financially. In Marcobruno, Vincenzo had found his match. The duke's dream had become the apothecary's.

Given that there were fifty-four herbals in circulation in Europe by the late sixteenth century and that neither the supposed sophistication nor the variety of medicinal remedies for sexual enhancement existing in the West had resolved the latent demand of a male population complaining of sexually related ailments, one wonders what novel therapies the New World was precisely offering to address male disorders, beyond the unidentified *gusano* that Marcobruno was committed to finding.[55] As usual, what stimulates trade is demand, and demand was soon such that the drug trade quickly became rewarding, to the point that a good number of biostimulators known today as coming from the Caribbean, Mexico, and South America were already being imported by the early seventeenth century. Maca root (*epidium meyenii*), for example, which boosted sexual stamina and increased performance, provided the most familiar relief. Maca's myth as an aphrodisiac and enhancer of fecundity and strength was furthered by the descriptions of Spanish soldiers who found themselves rendered infertile by the soaring Andean elevation. According to popular lore, the Incas, who were initiated to the strength of this root by the Yaro tribes, found it so powerful that only royalty were allowed to use it. Introduced to the Spanish conquistadores in due course, by the mid-sixteenth century more than 15,000 pounds of maca per year were being shipped from the Andean highlands to European ports.[56] In addition, catuaba, an Amazonian tree, revealed its virtues 500 ago, when it began to be used to enhance virility, increase sperm activity, and treat fatigue. A decoction of its bark was thought to stimulate the nervous system and increase sexual performance. Sarsaparilla, which was present in both Mexico and Peru, was mostly used to treat syphilis and had already hit the European markets by 1563, but is was also known as a stamina enhancer, and thus was used to prolong performance. Yerba maté (*ilex paraguariensis*), another ancient New World plant with immunostimulating properties, was thought to invigorate the body, increase staying power, and constitute a spirited tonic. Damiana, appropriately referred to as *turnera aphrodisiaca*—a shrub with tiny yellow flowers growing in rocky terrain, which Mayans and Aztecs employed as a stimulant for circulation—was also used for arterial erectile impotence: it was thought that, taken as an energy tonic before making love, it brought oxygen to the genital area. *Macuna pruriens*, commonly known as "velvet bean," was used in Brazil and the nearby region to treat impotence, sterility, and sexual debility. A concoction made from its seed pods was considered a good aphrodisiac. Another remedy was the *uña de gato*, or cat's claw, a Peruvian vine used to blast the libido and relieve stress and pain. The roots of the muira puama from the Amazon forest were also known for enhancing one's sexual drive and increasing satisfaction; the everyday name of "common wood" explains the roots' effect as a restorer of sexual vigor. Guarana, a plant native to the Amazon forest, was thought to be an energy enhancer and stimulator, like caffeine today. Quinquefolia, the West Indian equivalent of ginseng, was also used to intensify erotic pleasure.[57]

Then there were the animal cures. The skin of the serpent *mazacoatl* drunk with water worked as an aphrodisiac; the opossum tail used in an infusion was quite effective when preparing for the pleasures of Venus; and nine burned spines of the porcupine of New Spain (*hoitztlacuatzin*) taken with wine and water increased the sexual drive.[58] Given the novelty of the American flora and fauna, the boundaries between the two were sometimes blurred.[59] How many of these herbal and animal remedies Marcobruno knew beyond maca, sarsaparilla, and catuaba is difficult to assess. Unlike us, however, he lived in a world in which every single herb had some value and was of interest to the physician and healer if it could be understood in terms of addressing and regulating excess and deficit in the body.

Researching the Unknown

Marcobruno mentions more than once in his letters that he knew where to go in the New World, because he had books, not to mention a mental map, and had read about the new places.[60] To be sure, his trip would repeatedly show him that knowledge based on established sources is worth little when what is seen is strikingly unfamiliar, yet we should not discount the immense importance of the Gonzaga library in Mantua as a source for Marcobruno's knowledge of therapeutic practices, travel, and geography.[61] Of course, our apothecary did not know, or knew only from references in other texts, what is today considered the most accurate herbal inventory of the New World, Francisco Hernández's survey of 1,300 or so plants in Mexico around the 1570s, which had been only partially published at the time.[62] In 1592, Fabio Colonna became the first scholar to incorporate material from Hernández's inventory into his *Phytobasanos sive plantarum aliquot historia*, a text that was known and could have very well been in the Gonzaga library.[63] But there were many other books in circulation, often partially edited, that Marcobruno most likely consulted, such as Juan Fragoso's text on aromatic medicaments or José de Acosta's encyclopedic *Historia natural y moral de las Indias* (1590), which contained information on geography, climate, plants, animals, minerals, and *exotica* from both Mexico and Peru.[64] There is no doubt that the Gonzaga library had at least one copy of Nicolás Monardes's *Delle cose, che vengono portate dall'Indie Occidentali pertinenti all'uso della medicina*, as it had already been translated twice into Italian.[65] If Hernández's aim was botanical and taxonomic, that of Monardes, the son of a Genoese merchant, was pharmaceutical. Even Vincenzo's doctor and secretary, Marcello Donati, began to translate in 1570 "l'opera del dottore Nicolosa."[66] And it is certain that Marcobruno had read the extensive *Summario della naturale et generale historia dell'Indie occidentali, composta da Gonzalo Ferdinando del Oviedo,* published together with Oviedo's *Della naturale e generale istoria dell'Indie a' tempi nostri ritrovate* in Giovanni Battista Ramusio's first edition of *Navigationi et Viaggi* (1556), the set of travel narratives that from the very beginning and for at least a century was obligatory reading for any educated traveler.[67]

Vernacular medical publishing in the Old World was sizable too, given the popularity of herbals, and we know that the Gonzaga library had them all, starting from the most respected, Mattioli's *Discorsi*. Marcobruno was also probably familiar with the popular *Herbario nuovo* of Castore Durante, which discussed all known plants of the Old and New World and contained approximately 1,000 woodcuts, as well as Durante's *Il tesoro della sanità*.[68] As for books of secrets, all following the Galenic humoral system, Marcobruno may have known a good number of them, from the work of Girolamo Ruscelli to that of Leonardo Fioravanti.[69] Being himself the son of an apothecary, Marcobruno knew specific druggists' texts too, for the apprenticeship of a pharmacist was, by all means, long, and local statutes required training of five to eight years.[70] He quite certainly consulted Prospero Borgarucci's *La fabrica degli speziali* (1567) and Antonio Brasavola's *Examen omnium simplicium medicamentom* (1539), because they were widely used in pharmacies.[71]

Finally, there were travel books specifically describing Peru, its people, and its geography that Marcobruno may have consulted, books such as Pedro Cieza de Léon's *Crónica del Peru*, which appeared in Rome in 1555 and was translated into Italian in 1556 as *Prima parte dell'istorie del Peru;* Francisco López de Gomara's *Historia General de las Indias* (1557 and 1559), which recounted Cortez's and Montezuma's conquests and also detailed native customs; and Agustín de Zárate's *Historia del descubrimento y conquista del Peru,* which came out in Italian in 1563.[72] Then there were the encyclopedic books written by the Italians themselves, such as Giovanni Lorenzo d'Anania's *L'universale fabrica del mondo,* and Gioseppe Rosaccio's *Il mondo e sue parti,* both published in 1596.[73] Last but not least, Marcobruno could have found information on the New World through the popular *Avisi* or *Nuovi Avisi*—that is, informal, often didactic, letters sent by Jesuit missionaries, translated from Spanish or Portuguese, on anything worth remarking on in the newly evangelized lands.[74]

The Aphrodisiac Sting

We do not know what American pharmaceutical panacea under the appellative *gusano* Evangelista Marcobruno precisely had in mind when he started his journey, for the lore about the biostimulating properties of worms was well established at the time.[75] Years earlier, following his voyage along the coast of Brazil down beyond latitude 50° south to what he appropriately called a *Mundus Novus*, Amerigo Vespucci had described a nature-enhancing bug that shameless local women used to invigorate their men's genitals:

> Women have also another cruel custom, one far away from any human habit: since they are inordinately lustful, in order to satisfy their dishonest desire they use this cruel custom of giving their men the juice of a certain herb to drink, which, once drunk, makes their member swell and grow greatly. If this is not enough, they bring close to the member certain poisonous animals to bite it until it engorges, from which it comes among them that many lose their testicles and become eunuchs.[76]

It is easy to see through Vespucci's account the usual strategy of representing problematic male desire in early modern culture: in this reading, men's inability to satisfy their lust due to personal failures leads them to displace their frustration onto women, who are rendered aggressive in the exchange. By sadistically combining drinking, biting, and poisoning in their inordinate sexual craving, these women end up literally castrating their men, who lose both their masculinity and their manhood the very moment they put the other sex in charge of the sexual congress. Dangerously enough, local women were particularly eager to sleep with Christians, Vespucci warned, thus sounding an alarm bell for his unsuspecting readers back home.[77] It pays to point out that this may be a bogus account of male disempowerment, since many historians doubt that Vespucci actually made this particular trip.[78] However, Vespucci's strategy of linking men's loss of a portion of their sexual organ, which at the time of his writing was painfully and easily verifiable in a number of syphilitic men, to women's inordinate desire—foreign women, to be sure, so that the threat is one removed from a generalized female menace—tells us that such a predatory fantasy was present in the cultural imagination of the early modern man.[79]

The Florentine merchant Francesco Carletti, whose journey around the world in the years 1594–1606 as a private citizen is recounted in *Lettere dalle Indie Occidentali e dalle Indie Orientali,* also reports the story of the "most lascivious women" of the West Indies practicing their "diabolical invention" and having poisonous animals "bite or sting their [men's] member," a custom that he judges common knowledge.[80] The same assertion is made by the Florentine traveler Galeotto Cei, who in his *Viaggio e relazione delle Indie (1539–1553)* explains the custom used by some West Indian men to satisfy their women, described throughout as sexually demanding and insatiable:

> [These men enlarge] the crest of their sexual organ [by making] three or four cuts in it so that they can open it as if they were the fingers of one's hand, that is, in four or five parts. Then they juice it with a local herb, which makes it heal fast and also swollen. Their women derived great pleasure from these practices.[81]

As is typical with such narratives, the horror and the longing that these customs evoke work toward radically "othering" the foreign. This "libidinously eroticized" America (or Africa or Asia, for that matter) constitutes what Anne McClintock has called a "porno-tropics for the European imagination—a fantastic magic lantern of the mind onto which Europe projected its forbidden sexual desires and fears."[82]

To say that the early modern period was preoccupied with insects and larvae—mosquitoes, gnats, hornets, maggots, wasps, lice, bedbugs, earthworms, caterpillars, grasshoppers, spiders, tarantulas, snakes, ringworms, tapeworms, and all wormlike parasites—is an understatement. One should rather talk of an obsession. Even syphilis, the acknowledged scourge of the century, was connected to insects, worms, and serpents, not because they caused it but because, as in popular Spanish parlance, men who were supposed to suffer from syphilis were "bitten by the tarantula." The expression "Picado de la *tarantula*" in the *Diccionario de autoridades* makes it clear: "Vulgarmente se entiende de los que padecen [suffer] el humor galico."[83] Among the many fictitious stories of origin explaining the syphilis etiology—that it was caused, for example, by unnatural conjunctions and sodomitic acts—we know that some were attributing it to "the venomous Bite of a Serpent."[84]

Spiders seemed to have had a special preference for the female gender, so much so that after being bitten on their legs or on their sexual organ, chiefly during puberty, young women became hysterical and feverish, and offered themselves wantonly to men. Men nibbled by the tarantula were "filled with so much luxury and libidinousness," a sixteenth-century treatise on dance informs, that "in seeing women, they assault them with such a rage as if they were beasts."[85] The only relief from a spider's bite was dancing to music with a sexual content. That dance is still known today as the "tarantella."[86] Contemporary painting likewise delighted in showing worms coming out of rotten fruits, plays became obsessed with fleas and bedbugs, and poems lingered over minuscule parasitic animals gnawing the flesh. "Decaying beauty became an aesthetic category," Piero Camporesi argues, and "painting supplied the figurative equivalent of the insect's victory over human life (for instance in Guercino's *Et in Arcadia Ego*)."[87] Well into the eighteenth century, well beyond the moment in 1688 when Francesco Redi demonstrated with the discovery of the ovum that every living being is produced from two parents, worms were thought to be autogenous, born without seed from corrupted matter.[88] People believed that lower animal beings, such as lizards, bees, horseflies, serpents, bedbugs, toads, and mice, were born spontaneously with the help of the sun—and this was not the folk belief of the uneducated, for Aristotle was among them. Oviedo accepted as true that the mice and rats of the New World were not brought "when Admiral Christopher Columbus came to discover these islands" but were everywhere "because they do not multiply through coitus but are generated through putrefaction."[89] Self-generating worms were also supposed to live parasitically inside human bodies; thus, a strict cleansing diet was encouraged for the sake of keeping their propagation in check. Worms were also rumored to cause a mind-boggling array of diseases, such as "epilepsy, dizziness, drowsiness, delirium, convulsions and headaches, loss of consciousness, palpitations, depression, terror, cough, vomiting, nausea, diarrhea, hiccup pains, stomach colic, restlessness, outbreaks, wasting away, chronic and acute fevers."[90] For the clerics, worms and men were closely linked, for human flesh was to become worm food. Adults, moreover, had to be vigilant at all times, for the devil could enter the human body in the form of vermin. The concern about worms was so high at the beginning of the seventeenth century that Giovan Battista Codronchi wrote an entire book addressing the violence with which a battalion of worms infested the wretched city of Imola.[91] And a treatise on worms, Fernando Salando's *Trattato sopra li vermi, cause, differenze, pronostico e curatione,* was dedicated to Vincenzo's wife, Eleonora, four years later, in 1607—the year that preceded Marcobruno's journey.

Reports from America put the whole New World under the spell of bugs. The women of Cueva, Oviedo offered, liked to eat the lice they picked from their bodies—a custom so common that it was hard to restrain them when they were employed in a Spanish household.[92] He also describes the venom of some ants in the New World used to poison arrows, a toxin so deadly that only four out of one hundred wounded men survive the ordeal.[93] Acosta mentions a Mexican and Peruvian custom in which men smear on themselves an ointment made of spiders, scorpions, centipedes, lizards, and vipers—all mixed with tobacco leaves—in order to become sorcerers; in fact, he adds, "this ointment also served to cure the sick and the children and so everyone called it divine medicine."[94] Fortunately worms could be expelled through pills of tobacco, a New World medicine that was recommended at the time to address problems as varied as ringworm of the scalp, poisonous bites, sores, abscesses, carbuncles, rheumatism, headache, and colic.[95]

Following the popular understanding that what causes a problem also providentially offers a solution, a number of immunostimulating therapies involving worms, bugs, and even parasitic larvae were available in the marketplace to promote good health. "Collect . . . a great abundance of volatile salt from insects, such as earthworms, millipedes, ants . . . toads, frogs and also the excrements thereof," Paolo Boccone suggested in the late seventeenth century. "The strength and efficacy of the effluvia of these insects, of the Spanish fly, of bedbugs, of scorpions is common knowledge."[96] Earthworm oil was highly recommended by Giambattista Morgagni (he is known today as the father of modern anatomical pathology) for one's well-being, together with viper's fat, powdered human cranium, woman's milk, viper flesh, and mouse blood—all in a decoction made with chicken broth. And he endorsed millipede powder, a diuretic par excellence, for the lungs.[97] Monardes wrote of an unknown worm with curative powers that people in the New World used as a cake to apply topically in cases of herpes zoster (*fuoco di Sant'Antonio*), an immunological disease that may also have afflicted Vincenzo.[98] Millipedes were advocated for throat trouble when taken with honey, whereas powdered cockroaches kept in oil were used for earache. In Mantua, for example, the recipe for the oil of scorpion—which required 300 live scorpions, 100-year-old oil, and 29 other substances—is described in a book by Antonio Bertioli (Berthioli), a pharmacist who operated in the city during Vincenzo's time.[99] Dried spiderwebs, salves of the excrement of millipedes, pickled frogs, pills of scorpion fat, water of butterfly, cakes of bedbugs, and electuaries of horny excrescences could be found in any well-stocked apothecary shop. The life of the early modern man was firmly under the sign of the worm.

The Land of Marvels

Before leaving Spain, Marcobruno had learned exactly where his prized poisonous worms were to be found: 400 leagues inside Peru.[100] His departure from Cádiz on February 6, 1610, on the galleon *Jesus Maria Joseph* was, everything considered, less eventful than the boating experience from Marseille to Barcelona at the start of his journey had proven to be. On that occasion, his vessel was ambushed by the Barbary corsairs ("una Galeotta de Barbari"), who abducted three Capuchin friars for eventual ransom.[101] Marcobruno journeyed on the southern route that Spanish convoys usually followed in making their way to either Portobelo in the Panama Isthmus or Cartagena in the Tierra Firme (now Colombia).[102] Upon arrival in either city, people and goods usually proceeded on llamas or mules to the Pacific side of the Panama Isthmus, and from there back on boats to Callao, where they disembarked, and then again mules or llamas were employed to reach the final destination of Lima or Potosí.[103] Marcobruno arrived in Cartagena forty-seven days after his departure from Cádiz, on March 25, 1610. Writing to Vincenzo on April 6, he describes a stop on the way in Guadalupe to get water and food (and does not fail to notice the large number of African slaves the Spanish kept in the area, all made to go around naked but for their shameful parts). He also marvels at the delicacy of the different fruits he found, such as bananas, pineapple, and variously shaped melons.[104] Next he wrote from Panama on May 27 to confirm that he was still collecting information on the American worm.

Marcobruno's next letter to the duke, seventeen months later, on October 25, 1611, is from Seville. This letter, Marcobruno's last one, details all the vicissitudes of the long-dreamed expedition. It took one month on board a large galleon, the apothecary noted, to go from Panama to Manta in Ecuador. Here he disembarked, together with some fifty passengers, to proceed on foot to Lima. From there he went well into the Andes to Cuzco, where he was able to get seven *gusanos*. Wanting more, he proceeded to Chuquiabo but was told that they were out of season, since the best time to acquire them was around Easter. So he went to Potosí, because he got assurance that the locals brought *gusanos* there from the Terra Caliente—indeed where else than in the subtropical Terra Caliente, an erotized virgin land, should this therapy be found? But he could locate no worm on sale there. Pressed for time, he left his *gusanos* in Chuquiabo with some merchants and the order to send them right away to Lima, and then embarked with the first departing ship. Resigned and in need of catching the convoy back to Spain, he went to Arica on the coast and subsequently took a boat headed to Lima, where he arrived eight days later. He ultimately made it to Cartagena, the departure point for any merchant's return trip to Europe. Here he found a letter from the ducal ambassador Bonatti, who was asking for a few more items that Vincenzo wanted from those far-away lands.[105]

Besides the *gusano*, Marcobruno may have also obtained the *contrayerba* (or *contrahierva*), a general Indo-Spanish term meaning literally "anti-poison." This might be a plant of Peruvian origin, probably the *Dorstenia contrayerva* of the family Urticaceae, present in the tropical parts of South America, whose roots were considered antidotes to poison.[106] Monardes wrote that the *contrayervas* "look like the roots of an iris, and are a marvelous remedy when they are powdered and taken with white wine."[107] The female *contrayerba* (*Contrayerba del Perù feminina*) was thought to be powerful against bites of animals that release poison, such as vipers, snakes, aspic, serpents, frogs, toads, and similar creatures.[108] If the side effects of the Peruvian *gusano* were in any way similar to those caused by the Spanish fly—cramps, extreme thirst, bloody urine, vomiting, loss of muscle control, and convulsions—the *contrayerba* was indeed the sine qua non needed to survive the experiment.[109]

The rest of Marcobruno's time was spent collecting curiosities to bring back to Mantua, such as stones, gums, and unusual animals. As he writes from Seville in a revealing moment of economic lust for the exotic and the antiquarian, he had bought four little local hawks; some birds that were similar to peacocks (but two died on the way); two more plumed birds; a large parrot (*guacamaya*), which unfortunately flew away; and three small green parrots (*catalincas*). Other unidentified parrots died during the crossing. He also bought medicaments as well as resins, oils, and dried paste (*conserva*).[110] Finally, before leaving Spain for Genoa, he bought two barrels of large olives, which he thought the duke would greatly appreciate.[111]

As for the *gusano,* we do not know whether the package that Marcobruno left in Chuquiabo to be sent to Mantua in the late summer of 1611 ever made it to Europe. Those months were tragic ones for the House of Gonzaga. In September Eleonora died of fevers; a few months later Vincenzo took to his bed and died. In that very month, Marcobruno, who had insisted on returning by boat rather than overland from Barcelona to Genoa because of the large number of curiosities he was bringing home, was captured by corsairs at sea and brought to Algiers as a slave. Not knowing that the duke had died, Filippo Soles, the secretary to the Gonzaga's ambassador Bonatti in Spain, sent a letter to Vincenzo from Seville on February 21, 1612, soliciting his goodwill in arranging for the apothecary's ransom. He was a good man, he wrote, and well deserved his freedom.[112]

The new Gonzaga ruler, Francesco, was not particularly interested in rushing to free Marcobruno from captivity. He had little time in any case, for he died of smallpox a few months later. His successor, Ferdinando, however, was a chemist in his own right and had kept up a correspondence with Marcobruno during his trip to the Indies.[113] Duke Ferdinando's letter of June 11, 1613, constitutes the last chapter of our apothecary's adventure. In promising three hundred *ducatoni* for Marcobruno's ransom, plus an imprecise amount for the commodities (*robbe*) he was carrying at the time of his capture, which he may have still had with him, Ferdinando seems to be declaring, upon his princely faith ("in fede di Principi"), that any scientific adventure should be supported dutifully by the court.[114] We do not know whether Marcobruno ever made it back to Mantua.[115]

Was this early modern journey to the neverland of Peru useless then? Was Duke Vincenzo's idea of sending a twenty-eight-year-old underling across the Atlantic early in the seventeenth century just the fantasy of a man with a large purse and a tomcatting problem? And along the same lines, was the apothecary's search for curiosities—be they a therapy for impotence or some *mirabilia* for the ducal cabinet—worth dying for, or even, as eventually happened, worth the risk of being enslaved in Algiers? To listen to Marcobruno, the trip was worth every minute of it, for the apothecary's curiosity matched the scientist's enthusiasm. Marcobruno turned out to be a go-getter, a new-age explorer who had been bit, just like Vincenzo, by his own far-reaching aspiration: that of dying, if necessary, in the process of furthering scientific knowledge.[116] If, as Mary Louise Pratt writes, the scientific exploration of the overseas territories and the classification of their natural products marked a new sense of the self for Europeans that led to "constructing modern Eurocentrism, that hegemonic reflex that troubles westerners even as it continues to be second nature to them,"[117] then our herbalist's dogged search for scientific curiosities while sending full accounts of the colonial geography and even of the colonial trade he witnessed back home to his duke constitutes a remarkable early moment of frontier imaginings. As the letters show, whenever there was any question about his expedition being limited to Spain, Marcobruno fretted. East or West Indies, these phantasmal scenes of longing were the same to him, as long as he could pursue his dream. Marcobruno took time not only to hunt for worms, herbs, and various curiosities but also to annotate the colonial geography and the colonial trade.[118] We are at the start of a new era as even an herbalist from Mantua has ambitions to emerge from the fog of obscurantism to participate in the understanding, ordering, and mapping of nature. The year Marcobruno journeyed to the New World, 1610, coincidentally was the same year in which Galileo published his *Sidereus Nuncius,* which in effect launched, without looking back, the study of nature through observation and experimentation.[119] Marcobruno's achievement is by all means dwarfed by that of Galileo, in fact cannot even be put on the same scale, and yet his journey can be understood as a manifestation of that hunger for knowledge that was coursing through the veins of many early seventeenth-century pharmacists, chemists, doctors, scientists, and academicians.

As the years since the 1610s have shown, the search for an invigorating *gusano* has at times been no less important to men, or at least to some men, than Galileo's heliocentric theories, which effectively recast mankind's position in the world. This search has known no geographical or temporal boundaries and has extended well beyond Marcobruno's lowlands of the Tierra Caliente. Some men thought they found their dream therapy in the cocoa bean from the tropics, for the Aztec king Monteczuma was known to drink fifty cups a day to ensure his sexual stamina; others have sworn by the power of the *yohimbine*, the bark of an African tree. Still others have looked for answers to the dictates of the flesh on the psychoanalyst's couch, or have rushed to undergo vascular surgery, penile implants, and vasodilating therapies. And then in 1998 Viagra was introduced to the world.

Surprisingly, my story ends well, even with a dead duke and an enslaved apothecary, for we know now that Marcobruno may have found the right stuff after all. If anything, his problem was that he had looked too prematurely for a cure, for as we are learning these days, early modern pharmacopoeia has still a lot to offer to drug manufacturers' scientific inquiries.[120] The worms that Marcobruno so doggedly tried to find in Peru and Bolivia were called locally what sounds onomatopoeically like *pullo pullos*. In Quechua, *pullo* means "hairy," so *pullo pullos* may mean "very hairy." Or perhaps the native word was *puyu*, which in Quechua refers even today to the moth that feeds as it burrows into fabric. Recently Giuseppe Ostino has suggested that the *gusano* is a worm well known in the Andes called *gusano de pollo*, probably a larva of the family Megalopygidae (flannel moths). He cites a Venezuelan doctor, Ramon Briceño, who describes the larva of this lepidopteran as having an oval form, a black head, and a body covered with hair. Upon contact with the human body, the hair causes a visible inflammation accompanied by vertigo and heart complications. The irritating action lasts for a long time following the creature's death. Today the larva is used by locals to cure rheumatism.[121] Along the same lines, Stefano Scansani has proposed that the *gusano* could be the *Megalopygidae lanata*, whose sting has an irritating and inflammatory effect on human skin and causes fever.[122] We do not know whether this bug (the larva is called puss caterpillar because it is hairy) was ever used for sexual enhancement.

There is also another animal that locals in Peru, Bolivia, and Chile were calling at Marcobruno's time *pallú* (or presently *pulu*, as in the Mapuche region of Chile), which we know today works to boost sexual performance. This animal has recently become the subject of scientific investigation in the laboratories of the Chilean Universidad de la Frontera, under the direction of Dr. Fernando Romero. Monardes had written about its poisonous bite and described it as very large, "at times like an orange."[123] I am referring to the *viuda negra,* also called *araña del trigo* (*Lactrodectus mactans*)—that is, the black widow spider, an arachnid actually not rare in the region and also present in Europe. It has been known for a while that the black widow's sting produces prolonged and painful priapism as well as heart trouble. The neurotoxic venom the spider injects is now being tested under the auspices of the Chilean government because its effects mimic those of Viagra, but without acceleration of the heart rate, and because the poison makes sperm infertile, thus offering a contraceptive effect.[124]

But if the black widow spider is present in Italy too, why go to the New World to find it? Was there another comparable and yet specifically American spider that could work as an erectile enhancer? Indeed, there is one present in the general area that belonged to the viceroyalty of Peru (North Argentina, Paraguay, Uruguay), as well as in Brazil, that fits the characteristics of Marcobruno's hairy and velvety *gusano* (or even of Vespucci's "Brazilian" bug) and that has become a subject of feverish research and excited reporting in the last few years. This tiny animal, which is "no longer than a finger's nail, is hairy, is variously colored, [and] has a head like that of a large fly," to describe it in Marcobruno's words, is the so-called Brazilian wandering spider (*Phoneutria nigriventer,* also known as the banana spider because it hides and travels in this fruit), which is being seriously studied these days because it appears to possess a natural Viagra-like chemical in its venom. Romulo Leite, Kenia Pedrosa Nunes, and other neurologists and scientists at the Medical College of Georgia, working with the Instituto Butantan of São Paulo, have recently reported the results of their testing on rats of a carnal compound (Tx2-6) present in the spider's poison, which boosts the level of nitric oxide (NO), which in turn causes blood vessels to relax and open up. Their hope is that it can be used to correct vascular disorders as well as problems with impotency.[125]

For a duke whose prized apotropaic family emblem was a scorpion—the arachnid that, according to natural history, arose from putrefaction, but also, and more to the point, the opportunistic predator that brutally captures or stings, even itself, but rises again—the toxic, cannibalistic touch of a *gusano* could indeed be imagined as a tonic, if voracious, energizer.[126] Vincenzo died still fixed in his longing for eternal youth and vigor, and he famously refused, even when dead, to be seen any way other than "alert and erect," as he spelled out in his last will. No worshiper—male or female—was allowed to see Duke Vincenzo Gonzaga, the Mantuan stylish trendsetter, without the fetishistic instruments of phallic potency that had defined his identity—and his desires—in the abundantly lived fifty-year span of his life.

Epilogue

Unwrapping the Body

UPON HIS RETURN to Mantua from his third crusade in 1601, Vincenzo Gonzaga had the wooden ceiling of a hall in his apartment within the Ducal Palace readapted with the carved emblem of a blue-and-gold labyrinth and a motto. The work started before his return home, under the supervision of his wife, Eleonora, and was perhaps initially meant to celebrate with a maxim, which is on purpose incomplete, the fact that the Duke of Mantua had journeyed as far as Hungary to crush the "Infidels'" arrogance: "While he was fighting the Turks under the rock of Canissa" (Dum sub arce Canisiæ contra turcas pugn).[1] The decorator/artist was asked to add a cryptic sentence that runs ten times throughout the web decoration, a sentence that has for centuries left onlookers dumbfounded as to its meaning: "Forse che sì forse che no" ("Maybe yes, maybe no") (Fig. 17). The simplest hypothesis critics have advanced is to read the label as replicating the title of a known *frottola*, a musical composition made in 1509 for Isabella d'Este by Marchetto Cara, the leading composer at the time in the Mantuan court.[2] For other critics, Vincenzo was instead registering with the motto exactly what was going on in his war offensive, that is, the psychological state of a small army unsure of victory outside the walls of the besieged Canissa.[3] On a more speculative approach, the caption could refer, as Maria Bellonci has hypothesized, to a Gonzaga woman named Francesca, with whom Vincenzo had at the time a son, whom he never recognized.[4] The script in the appropriately named Sala del Labirinto (Hall of the Labyrinth) is now mostly remembered because it has been recycled

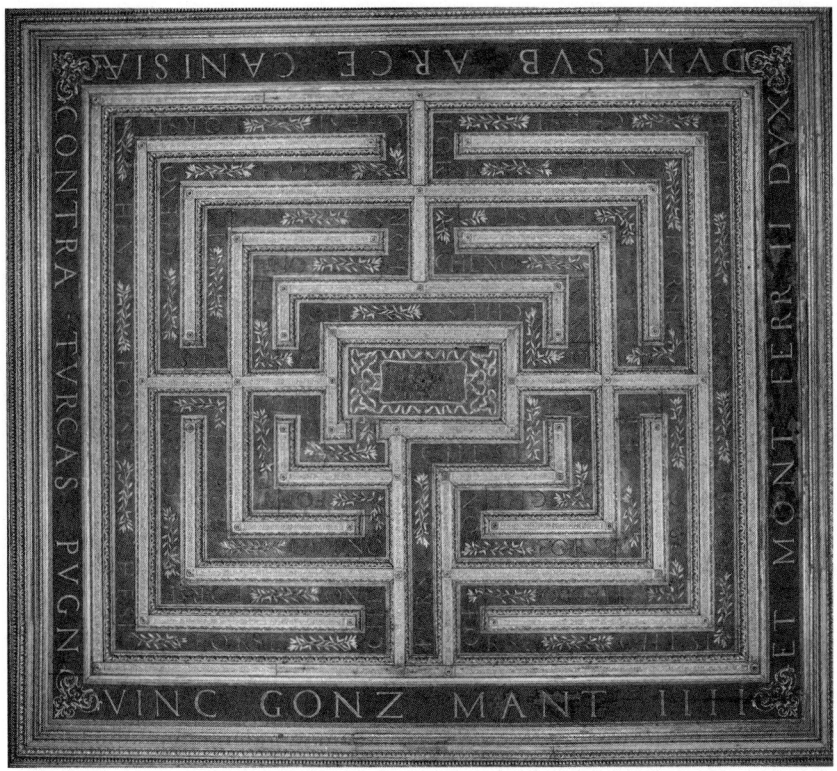

Fig. 17. "Forse che sì forse che no." Ceiling of the Hall of the Labyrinth, Palazzo Ducale, Mantua. (Photo: Art Resource.)

in the torrid and incestuous love story of the late nineteenth-century decadent writer Gabriele D'Annunzio, *Forse che sì forse che no* (1910).

At the center of the Mantuan labyrinth are two hearts laced together by string, followed by the words: "Dedalee industrie et teseie virtutis." Here the enigma seems to recall the myth of Daedalus, who was put in charge of building a labyrinth to imprison the man-eating Minotaur but was himself imprisoned in it when King Minos, his employer, found out that he had revealed the secret of its course to his daughter, Ariadne. She in turn had told Theseus, the Athenian founding hero, with whom she had fallen in love. Without looking left or right, Theseus entered the labyrinth to slay the Minotaur and was able to get out with all the young Athenians as well as Ariadne. The myth implies that by thinking through issues and engaging in crucial deeds—that is, by attempting to know oneself—it is possible to get out of the maze of life. Or is it? Maybe yes, maybe no!

It pays to note that by the middle of the sixteenth century, the "know thyself" motto, *nosce te ipsum*, was mostly used in anatomical illustrations, fugitive sheets, and atlases of the human body, printed predominantly in Venice but also appearing frequently elsewhere in Europe. The phrase thus meant that exploration inside the body to know human nature—by medical practitioners and surgeons—was just as important as psychological inquiries of inner behaviors and motivations. In the dedication of his book *De humani corporis fabrica* to Emperor Charles V, Andreas Vesalius had indeed claimed that we can know the inner man through anatomy ("et nosmetipsos denique [quod vere hominis est] cognoscimus"). Vesalius had also coupled his structural studies with aesthetic strategies (illustrators of his human atlas were artists from Titian's studio in Venice) meant to assuage the cultural fear that by "seeing" deep below one's flesh the anatomist strives for the knowledge that only God should have.

This book has delved into the life of an iconic early modern figure not to demythologize him through a voyeuristic look into his physical problems, nor to find a private persona by examining his most personal documents. Rather, it has aimed at exploring pertinent, often fascinating, preoccupations of the medical culture of the late sixteenth and early seventeenth centuries regarding function and meaning—a culture that privileged empiric observation but was still mired in Galenic humor-driven guidelines and often felt uneasy about violating taboos associated with cutting into the body and piercing the skin. As a man of means with an aesthetic bent, the attention-grabbing Vincenzo would perhaps not have been against remedial procedures that could have better aligned his private self with the medical technologies of his time, allowing him to project the public identity of a healthy, vigorous statesman. But an engineered body made through demisurgery was hardly his predisposition, and more to the point, such a possibility was not in the realm of medical undertakings in an era when only emergency medicine was practicable. What this book shows is that the stories that Vincenzo's body unwraps tell us something about the successes and limitations of the technologies of health care at a time when affluent patients demanded assistance for their afflictions when a cure, perhaps a panacean one, was rumored to exist somewhere or somehow, and legal medicine was routinely called on to assist in canon regulations.

In the end, no matter the archival resources that have moved this study along and the popularity through the centuries of its main character—Vincenzo has turned into a sort of pop-cultural totem of his era—we are left with the mysteries of a duke who both flamboyantly played on his legend while alive and took great pains to hide his body at death from the malevolent scrutiny of future generations. Or even from a benevolent scrutiny, as in this reading. Vincenzo's tomb has yet to be discovered, and thus with no autopsy, paleopathological examination, genetic analysis, radiocarbon testing, or computer tomography scan, we cannot know for certain the extent of his afflictions, and we are left speculating on his health and his illnesses: "forse che sì forse che no."

Lying on what turned out to be his deathbed at the dusk of his life, Vincenzo experienced a few hours of relief from his ailments. Rejoiced, the doctors allowed him to be fed and ordered wine. Thanking God for the seemingly happy outcome, he asked to be clothed in the shabby penitentiary garments of the Franciscan order. Perhaps he had escaped the grim reaper one more time, this energetic survivor must have hoped as he humbled himself before the cross.[5] He instructed his servants to distribute 2,000 scudi to the city's poor, although the order had to be soon rescinded because, forward-thinking as usual, Vincenzo felt he needed the money for his upcoming trip to Germany.[6] But then the fever returned, and the end came: "As he sighed for the third time the most sweet name of Jesus, his soul expired toward the second hour in the night of February 18. His cadaver was embalmed . . . and with this funeral accompaniment he was transferred to the church of St. Andrea."[7] Here a catafalque was constructed for the purpose of having the casket lie in state for the ceremonial memorial, a superbly staged event for which Francesco Gonzaga, the new *Dux Mantuae*, leaving aside any restraint, spent the sum of 50,000 scudi.[8]

Embalming the body of a prince meant evisceration as well as removal of the blood before filling the cavities with vegetable material, such as rosemary, sage, foxtail, wormwood, myrtle, mint, and thyme.[9] Embalming required one final change of clothing for Vincenzo, as his friar's tunic was exchanged for the sumptuous mantle and crown of the Duke of Mantua. The lowly and decaying body of the dead man thus metamorphosed into the body of the prince, as inscribed in the register obituary: "Serenissimus Vincentius Gonzaga Dei Gratia Optimus Dux Mantuae Quartus, Monferratus Secundus." Whereas as a man Vincenzo was wide open to disease and decay, as a ruler it was another story, for "the Majesty of God appears in the Prince externally, for the utility of the subjects," as the legist Pierre Gregoire wrote in those very years.[10] In the end Vincenzo may have proven that in screening through flamboyance his masculine vulnerabilities and flaws, he deftly navigated not only the art of living well—going always forward and never left or right, just like Theseus—but also the art of dying well. His remains, placed "forse che sì forse che no" in the church of St. Andrea, have stayed concealed—400 years now and counting—from the scrutiny of all inquiring minds, "for Jesus sake," just as Shakespeare had intimated on his grave in the Holy Trinity Church of Stratford-upon-Avon:

> Good friend for Jesus sake forbear
> To dig the dust enclosed here!
> Blest be the man that spares these stones,
> And curst be he that moves my bones.

NOTES

SELECTED BIBLIOGRAPHY

ACKNOWLEDGMENTS

INDEX

Notes

Introduction

1. Eleonora de' Medici Gonzaga died on September 9, 1611.
2. "Quod quidem cadaver sepeliatur et sepeliri voluit et mandavit, non quidem ut moris est, iacendo sed sedendo cum suo ense apposito super chatedra marmorea ad hoc parata nullo autem modo in arca lignea includetur et reponetur, in camerino in quo iacet corpus Ser. me D. D. Eleonorae Ducisse Mantue, eius coniugis dilectissimae." The will is in Archivio di Stato di Mantova (hereafter ASM), Archivio Gonzaga (hereafter AG), busta 330, fols. 297r–298r. Unless otherwise indicated, all translations from Latin and Italian here and throughout are mine. Vincenzo also asked that the crypt be enlarged, that marble also be used on the walls, and that the remains of earlier Gonzaga princes be transferred there.
3. On the sacrality of the body of the prince, see Giovanni Ricci, *Il principe e la morte: Corpo, cuore, effigie nel Rinascimento* (Bologna: Il Mulino, 1998); and the classic study of Ernst H. Kantorowicz, *The Prince's Two Bodies: A Study in Mediaeval Political Theology* (Princeton: Princeton University Press, 1957).
4. The crypt was hidden behind the inconspicuous grave marker of a Gonzaga counselor, Gregorio Carbonelli, who died in 1624, and came to light as a new heating system was being put in place. Tombstones give the names of the buried, including that of the child Guglielmo Lungaspada (1589–1591), presumed to be buried until now in the Church of Sant'Andrea. See *La Repubblica*, December 4, 2007.
5. The burial chambers were sacked in the Napoleonic era; in one instance the year 1740 had been chalked on a wall. See *La Repubblica*, December 4, 2007.
6. According to the lore, Charlemagne too was buried sitting on a throne. When his tomb was opened by Emperor Otto III, one source, Thietmar of Merseburg, stated that Charlemagne's corpse "haec in solio inventa sunt

region." There has been much discussion among medievalists as to whether this could be translated as "royal throne" or not. The idea of burial in a sitting position is further fueled by another, although less trustworthy, account, given by Ademar of Chabannes: "Et peracto triduano jejunio, inventus est eo loco quem per visum cognoverat imperator, sedens in aurea cathedra intra arcuatam speluncam infra basilicam Marie, coronatum corona ex auro et gemmis, tenens sceptrum et ensem ex auro purissimo, et ipsum corpus incorruptum inventum est." See Pascale Bourgain, ed., *Ademari Cabannensis Chronicon*, Corpus Christianorum Continuatio Mediaevalis 129 (Brepols: Turnhout, 1999), 153–154. I would like to thank Romedio Schmitz-Esser for this reference. For some reflections on Vincenzo's desire to sit, at least when dead, on the throne he always wanted in his lifetime but was unable to get, see Giancarlo Malacarne, "Il trono di pietra," in his *La luna rotta: Racconti mantovani* (Mantua: Rossi, 1997), 143–151.

7. Vincenzo sent a couple of ambassadors to Ragusa (now Dubrovnik, Croatia) to check the feasibility of the whole Albanian enterprise, but it was soon understood that the offer was a ruse, and the idea was shelved. See Giuseppe Coniglio, *I Gonzaga* (Milan: Dall'Oglio, 1967), 392–393. Actually the Gonzaga line could make some (feeble but legal) claim to Byzantium too, since the Paleologus line, descended from one of their female ancestors, had the right to the crown of Byzantium if the area were to be freed from Ottoman domination.

8. Bernardino Ramazzini, *La salute dei principi ovvero come difendersi dalle malattie e dai medici*, ed. Francesco Carnevale (Florence: Tosca, 1992), 25.

9. Edmund Plowden (1518–1585), *The Commentaries or Reports* (London: S. Brooke, 1816), cited in Kantorowicz, *The King's Two Bodies*, 7.

10. Plowden, *The Commentaries*, in Kantorowicz, *The King's Two Bodies*, 7.

11. On this social and anthropological aspect of medicine, see Gianna Pomata, *Contracting a Cure: Patients, Healers, and the Law in Early Modern Bologna* (Baltimore: Johns Hopkins University Press, 1998); Roy Porter, ed., *Patients and Practitioners: Lay Perspectives of Medicine in Pre-industrial Society* (Cambridge: Cambridge University Press, 1985); and Roy Porter, "The Patient's View: Doing Medical History from Below," *Theory and Society* 14 (1985): 175–198.

12. Roy Porter and G. S. Rousseau, *Gout: The Patrician Malady* (New Haven: Yale University Press, 1998), 2. In using the word "pathological," I am of course aware that there are disputes as to whether aging and sexuality could be viewed as pathological states.

13. The Gonzaga studied also in Bologna, as in the case of Cardinal Ercole, or in Pisa, as in the case of Vincenzo's son, Cardinal (later Duke) Ferdinando. They usually did not end their university years with an official degree.

14. The greatest pandemic to hit Italy was the Great Plague that swept through Europe in the fourteenth century, hitting most places in the peninsula in 1348–1350. Almost as deadly was the plague of 1575–1577, which greatly reduced the population of cities like Venice, where 50,000 people died. The plague of 1629–1631, also called by many "the plague of Milan," killed about one million people in northern and central Italy and slowly progressed in the following years through the South to kill an additional one million. Material on Italian plagues is extensive. For the seventeenth century, see Carlo Cipolla, *Fighting the Plague in Seventeenth Century Italy* (Madison: University of Wisconsin Press, 1981).
15. Today these abscesses do not require surgery. They are first drained and then treated with antibiotics. See Y. T. Lee et al., "Psoas Abscess: A 10 Year Review," *Journal of Microbiology, Immunology and Infection* 31.1 (1999): 40. No such knowledge was available at the time. Bone tuberculosis is not considered contagious, and once diagnosed, it can be easily treated at home.
16. Not that Leonora's pious leanings mattered: the Gonzaga/Habsburg marriage was a political one. Still, the couple's pious inclinations were recorded by contemporary observers. The judgment of historians regarding Guglielmo Gonzaga's ability to run the Mantuan duchy varies: for some he should be praised because he left the state's finances healthy; as a lover of music he fostered important musical innovations. For others he should be judged negatively, since out of unbridled ambition he cunningly recurred to skirmishes with his subjects, especially at Casale, in the newly acquired land of Monferrato, and imposed excessive taxation that made him despised. For Coniglio, Guglielmo was an unredeeming miser and a sanctimonious ruler (*I Gonzaga*, 337).
17. "Sperando che questo mio procedure humile et obediente dovesse trovare nell'animo di S. A. qualche recognizione delli molti torti che da lei [Guglielmo] mi sono fatti, così nel trattarmi in tutte le mia ationi da putto, ancorché mi ritrovi 19 anni come ella sa meglio di me, età che in tutti gli altri suol apportare libertà e credito, come nel negarmi quello che le genti basse non che pari nostri sogliono concedere a suoi figlioli il vivere et vestire." Letter of September 13, 1580, in G. B. Intra, "Una pagina della giovinezza del principe Vincenzo Gonzaga," *Archivio storico italiano* 18 (1886): 197–230, at 205.
18. "Ho detto che se non viene preso qualche partito dalla prudenza del S.r Duca alle cose di questo figliolo . . . dubito un giorno di peggio, poiché vive una vita così fatta, et sia detto con ogni riverenza et humilità, . . . è pubblica opinione, et qui et fuori che si lasci occupare troppo il S. Prin. in quello che non si deve, et niente in quello che si doveria." Letter of July 5, 1582, to the ducal counselor, Aurelio Zibramonti, now in Intra, "Una pagina della giovinezza del principe Vincenzo Gonzaga," 219. A few years

later, on May 10, 1587, Vincenzo killed again, perhaps in a brawl determined by jealousy over a love affair. The victim was a church organist, Rogero Detroffeis. Here too it is unclear who did what, but in any case the two Gonzaga courtiers accompanying Vincenzo the night of the melee fled to Bologna. Later they had to return to Mantua to be put on trial. See Coniglio, *I Gonzaga*, 355.

19. Ferdinando had one illegitimate son, Giacinto, born from his morganatic marriage (later deemed unlawful) to Camilla Faà (1599–1662). The son was never legitimized and died in the pandemic of 1629–1631. See Valeria Finucci, "Re-membering the 'I': Faà Gonzaga's *Storia* (1622)," *Italian Quarterly* 28 (1987): 21–32.

20. We also know of another child who died at birth and of a miscarriage, as Vincenzo informs his wife's uncle, Ferdinando de' Medici: "Dopo il ritorno nostro da Vinegia et da Ferrara . . . si è sentita la S.ra Duchessa travagliata da un poco di febre . . . hieri le sono sopragionti dolori, nella terminatione de' quali la notte passata Sua Alt.a, la quale doveva esser nel quarto mese della gravidanza ha disperso una creatura." Letter of July 18, 1596, in Archivio di Stato di Firenze (hereafter ASF), Mediceo del Principato (hereafter MDP) 2942, DocID 4968.

21. "Poiché a casa non posso acquistare né honore né riputatione ma piuttosto perdere di continuo, ho risoluto di andar in luogo dove me ne possi acquistare colla persona mia." Letter of Vincenzo to Aurelio Zibramonti, February 28, 1587, in Intra, "Una pagina della giovinezza del principe Vincenzo Gonzaga," 227.

22. A full account of the lavish coronation ceremony is in Federico Amadei, *Cronaca universale della città di Mantova* (Mantua: CITEM, 1953), 3:7–17. The full regalia as described by Amadei was also painted by Johan Bahuet. His work has been recently identified (1999) and is now in Bath, England.

23. Torquato Tasso, "Canzone 10," in *Scelta di poesie liriche dal primo secolo della lingua al Novecento* (Florence: Le Monnier, 1839), 574.

24. "Per l'imprestito fatto al re di Spagna [Philip II] con tanta prontezza e liberalità, possede ottimamente la grazia sua, onde che . . . si può permettere il signor duca ogni onesta dimanda." In Arnaldo Segarizzi, ed., *Relazioni degli ambasciatori veneti al Senato*, vol. 1 (Bari: Laterza, 1912), 84. Vincenzo also received the "stocco benedetto" from Pope Sixtus V in 1588.

25. According to the Venetian ambassador Giovanni da Mulla, "il duca Vincenzo non solo alienò in vita sua una grande quantità di beni, ma spendeva in tutte le cose tanto profusamente che non è da maravigliarsene. Oltre che la costruzione della cittadella di Casale gli costò tanto, che sarebbe stata spesa grandissima anco per un re di Spagna, affermando alcuni che gli costasse un million d'oro; onde si può attribuire in gran parte a questo particolare ancora la causa de' debiti che lasciò." In Segarizzi, ed., *Relazioni degli ambasciatori veneti al Senato*, 1:134. The fortress, which

occupied a polygonal perimeter and was defended by a moat outside, effectively checked invasions for a number of years. It was put under siege when the war of succession began in 1628, following the death of Vincenzo II Gonzaga.

26. Letter of October 28, 1608, to the ducal secretary, Annibale Chieppio, in Peter Paul Rubens (1577–1640), *Correspondance de Rubens et documents épistolaires concernant sa vie et ses oeuvres*, vol. 1 (Anvers: Veuve de Backer, 1887).

27. For an inventory, see Raffaella Morselli, *L'elenco dei beni del 1626–27* (Milan: Silvana Editoriale, 2000). See also Alessandro Luzio, *La Galleria dei Gonzaga venduta all'Inghilterra nel 1627-28: Documenti degli archivi di Mantova e Londra raccolti ed illustrati* (Milan: Cogliati, 1913).

28. Gazetteers eagerly documented some of Vincenzo's expenses as in this "Avviso" of June 13, 1590, from Milan: "Il Ser . . . mo di Mantova [Vincenzo] hiersera arrivò qui in Milano, et hoggi se n'è andato per Milano a spasso per li orefici, et altri luoghi, dove ha speso molti scuti in gioie et vasi di cristallo per bevere." In ASF, MDP 3255, DocID 11140.

29. On the wide net of intercontinental communication that the Gonzaga court had established to feed Vincenzo's "omnivorous collecting," see Michaela Sermidi, "Vanità, lusso, arte e scienza: Il collezionismo onnivoro di Vincenzo I Gonzaga a Venezia," in *Le collezioni Gonzaga: Il carteggio tra Venezia e Mantova (1588–1612)*, ed. Michaela Sermidi (Milan: Silvana Editoriale, 2003), 13–72, esp. 26. In his trip to Spa, Belgium, in 1599, for example, Vincenzo acquired not only precious local artifacts but also a variety of relics, such as the head of St. Bona, two heads of St. Maurice's companions, eighteen heads of holy virgins of the order of St. Ursula, and sixteen arms of various saints, all of which, together with other relics given to him, he donated later that year to the ducal church of St. Barbara. See Amadei, *Cronaca universale della città di Mantova*, 3:181.

30. For a sense of Vincenzo's drive in selecting the most intriguing material, see Roberta Piccinelli, "Le *facies* del collezionismo artistico di Vincenzo Gonzaga," in *Gonzaga, la Celeste Galeria: L'esercizio del Collezionismo*, ed. Raffaella Morselli (Milan: Skira, 2002), 341–347. Illustrations of many works of art belonging to the Gonzaga are now in a splendid book edited by Raffaella Morselli, *Gonzaga, la Celeste Galeria: Le raccolte* (Milan: Skira, 2002), which gives a sense of what level of refinement was being displayed in the Mantuan court at the start of the seventeenth century.

31. Plenty has been written on the beginning of opera in Mantua. See, for example, Tim Carter, *Monteverdi's Musical Theatre* (New Haven: Yale University Press, 2002); and Nino Pirrotta, *Music and Culture in Italy from the Middle Ages to the Baroque* (Cambridge: Harvard University Press, 1984).

32. For a list of female singers and instrumentalists he employed at court (playing lute, Spanish guitar, trombone, and lyre), see Don Harrán, "Madama Europa, Jewish Singer in Late Renaissance Mantua," in *Festa Musicologica:*

Essays in Honor of George J. Buelow, ed. Thomas Mathiesen and Benito Rivera (Stuyvesant: Pendragon Press, 1995), 197–230, at 225. More generally, see Alessandro Ademollo, *La bell'Adriana ed altre virtuose del suo tempo alla corte di Mantova: Contributo di documenti per la storia della musica in Italia nel primo quarto del Seicento* (Città di Castello: Lapi, 1888).

33. Don Harrán, *Salamone Rossi: Jewish Musician in Late Renaissance Mantua* (Oxford: Oxford University Press, 2003).

34. On Vincenzo's repeated attempts to stage Guarini's play, see Iain Fenlon, "Vincenzo Gonzaga and the New Arts of Spectacle" in *Music and Patronage in Sixteenth-Century Mantua* (Cambridge: Cambridge University Press, 1980), 1:119–161; and Alessandro D'Ancona, *Origini del teatro italiano* (Turin: Loescher, 1891), 2:535–575. For a contemporary account, see Ferrante Persia, *Relatione de' ricevimenti fatti in Mantova alla Maesta della Regina di Spagna Dal Sereniss. Sig. Duca, Anno MDXCVIII del Mese di Novembre* (Ferrara: Baldini, 1598). On Vincenzo as illuminated patron, see Anne MacNeil, "The Nature of Commitment: Vincenzo Gonzaga's Patronage Strategies in the Wake of the Fall of Ferrara," *Renaissance Quarterly* 16.3 (2002): 392–403.

35. On Commedia dell'arte and its many ties to the Gonzaga court, see Robert Henke, *Performance and Literature in the Commedia dell'Arte* (Cambridge: Cambridge University Press, 2002); Ferdinando Taviani and Mirella Schino, *Il segreto della Commedia dell'Arte: La memoria delle compagnie italiane del XVI, XVII, e XVIII secolo* (Florence: Usher, 1986); and Ferruccio Marotti and Giovanna Romei, eds., *La commedia dell'arte e la società barocca: La professione del teatro* (Rome: Bulzoni, 1991).

36. "Eseguiva spesso delle pantomime, ballava, cantava e recitava in maschera sul palcoscenico," in Kate Simon, *I Gonzaga: Storia e segreti* (Rome: Newton-Compton, 1990), 262. On court performances in Mantua by commedia dell'arte troupes, see the excellent study of Claudia Burattelli, *Spettacoli di corte a Mantova tra Cinque e Seicento* (Florence: Le Lettere, 1999).

37. For a thorough study of this new, short-lived university (it ceased to exist after the sack of Mantua), see Paul Grendler, *The University of Mantua, the Gonzaga and the Jesuits* (Baltimore: Johns Hopkins University Press, 2009).

38. See Antonio Favaro, *Galileo Galilei e lo studio di Padova* (Florence: Le Monnier, 1966), 1:158, 177; and Mario Biagioli, "Galileo's System of Patronage," *History of Science* 28 (1990): 1–61.

39. Among historians defending Vincenzo, see Coniglio, *I Gonzaga;* Riccardo Braglia, *I Gonzaga: Il mito, la storia* (Cerese di Virgilio: Rossi, 2002); Giancarlo Malacarne, *Splendore e declino: da Vincenzo I a Vincenzo II (1587–1627),* vol. 4 of *I Gonzaga di Mantova: Una stirpe per una capitale europea* (Modena: Il Bulino, 2007); and Maria Bellonci, *Segreti dei Gonzaga* (Milan: Mondadori, 1947), a remarkable, historically accurate, and sensibly written best seller centered on Vincenzo's psychology. A balanced historical assessment of Vin-

cenzo's strengths and weaknesses is in Cesare Mozzarelli, *Mantova e i Gonzaga dal 1382 al 1707* (Turin: UTET, 1987).

40. "Con gran ragione si può dire essere verissimo il detto del signor granduca di Toscana: che la gioventù del signor duca sia lunga, poiché non intermette ora niuno delli gusti e piaceri che pigliava nelli suoi primi anni. È principe di spirito grande, di generosi pensieri e così largo nello spendere che sempre si trova in bisogni e necessità; affabile, benigno e clemente con suoi sudditi, gli animi de' quali si ha conciliati talmente con questa umanità che, se bene alcuna volta li aggrava più dell'ordinario sopportano il tutto volentieri per il particolare amore che gli portano." In Segarizzi, ed., *Relazione degli ambasciatori veneti al Senato,* 1:91.

41. See Bellonci, *Segreti dei Gonzaga,* 162. Vincenzo also established a new Monte di Pietà in 1596, provided for the construction of a dyke for the river Mincio in 1610, and earlier funded a new mill bridge. See Pompeo Litta, *Celebri famiglie italiane* (Milan: Giusti, 1919–1985), vol. 3.

42. "La seguente settimana se le manderà il vasettino dell'unguento ch'ella disidera per il mal caduco, facendone fare di presente il S.r Duca mio per esser finito quello che v'era di fatto, distribuendone ogni dì per la continova richiesta che ne vien fatta a S. A." Letter of Elenora de' Medici to Belisario Vinta in Florence, April 4, 1608, in ASF, MDP 2944, DocID 5097.

43. For example, he asked his father-in-law, Francesco de' Medici, to send a remedy for breast cancer for an unnamed noblewoman: "Una Gentildonna amica mia d'età d'anni cinquanta ha un cancaro ulcerato in una Popa. Se V. A. havesse qualche rimedio per questo male, mi farebbe grazia a mandarlomi." Letter of December 14, 1585, in ASF, MDP 2940, DocID 4566.

44. See Ippolito Donesmondi, *Dell'historia ecclesiastica di Mantova* (Bologna: Forni, 1977), 1:471–472.

45. The Jewish population in Mantua amounted at the time to circa 3,000 people. They had traditionally been treated well, to the point that Jewish merchants were satirized as untouchable and fully enjoying the protection of a Gonzaga duke in Pietro Aretino's play *Il Marescalco* (1539). Indeed, in 1545 Vincenzo's grandfather, Federico II, had issued a decree of full integration. Although he approved the institution of the ghetto, Vincenzo did not ask for any recognizable and distinguishable sign to be worn by the Jewish population. He commissioned a comedy from Leon Ebreo to be performed for his first wedding (see letter by Revere, a court functionary, to Ebreo in ASM, AG, busta 2210). The "Università degli ebrei" also performed a play for his second wedding, *Gli ingiusti sdegni,* on May 2, 1584. Masked at Carnival time, he joined in Jewish evening entertainments as when he went to "the house of Isachino," a dancing master, to hear a boy soprano (see letter of Cesare Andreasi to Guidobono Guidoboni of January 15, 1594, in ASM, AG, busta 2665). Yet the first act of his son, Francesco, when he became duke was to ask the Jews to add a

three-inch yellow ribbon to their hats. Francesco originally wanted the Jews to wear a yellow hat, as it was customary in other parts of Italy, but then changed his mind. See Donesmondi, *Dell'Historia ecclesiastica di Mantova*, 1:474. For a more in-depth study of the local Jewish population, see Shlomo Simonsohn, *History of the Jews in the Duchy of Mantua* (Jerusalem: Kiryath Sepher, 1977).

46. "Mostrare al mondo che voglio vivere et morire soldato come hanno fatto li miei antecessori." Letter of February 28, 1587, to Aurelio Zibramonti, in Intra, "Una pagina della giovinezza del principe Vincenzo Gonzaga," 227.

47. Vincenzo's apartment in the Gonzaga palace, which he occupied until he became duke, was appropriately named "del Tasso."

48. This comment is in ASM, AG, busta 1091; cited in *Mantova: La storia, le lettere, le arti,* ed. Leonardo Mazzoldi, Renato Giusti, and Rinaldo Salvatori, 9 vols. (Mantua: Istituto Carlo d'Arco per la Storia di Mantova, 1963), 3:82.

49. The letters are in ASM, AG, buste 2699, 2702.

50. Vincenzo's last will had provisions for three out-of-wedlock children: Silvio, Francesco, and a daughter named Caterina, who had taken vows as Anna Eleonora. Another illegitimate child, Giovanni, was conceived just before Vincenzo's death in 1612. He died in Paris in 1679. See ASF, MDP Person ID 9335. True to Vincenzo's starring relationships with the opposite sex, in Henry Reed's 1955 radio play *Vincenzo,* broadcast on BBC's Third Programme, a good example of radio literature, Vincenzo's Casanova-style life is narrated directly by his wives (the first and the second) and mistresses in what has been called a "choric narration."

51. On Martinelli, see Edmond Strainchamps, "The Life and Death of Caterina Martinelli: New Light on Monteverdi's 'Arianna,'" *Early Music History* 5 (1985): 155–186.

52. "In alcun conto non accetteremo questo obligo di promettere con voto solenne et giurato la castità coniugale, sapendo molto bene noi . . . quanto più grave si renderebbe per sì fatta circostanza il peccato in caso di trasgressione." Letter of May 27, 1608, to the Mantuan resident to the Holy Seat, Giovanni Magni, in ASM, AG, busta 2269. In the end, the pope did not sign a bull authorizing the order but simply gave a brief. For more on the correspondence, see Malacarne, *Splendore e declino,* 150–155.

53. Victor Hugo's play *Le Roi s'amuse / The Prince's Play* (1832, London: Faber and Faber, 1996) cast the king of France, Francis I, as the seducer of Blanche, the daughter of his buffoon, Thibaulet. The play was banned in France because censors saw similarities between the early modern king and the current one, Louis-Philippe. In order to have permission for the play to be staged, Hugo launched a lawsuit that made him famous as a defender of free speech. It did not help, however, because the play was banned for another fifty years.

54. Giuseppe Verdi, *Rigoletto* (New York: Riverrun Press, 1982). In writing music from Hugo's play, Verdi moved the story to a superficially identified Mantua. The opera had its premiere in complete triumph in 1851 at La Fenice opera house in Venice.
55. "We are right to note the license and disobedience of this member which thrusts itself forward so inopportunely when we do not want it to, and which so inopportunely lets us down when we most need it; it imperiously contests for authority with our will; it stubbornly and proudly refuses all our incitements, both of the mind and hand." See Michel de Montaigne (1533–1592), "On the Power of the Imagination," in *The Complete Essays,* ed. M. A. Screech (London: Penguin, 1993), 115.
56. Giambattista della Porta, *Della fisionomia dell'uomo,* ed. Mario Cicognani (Milan: Longanesi, 1971).
57. "Si ammalò nel febbraio di una febbre così acuta accompagnata da gagliardo dolore di fianco e da una sì ostinata massa di catarro, che in meno di quattro giornate già era ridotto agli estremi. Tutta la città umiliò preci pubbliche e fervorose davanti a Dio per la salute dell'ottimo suo sovrano; ed infatti si migliorò a segno tale che li medici, giudicandolo fuori pericolo, permisero a questo convalescente l'uso del vino e del suo consueto pranzo. . . . Ed ecco nuova frebbre lo assalisce, ed eccolo in breve ridotto di bel nuovo agli estremi. Egli allora . . . dispose delle temporali sue cose; poi preparossi alle eterne." In Amadei, *Cronaca universale della città di Mantova,* 3:279.
58. "Il ventiotto di genaro del corrente [1611] a hore 15 e tre quarti la Ser.ma Duchessa, stando ancora in letto fu sopraresa da un accidente apopletico . . . restò priva di moto e di senso; onde portata dal letto al fuoco ivi cominciò, interrogata, a parlar balbutiendo, e si querelava, che dal canto destro dal capo sino a' piedi si sentiva torpida con un sentimento per le sodette parti formicante. . . . Furono da principio et incontinente fatte fricationi e legature gagliarde e replicati due suppositorii, e datagli a bere acqua di cannella sallata , et appresso fricandole la radice della lingua et il palato con confettione anacardina si passò a servitiali acri e potenti . . . li si diede l'acqua di rosmarino con l'elisir vitae, come liquida teriaca, e tuttavia perseverando li sodetti accidenti, si giudicò espediente il darle un botton di fuoco nella nucha e porle i vessicatori nella parte manca . . . la notte del secondo giorno . . . le diedero . . . alcune giocciole d'oglio di cranio humano . . . due o tre cucchiari d'ossimele di miele di spagna. Appresso i sopradette rimedi si è sempre continovata . . . innanzi al cibo di rasura di corno di rinoceronte, d'unicorno, d'ossi di [proposed reading: cru] di cervo, di cranio humano, e dell'ugna dell'alce, e per due volte le si è dato un poco di sal volatile di coralli passato per lambico e fatte più volte ontioni ordinarie e straordinari alla nucha. . . . Dopo la già detta artificiale purgatione e naturale della quarta [giornata], procurassimo d'evacuar per il naso con uno sternutatorio la materia contenuta nella testa . . .

Passata la settima [giornata] habbiamo risoluto questa mattina di provocar il ventre con un servitiale . . . e per aiutare l'espulsione delle sodette escere . . . le si sono applicate parimente al dorso ventose non scarificate ma con molta fiamma, non havendo voluto l'A.S. tolerar la scarificatione." In ASF, MDP 2951, DocID 5428.

59. In his "Memorie dei quattro ultimi duchi di Mantova" (Cod. 162, Fondo D'Arco, Archivio Storico, Mantua), Lodovico Andreasi states that Vincenzo had already received the passport from the Ottomans. See Vincenzo Errante, "Forse che sì, forse che no: la terza spedizione del duca Vincenzo Gonzaga in Ungheria alla guerra contro il Turco (1601) studiata su documenti inediti," *Archivio storico lombardo* 42.1 (1915): 15–114, at 22.

1. The Virgin Cure

1. When Ottavio died, Margherita's father did not return to Parma and nominated his young son, Ranuccio (1569–1622), as the duchy's regent in his absence.
2. "Sua altezza mi ha chiamato mentre magnava et dettomi all'orrecchio che sua altezza resta soddisfattissima della signora sposa, piacendole infinitamente et amandola in estremo, in maniera che la presenza ha superato il ritratto." Letter of Zibramonti to Guglielmo, February 25, 1581, in ASM, AG, busta 1379, fol. 1, cc. 13–16.
3. Information on the sumptuous nuptial banquet was later recorded by Fusorito Reale da Narni in "Convito nuziale alla corte dei Gonzaga (Banchetto reale nelle nozze dell'Ecc.mo signor Principe di Mantova, et ora Duca di Mantova, l'anno 1581 del mese di maggio)," in Vincenzo Cervio, *Il trinciante* (Rome: Nella stampa del Gabbia, 1593), 88–93.
4. "Entrata chi fu l'Altezza sua in litto, mentre stava aspittando il Signor Principi suo, chiamò la signora Bianca . . . et li dissi chi ringratiava infinitamente il Signor Iddio, qual dopo l'haverli conciso un marito tanto grandi, et tanto a gusto suo." Letter of Cesare Cavriani, master of dance at the Gonzaga court, to the Duke of Mantua, April 3, 1581, in ASM, AG, busta 201, fol. 45.
5. "Married folk have time at their disposal: if they are not ready, they should not try to rush things. Rather than fall into perpetual wretchedness by being struck with despair at a first rejection, it is better to fail to make it properly on the marriage-couch, full as it is of feverish agitation, and to wait for an opportune moment, more private and less challenging. Before possessing his wife, a man who suffers a rejection should make gentle assays and overtures with various little sallies; he should not stubbornly persist in proving himself inadequate once and for all." In Michel de Montaigne, "On the Power of the Imagination," in *The Complete Essays*, trans. M. A. Screech (London: Penguin, 1993), 114–115.

6. Since history uncannily repeats itself, it pays to point out that Ottavio's own marriage to Margaret, contracted when both bride and groom were adolescents (he was thirteen and she was sixteen and already a widow), remained unconsummated for a good number of years, no matter the pressures at court. See the relative documents of May 13, 1540, in ASF, MDP 3263, DocID 19030.
7. "Insomma il membro del maschio è più grosso di quello che possa comportare la natura della femmina che è picciola fuor di l'ordinario, per quanto ne dice il Sig.r Principe . . . né ancor le é fiorito Maggio." Letter of March 11, 1581, in ASM, AG, busta 1379, now in Attilio Zanca, *Notizie sulla vita e sulle opere di Marcello Donati da Mantova (1538–1602), medico, umanista, uomo di stato* (Pisa: Tip. Editrice Giardini, 1964), 14.
8. I use the terms "vaginal" and "vagina" to properly refer to this female anatomical part, conscious of the fact that we have to wait until much later—that is, 1775, according to a historical dictionary of sexual terminology—for the terms to enter the Italian language. See Valter Boggione and Giovanni Casalegno, *Dizionario storico del lessico erotico italiano* (Milan: Longanesi, 1996), 212.
9. "Se bene sono molte le cagioni che possono impedire la donna a vicinarsi il membro dell'huomo, non dimeno io, lasciate l'altre, mi restringerò a quella che nel caso nostro con la fede dell'occhio è stata giudicata propria et particolare cioè che sia una escrescenzia di carne; questa Signor mio è necessaria che sia levata perché essendo forata concludono tutti i nostri dottori che in tutto et impedisca l'entrata del membro dell'huomo." Letter of March 15, 1581, to the ducal counselor, Zibramonti, in ASM, AG, busta 1379, now in Zanca, *Notizie sulla vita*, 15.
10. The letters by Zibramonti relative to these manual interventions are of March 10, 1581, and March 25, 1581, in ASG, AG, busta 1379, fol. 97r and fol. 135r–v.
11. Mozart's *Così fan tutte* was first performed in Vienna in 1790; the libretto was by Lorenzo Da Ponte.
12. John Chrysostom, *On Virginity, Against Remarriage*, trans. Sally Reiger Shore, with an introduction by Elizabeth A. Clark (Lewiston: Mellen Press, 1983), V. I. See also Ambrose, *De institutione virginis*, in *Verginità e vedovanza*, ed. Franco Gori, 2 vols. (Rome-Milan: Città nuova editrice, 1989), 2; and, more generally, Elizabeth Clark, "Sex, Shame and Rhetoric: En-gendering Early Christian Ethics," *Journal of the American Academy of Religion* 59.2 (1991): 221–245. On the pervasive cultural need to keep the female body enclosed in order to preserve bodily purity, see Peter Stallybrass, "Patriarchal Territory: The Body Enclosed," in *Rewriting the Renaissance: The Discourses of Sexual Difference in Early Modern Europe*, ed. Margaret Ferguson, Maureen Quilligan, and Nancy J. Vickers (Chicago: University of Chicago Press, 1986), 123–142.

13. Giambattista della Porta (1535?–1615), *Magiae naturalis* (Palermo: Il Vespro, 1979), 115.
14. See Helen Lemay, "Human Sexuality in Twelfth- through Fifteenth-Century Scientific Writings," in *Sexual Practices and the Medieval Church*, ed. Vern Bullough and James Brundage (Buffalo: Prometheus Books, 1982), 187–205, at 195; and Valeria Finucci, *The Manly Masquerade: Masculinity, Paternity, and Castration in the Italian Renaissance* (Durham: Duke University Press, 2003), 86–87.
15. See Michael Stolberg, "The Decline of Uroscopy in Early Modern Learned Medicine, 1500–1650," *Early Science and Medicine* 12 (2007): 313–336.
16. Giulio Mancini (1558–1630), the personal physician of Pope Urban VIII, was a Galenist and an art collector. His book, *Della sanità*, is still in manuscript at the Biblioteca Apostolica Vaticana, Barb. Lat. 4315.
17. Laurent Joubert, *Popular Errors*, trans. Gregory David de Rocher (Tuscaloosa: University of Alabama Press, 1989), 210, 211. Joubert (1529–1583) was well known in Italy as Lorenzo Gioberti.
18. On the easiness with which sexual pleasure could be simulated, see Marjorie Garber, "The Insincerity of Women," in *Desire in the Renaissance: Psychoanalysis and Literature*, ed. Valeria Finucci and Regina Schwartz (Princeton: Princeton University Press, 1994), 19–38.
19. Monica Green, "The Development of the *Trotula*," in *Revue d'Histoire des Textes* 26 (1996): 118–203, at 195.
20. "Delle furbe donne che corrugano il collo della matrice con astringenti, di poi con un mezzo fraudolento fingono emettere del sangue, per apparire inviolate ai babbei." In Jacopo Berengario da Carpi (ca. 1480–ca. 1530), *Carpi commentaria cum amplissimis additionibus super Anatomia Mundini*. Cited in Felice La Torre, *L'utero attraverso i secoli: da Erofilo ai giorni nostri* (Città di Castello: Unione Arti Grafiche, 1917), 189.
21. "Fare devenir strettissima per modo che ogne persona che experta che sia altramente che vergine non la reputarà quella cosa che tra noi donne cusì ce tenemo nominare id est la natura." In Caterina Sforza (1463?–1509), *Experimenti de la Ex.ma S.ra Caterina da Furlj matre de lo Inllux.mo Signor Giovanni de Medici* (Imola: Tip. d'Ignazio Galeati, 1894), 71.
22. In Helen Lemay, "William of Saliceto on Human Sexuality," *Viator* 12 (1981): 165–181, at 176.
23. Such concerns seem to have increased from the Middle Ages on, according to Joan Cadden, *Meanings of Sex Difference in the Middle Ages: Medicine, Science, and Culture* (Cambridge: Cambridge University Press, 1993), 260–265. Yet they have not totally disappeared. A Chinese online retailer, Gigimo, has, for example, just put on the market a fake-blood-squirting hymen, with an eye to the Middle East conservative community. It costs approximately $40 and works exactly as the medieval techniques described in the text: "A small plastic insert adheres to the sides of a woman's cervix. During sex, the pouch is punctured, releasing a red liquid

('not too much but just the right amount,' according to the website). The site also offers some free advice: A woman should add 'a few moans and groans' to make her case more believable to her partner. What happens to the fake hymen after the deed? It will simply 'melt inside the vagina,' the site says." In *Marie Claire,* January 20, 2010.

24. Albertus Magnus (1206?–1280), *De animalibus libri 26* (Munster: Aschendorff, 1916–1922), ch. 24, 164. See also Danielle Jacquart and Claude Thomasset, *Sexuality and Medicine in the Middle Ages* (Princeton: Princeton University Press, 1988), 44.

25. "Le piccole labbra, per il freddo, e più all'interno, all'altezza della cervice, un velo sottile." In Mondino de' Luzzi (1275–1326), *Anatomia* (1316), cited in La Torre, *L'utero,* 171.

26. Michele Savonarola (1385?–1466?), *Practica major* (Venice: Giunta, 1547), ch. 21. See also Jacquart and Thomasset, *Sexuality and Medicine,* 44. For the etymology of the word, see Kathleen Coyne Kelly, *Performing Virginity and Testing Chastity in the Middle Ages* (New York: Routledge, 2000), 150, n. 67.

27. Cynthia Klestinec, *Theaters of Anatomy: Students, Teachers, and Traditions of Dissection in Renaissance Venice* (Baltimore: Johns Hopkins University Press, 2011); and Klestinec, "Medical Education in Padua: Students, Faculty and Facilities," in *Centres of Medical Excellence? Medical Travel and Education in Europe, 1500–1789,* ed. Ole Peter Grell, Andrew Cunningham, and Jon Arrizabalaga (Aldershot: Ashgate, 2010), 193–210.

28. Andreas Vesalius (1514–1564), *Epistola rationem modumque propinandi radicis Chynae decocti* [Letter on the China root] (Brussels: Oporini, 1546): "In the presence of a few students I examined the uterus of the girl since I expected her to be a virgin because very likely no one had ever wanted her. I found a hymen in her as well as in the nun, at least thirty-six years old, whose ovaries, however, were shrunken as happens to organs that are not used" I cite from the English translation by Charles D. O'Malley, *Andreas Vesalius of Brussels* (Berkeley: University of California Press, 1964), 201.

29. "I had never dissected a virgin, except a child of perhaps six years, dead of a wasting disease, which I had obtained in Padua . . . from a student who had secretly removed it from a tomb." In O'Malley, *Andreas Vesalius of Brussels,* 201.

30. "I dissected the uterus solely for the sake of the hymen; although I found it just as I have seen it recently since the publication of my books, I did not dare make any definite statement about it since I had observed it to be lacking in animals, and furthermore because I am not accustomed to saying anything with certainty after only one or two observations." In O'Malley, *Andreas Vesalius of Brussels,* 201.

31. Gabriele Falloppio (1523–1562), *Observationes anatomicae,* ed. Gabriella Righi Riva and Pericle Di Pietro (Modena: Mucchi, 1964), 2:370. See also

Giulia Sissa, "La verginità materiale: Evanescenza di un soggetto," *Quaderni* storici 25 (1990): 739–756, at 751.
32. Joubert, *Popular Errors*, 217.
33. Midwives were routinely called in to digitally examine women in court cases regarding rape, fallen maids, unconsummated marriages, pregnancies, and even stopped menses. See Jacqueline Murray, "On the Origins and Role of 'Wise Women' in Causes of Annulment on the Grounds of Male Impotence," *Journal of Medieval History* 16 (1990): 235–249; Thomas Benedek, "The Changing Relationship between Midwives and Physicians during the Renaissance," *Bulletin of the History of Medicine* 51 (1977): 550–564, at 562; Monica Green, "Women's Medical Practice and Health Care in Medieval Europe," *Signs* 14 (1989): 434–473; and Silvia De Renzi, "Witnesses of the Body: Medico-Legal Cases in Seventeenth-Century Rome," *Studies in History and Philosophy of Science* 33 (2002): 219–242, esp. 229–232. More generally on the issue, see Catherine Bicks, *Midwiving Subjects in Shakespeare's England* (Aldershot: Ashgate, 2003); and Alessandro Pastore, *Il medico in tribunale: La perizia medica nella procedura penale d'antico regime* (Bellinzona: Edizioni Casagrande, 1998). By the early seventeenth century, midwives started to be put under a stricter medical control, and civic entities began requiring that they pass specific exams. By 1624, for example, midwives in Venice were asked to enroll in a corporation. See Nadia Maria Filippini, "Levatrici e ostetricanti a Venezia tra sette e ottocento," *Quaderni storici* 58 (1985): 149–180, at 152. The same happened in Bologna, where not only were women not allowed to practice as barber-surgeons but, by the second half of the seventeenth century, they could no longer "establish the loss of virginity testifying on the matter of rape and deflowering, without the advice of a licensed physician." See Gianna Pomata, *Contracting a Cure: Patients, Healers, and the Law in Early Modern Bologna* (Baltimore: Johns Hopkins University Press, 1998), 227.
34. The sentence was preceded by a similar categorical denial: "Ostenditur virgines foeminas eam non habere ex natura membranam, quam nonnulli interseptum, alii claustrum virginale, alii hymen vocant. . . . Virgines non habent aliquam corporis partem qua sint destitutae mulieres. Deinde." In Orazio Augenio (1527–1603), *Epistolarum et consultationum medicinalium alterius tomi libri XII* (Venice: Zenarium, 1592), bk.1 (dated July 6, 1587), fol.1r–v.
35. Realdo Colombo (1494–1559), *De re anatomica libri XV* (Venice: Bevilacqua, 1559). For more on Colombo, see Sissa, "La verginità materiale," 753.
36. "Dalla parte vicina alla natura della donna si veggono due pezzetti di carne, ineguali a punto come le creste dei piccioli polli, dette ninfe o imeneo, i quali mentre stanno congiunti insieme, sono segno della virginità, e quando nella congiunzione con l'uomo si rompono e separano, spesse volte con molto sangue, danno segno della virginità perduta." In Girolamo

Mercurio (Scipion Mercurii, d. 1615), *La commare o riccoglitrice* (Venice: Ciotti, 1596), 7. Cited in *Medicina per le donne nel Cinquecento. Testi di Giovanni Marinello e di Girolamo Mercurio*, ed. Maria Luisa Altieri Biagi et al. (Turin: UTET, 1992), 72–73.
37. Ambroise Paré (1510?–1590), *The Workes of That Famous Chirurgion Ambrose Parey*, trans. Thomas Johnson (London, 1638), 937–939.
38. Nicholas Culpeper (1616–1654), *A Directory for Midwives; or, A Guide for Women in Their Conception, Bearing, and Suckling Their Children* (London: Cole, 1651), 29.
39. Joubert, *Popular Errors*, 20. On the scarce physical contact between male doctor and female patient in the early modern period, see Eve Keller, "The Subject of Touch: Medical Authority in Early Modern Midwifery," in *Sensible Flesh: On Touch in Early Modern Culture*, ed. Elizabeth Harvey (Philadelphia: University of Pennsylvania Press, 2003), 62–83.
40. "Una certa Serva, la quale molti scolari tentarono di sfiorare; mà io . . . gli dissi, che quando avesse voluto maritarsi, se ne venisse da me, ch'io ce l'avrei resa abile. Non venne però, perche credo, ch'ella trovasse qualchedun altro più anatomico di me, che le ruppe l' Imeneo." I cite here and throughout from bk. 2 of the Italian translation of Girolamo Fabrici d'Acquapendente (1537–1619), *L'opere cirurgiche del signor Fabritio d'Acquapendente . . . divise in due parti. Nella prima si tratta de' tumori, ferite, vicere, rotture, e slogature. Nella seconda dell'operationi principali di cirugia* (Bologna: Stamperia del Longhi, 1709), 208. The original version, *Opera chirurgica in duas partes divisas* (Venice: Megliettum, 1619), appeared in Latin. Fabrici was well paid for his position, with a salary of 400 florins for his annual public anatomy and 200 florins for his surgery lessons. His younger rival, Giulio Casseri, soon took charge of the less prestigious surgery lessons while Fabrici performed the well-attended public anatomies, which, starting in 1594, he was able to perform in an anatomy theater, built for him within the university and still perfectly standing. See Giuseppe Sterzi, "Giulio Casserio, anatomico e chirurgo (c. 1552–1616)," *Nuovo archivio veneto*, ser. 3, 18 (1909): 207–278; 18 (1910): 25–111; and Cynthia Klestinec, "Private Anatomies and the Delights of Technical Expertise," in *Theaters of Anatomy*, 142–166.
41. Fabrici understood how blood circulates but failed to draw the correct conclusions from his reasoning. This was left to his student William Harvey (1578–1657) upon his return to England. As far as it concerns gestation and fetus, he was historically the first surgeon to correctly describe the placenta.
42. Both "tabulae anatomicae" come from *De anatomia abdominis et partium in eo contentarum*, a set of precise human and animal anatomical illustrations, never published in the past and housed at the Marciana Library, Venice. They have been recently restored and are now printed in Maurizio Rippa Bonati and José Pardo Tomás, eds., *Il teatro dei corpi: Le pitture colorate*

d'anatomia di Girolamo Fabrici d'Acquapendente (Milan: Mediamed, 2004), 331. I would like to thank Alessandro Riva for guiding me through the female anatomical sexual apparatus. Comparable figures are at 74–75 (woman with hymen) and at 209 (pregnant woman) of his *Flesh and Wax: The Clemente Susini's Anatomical Models in the University of Cagliari* (Nuoro: Ilisso Edizioni, 2007). Beside *De formato foetu,* Fabrici wrote another treatise on human and animal generation, *De formatione ovi et pulli* (Padua: Meglietti, 1621). During his many years of practice, he more than once described the anatomy of a pregnant woman. For example, in 1579 one of the three bodies he dissected belonged to a woman who had died during delivery, in 1586 he was able to show what the uterus and placenta of a pregnant woman look like, and in 1592 he examined the anatomy of a fetus. Thanks to his fame and his connections, Fabrici was also able in 1584 to raise the status of anatomy in Padua to that of "ordinary professorship" (lettura ordinaria) in an attempt to make the subject as important as theoretical medicine.

43. "Finalmente, essendo ella già vicina alla morte, v'andai, e con gli occhi propri, avendo veduto il male, con un semplice taglio, divisi la membrana, e subitamente essendo uscita gran quantità di sangue grossissimo, vischioso, rugginoso, e fetente, quasi per miracolo, rimase un tempo liberata da tutti i mali. . . . Questa adunque è la chirurgia, che sicurissimamente, e con felicissimo successo adoprai in quella vergine, e nell'imeneo non forato." In Fabrici d'Acquapendente, *L'opere cirurgiche,* 208–209. Abdominal back pain and difficulty with bowel movement are often the result of menstrual blood backed up into the vagina and the abdomen.

44. The information on the date is in a letter by Giambattista Pico, the bishop of Osimo, of April 3, 1581. In ASM, AG, busta 1379, fol. 228.

45. "Quella membrana chiamata himen che si trova in tutte le vergini che in questa è carnosa più dell'ordinario et che anco la natura è piccola per la poca età." In Zanca, *Notizie sulla vita,* 16. To be precise, Margherita was thirteen years and five and a half months old when she got married.

46. Letters of Zibramonti to Duke Guglielmo regarding Aranzi's (1530–1589) visit are of April 9 and April 20, 1581. See ASM, AG, busta 1379, fols. 148r–150v and 152r–153r. Aranzi's studies on generation made him a natural choice for such a consult. In the *De humano foetu libellus* (Bologna: Ioannis Rubii ad insigne Mercurii, 1564), Aranzi was the first anatomist to describe the deformed pelvis. See Raffi Gurunlouglu and Aslin Gurunlouglu, "Giulio Cesare Arantius (1530–1589), a Surgeon and Anatomist: His Role in Nasal Reconstruction and Influence on Gaspare Tagliacozzi," *Annals of Plastic Surgery* 60.6 (2008): 717–722. The opinion of doctors called two years later to check Margherita's apparatus was that Aranzi's and Fabrici's original intervention on the princess had put in motion a negative outcome: "[the doctors] vogliono che habbiano nociuti li tagli datile dall'Aranzo et Acquapendente, perché dopo la consolidazione loro

hanno reso il luogo calloso." Letter of Zibramonti from Parma, February 18, 1583, in ASM, AG, busta 201, cc. 346–347. Before leaving Parma, Aranzi sent Vincenzo a recently published historical treatise by the humanist Carlo Sigonio, *Historiorum de regno Italiae*: "Partendomi da Parma, restai con l'obligo di mandare al serenissimo signor principe l'Historie del Sigonio, de regno Italiae, le quali mando hora, doppo coteste nozze splendide e regali." Letter of May 8, 1581, to Zibramonti, in ASM, AG, busta 1161, fol. 7, cc. 350–351.

47. See letter of Aurelio Zibramonti to Duke Guglielmo, April 13, 1581, in ASM, AG, busta 1379 (1581), fols. 166r–167r.
48. For some examples of marriages annulled in Venice because they could not be consummated—usually the husband was deemed impotent—see Joanne Ferraro, *Marriage Wars in Late Renaissance Venice* (New York: Oxford University Press, 2001), 70–103. Ferraro presents the case of Lucieta Padoani, whose marriage to Giovanni Francisci was annulled in 1586 by the patriarchal court in Venice because she was "impotent," that is, impenetrable (91–97). Thirteen cases, from 1570 to 1700, are also examined in Daniela Hacke's *Women, Sex, and Marriage in Early Modern Venice* (Aldershot: Ashgate, 2004). More generally, see Angus McLaren, *Impotence: A Cultural History* (Chicago: University of Chicago Press, 2007). On marriage economics and regulations in the period, see Trevor Dean and K. J. P. Lowe, eds., *Marriage in Italy, 1300–1650* (Cambridge: Cambridge University Press, 2002).
49. "Tale che co'l membro virile se ben fosse di ferro non si potria penetrar." Letter of Cesare Pendasio, February 12, 1583, in ASM, AG, busta 1513, fol. 568v.
50. I cite from Kathryn Schwarz, "The Wrong Question: Thinking through Virginity," *differences* 13.2 (2002): 1–34, at 7. See also Marie H. Loughlin, *Hymeneutics: Interpreting Virginity in the Early Modern Stage* (London: Associated University Presses, 1997). On speculations about Elizabeth's physical problems, see Carole Levin, "Power, Politics, and Sexuality: Images of Elizabeth I," *Sixteenth Century Essays and Studies* 12 (1989): 95–110. On the problems that prolonged virginity is supposed to cause, as in the cases of women who choose not to marry or to have sex even though they are biologically capable, see also Theodora Jankowski, *Pure Resistance: Queer Virginity in Early Modern English Drama* (Philadelphia: University of Pennsylvania Press, 2000); and Kathleen Coyne Kelly and Marina Leslie, eds., *Menacing Virgins: Representing Virginity in the Middle Ages and Renaissance* (London: Associated University Presses, 1999).
51. According to Giovanni Marinello, women with a closed or inverted uterus cannot engender: "Impedisce . . . il generare figliuoli . . . la matrice chiusa, rivolta e torta." See *Le medicine partenenti alle infermità delle donne*, in Altieri Biagi et al., eds., *Medicina per le donne nel Cinquecento*, 51.
52. Either way, the Gonzaga of Mantua, who had ruled the territory since the early fourteenth century, would no longer rule Mantua. Moreover, their

Monferrato region could be easily lost, since the Savoia of Turin would take any occasion of a lack of apparent heirs to exercise a claim on it.

53. Traditionally, although not necessarily in aristocratic families, dowries were disbursed, partially or totally, within a few days of the consummation of marriage. See Julius Kirshner, "The Morning After: Collecting Monte Dowries in Renaissance Florence," in *From Florence to the Mediterranean and Beyond: Essays in Honor of Anthony Molho*, ed. Diego Ramada Curto et al. (Florence: Olschki, 2009), 29–61.

54. See Zanca, *Notizie sulla vita*, 15. In a later letter, dated April 8, Donati had made clear that it was possible to find information on this surgical procedure in the works of Arabic doctors and recommended caution, for if the womb were to be touched, he warned, there would be spasmodic pain, extremely dangerous blood fluxes, ulcerations, and abscesses—and they could all be deadly: "Nel tagliare . . . non si tocchi parte della matrice, atrimenti sopravvengono dolori spasmosi, flussi di sangue pericolosissimi, ulcere et apostemi della matrice effetti tutti mortali." The letter is addressed to Zibramonti. In Zanca, *Notizie sulla vita*, 15–16.

55. Colombo, *De re anatomica*, 268–269. More generally, see Bettina Mathes, "As Long as a Swan's Neck? The Significance of the 'Enlarged' Clitoris for Early Modern Anatomy," in *Sensible Flesh: On Touch in Early Modern Culture*, ed. Harvey, 104–124.

56. The words *hortus conclusus* were famously used in *Song of Songs*, 4:12: "Hortus conclusus soror mea, sponsa, hortus conclusus, fons signatus" (A garden enclosed is my sister, my spouse; a garden enclosed, a fountain sealed up).

57. The judgments of the Mantuan theologians Giovanni Pietro Barchi, Padre Don Floriano, and Padre Gregorio Capiluti, all solicited by the Gonzaga, are in ASM, AG, busta 201, D, II.

58. As in this letter of August 8, 1582, which Guglielmo sent to Rome (the correspondent's name is left blank): "Non potiamo mancare di metterle in consideratione quanto pericolosa cosa sarebbe che, mancando la nostra linea, venessero in questi stati [Mantua and Monferrato], che pur sono due porte d'Italia, li figliuoli del duca nostro fratello, che vi condurrebbono seco nationi pericolose del contagio." In ASM, AG, busta 201, c. 142.

59. The two families' cardinals were Scipio Gonzaga from Mantua and Alessandro di Pierluigi Farnese from Parma. For an interesting fictional rendering of the politico-clerical discussions taking place in Rome on the issue, see Roger Peyrefitte, *The Prince's Person* (London: Panther, 1964).

60. "Orificio della natura unito . . . come occorse alla moglie d'un certo tale, il quale volendo dappoi congiungersi con lei, trovò il luogo chiuso, né potè farlo, se prima con la cirugia non fossero separate le labbra." In Fabrici d'Acquapendente, *L'opere cirurgiche*, 209.

61. "In tal caso si amministra cotesta cirugia. Fatta voltar supina, ò rovescione la donna, e ritratte le gambe alle cosce, e legatele, ed allargate l'una dall'altra, e sottoposti li suoi gombiti sotto alle ginocchia, e legatele con funicelle aggiustate alla cervice, o collo, come ammonisce Paolo, indi con un siringotomo, o gamaut, acuto da un estremità, ò con un lunghissimo coltello, c'habbia il taglio da una parte, cioè dall'interna, e dall'altra sia rintuzzato, e moderatamente curvo nella punta, con un manico lunghissimo, e tagliamo la fessura, con uno, ò due tagli esquisitamente, facendo per mezzo alle labbra, una linea segnata prima con inchiostro, spiata, ed investigata di fuori col dito indice, e di dentro col ferro." In Fabrici d'Acquapendente, *L'opere cirurgiche,* 209. The position of a woman on her back in preparation for surgery, with her knees flexed and her legs widely separated—a position called lithotomy—was first described by the Greek surgeon Archigenes, who practiced in Rome at the time of the emperor Trajan.

62. One should recall in this context the famous cover of a book of anatomy by Andreas Vesalius, who a few decades earlier had put a female cadaver open at the womb in the frontispiece of his *De humani corporis fabrica* (Basilea: Johannes Oporinus, 1543). We know that this woman had tried to avoid execution by saying that she was pregnant, but in the drawing, a fatherly looking Vesalius, surrounded by his children/students, showed with the fingers of his hand pointed toward the empty uterus that such was not the case (the midwives who had previously examined the woman had reached the same conclusion). This female cadaver, the illustration seems to suggest, had no secrets for men of science—unlike indeed the living body of Margherita, which escaped control in the very place that seemed most controllable. See also Katharine Park, *Secrets of Women: Gender, Generation, and the Origins of Human Dissection* (New York: Zone Books, 2006), 211–221. On the increased use of the practice of physical examination in the period, see Roy Porter, "The Rise of Physical Examination," in *Medicine and the Five Senses,* ed. Roy Porter and William Bynum (Cambridge: Cambridge University Press, 2003), 79–97; and De Renzi, "Witnesses of the Body."

63. Carlo Borromeo (1538–1584) was canonized in 1610, and his feast day is celebrated on November 4. He was a learned cardinal, who advised both popes and foreign leaders. He was also a committed reformist in post-Tridentine Italy and founded seminaries for the education of priests after he came to the conclusion that abuses in the church were often the result of ignorance on the part of the clergy. He is often remembered for his fearless commitment to help the sick and poor when a particularly deadly bubonic plague hit Milan in 1576.

64. Borro (spelled "Boro" in documents) was a Milanese surgeon often consulted for syphilis. In 1578, for example, he compiled with other doctors a document addressing syphilitic therapies and their appropriate diets.

See Vincenzo Bevacqua, "L'ospedale del Brolo," *La Ca' Granda* 45.2 (2004): 30–37, at 37.

65. The list may be incomplete. I compiled it from an array of sources, including Stefano Scansani, *L'amor morto* (Milan: Mondadori, 1991), 97; Maria Bellonci, *Segreti dei Gonzaga* (Milan: Mondadori, 2000); and a letter from the Gonzaga ducal counselor, Zibramonti, February 18, 1583, in ASM, AG, busta 201, c. 346.

66. The marriage was annulled by Pope Alexander VI, and Jeanne de France later entered a convent. She died in 1505 and was canonized by Pope Pius XII in 1950, "a tardy reparation," as Desmond Seward puts it. See his *Prince of the Renaissance: The Life of François I* (London: Constable, 1973), 21.

67. Letter of Cavriani to the Duke of Mantua, August 29, 1582, in ASM, AG, busta 1380, fol. 74r–74v.

68. "Né fia maraviglia, che facilmente s'unisca la fessura ulcerata della natura, perche le donne, in particolare le più oneste, mostrano mal volentieri le sue parti esterne alli cirugici." In Fabrici d'Acquapendente, *L'opere cirurgiche,* 209. For this information, beyond my personal reconstruction made from ASM, AG, buste 1379 and 2615, I have followed Bellonci, *Segreti dei Gonzaga,* 44–72; Scansani, *L'amor morto,* 89–97; and Adele Bellù, "Margherita Farnese, sposa mancata di Vincenzo Gonzaga," *Archivi per la storia* 1–2 (1988): 381–420. The spell that a woman's uterus conjures is such that when many years later (1771) it was decided in Venice that lessons for obstetricians could be open to the public, so many people flocked to see dissections of the uterus, voicing their opinions on what was being dissected, that the Senate felt compelled to legislate that such lessons could only be done with doors closed. See Archivio di Stato di Venezia, Provveditori alla Sanità, Notatorio 765, c. 12, March 24, 1774.

69. The information on the visit of Madonna Antonia is in a letter from Cavriani to the Duke of Mantua, June 17, 1582, in ASM, AG, busta 201, D II, fol. 101.

70. The report is in a letter from Cavriani to the Duke of Mantua, February 12, 1583, in ASM, AG, busta 202, D II, fols. 117–118.

71. See ASM, AG, busta 201, D II, fols.119–122v.

72. Letter of Cavriani to Theodoro di San Giorgio, January 28, 1583, in ASM, AG, busta 202, D II, fol. 36.

73. Letter of Aurelio Zibramonti to Duke Guglielmo, February 5, 1583, in ASM, AG, busta 202, D II.

74. Bellonci, *Segreti dei Gonzaga,* 67.

75. "Le clausure over coperture che vengono nelle parti genitali delle femine, quali sono nominate dalli Greci *Phimosis,* dalli latini *clausure* et da Cornelio Celso *natura feminae impedita ad concubitum,* cotale dico clausure patiscono molte differenze, et prima patiscono differenza per conto della diversità delli luoghi, over parti genitali nelle quali provengono; perciò che

alcune si ritrovano nel *pudendo* over *vulva* detta dà vulgari; altre si ritrovano nella cervice dell'utero, et alcun'altre nel proprio orificio d'esso utero; et in due delle dette parti, cio è *cervice* et *pudendo*, si ritrovano anche diversamente poste." Letter of January 22, 1583, to Guglielmo Gonzaga, in ASM, AG, busta 1513, c. 563r. Pendasio wrote a total of three letters (Jan. 22, Jan. 29, and Feb. 12, 1583) that reveal, just as Fabrici will do in his later writings, how well developed was the medical knowledge at the time regarding malformed genitals.

76. "Alcune si curano colle sole mani, distrahendo le parti clause, et poi medicarle con unguenti et polvere. Alcune altre hanno bisogno del ferro et d'incisione sola; altre hanno bisogno et di sequestramento et distratione, et di diversi tagli, non di uno solo, fatti o in modo di croce prima, come insegna Cornelio Celso, et poi in modo circolare et transversale, come insegnano anco li Arabi. . . . Alcune altre sono anco quali si curano colli medicamenti corosivi soli, senza ferro, o con l'uno et l'altro." Letter of Pendasio, January 22, 1583, in ASM, AG, busta 1513, cc. 564r–564v.

77. Non "mancarà huomo sufficientissimo senza anche L'ecc.mo Aquapendente et Arancio." Letter of January 29, 1583, to Gugliemo Gonzaga, in ASM, AG, busta 1513, c. 566v.

78. Letter of Zibramonti to Duke Guglielmo, February 18, 1583, in ASM, AG, busta 201, c. 346–347.

79. "Alcuni di loro reputano la predetta S.ra non haver impedimento che non sia naturale, et che se il Ser.mo Prencipe havesse minor membro et più duro di quello che essi hanno veduto nelle due visite fatte a Reggio, ove non gli lo trovorono ben duro forsi come dicono, perché S. A. o non ebbe occasione che l'incitasse alla lussuria, o non si trovava in termine di perfetta erettione, come molte volte avviene a gli huomini, S. A. haverebbe di già consumato il matrimonio; ma che infatti troppo importa che il membro suo sia ben duro, et sia troppo sproportionato alla natura d'essa S.ra." Letter of Zibramonti to Duke Guglielmo, February 18, 1583, in ASM, AG, busta 201, cc. 346–347.

80. "Li due chirurghi di Milano et di Pavia affermano la cura potersi fare con bagni et altre cose emolienti per mollificare il luogo et dilatarlo poi con certi instrumenti chiamati passarij, et anco con le mani, il qual rimedio il predetto S.or Zacharia non ha per sicuro." Letter of Zibramonti from Parma, February 18, 1583, in ASM, AG, busta 201, c. 347.

81. On how canon law was enacted in these circumstances, see John McCarthy, "The Marriage Capacity of the *Mulier excisa*," *Ephemerides Iuris Canonici* 3,2 (1947): 261–285; and B. Lavaud, "The Interpretation of the Conjugal Act and the Theology of Marriage," *Thomist* 1 (1939): 360–380. In this particular case, annulment came only two years after the signing of the marriage contract. For how the church began to theorize on the issue of a husband's (but not a wife's) fertility just four years later, with Pope Sixtus V's bull "Cum Frequenter" (1587), see Finucci, *The Manly Masquerade*,

263–271. In Vincenzo's case, the notoriously rigid Cardinal Borromeo was against a notarial formalization of the deed regarding the marriage dissolution, but just four days after his death (and one year after the pope's pronouncement), Zibramonti was able to notify the Gonzaga ambassador, Aurelio Pomponazzi, that it was finally time to act on the issue: "Essendo passato di questa vita il ditto signor cardinal [Borromeo], potrebbe essere facile quello ch'è stato impossibile in sua vita, cioè l'haver il processo rogato dal signor Amato suo segretario sopra la dissolutione del matrimonio del serenissimo signor principe colla signora principessa all'hora di Parma." The letter, dated November 7, 1584, is in ASM, AG, busta 1701, now in *Le collezioni Gonzaga: Il carteggio tra Milano e Mantova (1563–1634)*, ed. Roberta Piccinelli (Milan: Silvana Editoriale, 2003), 144.

82. The Farnese even took away the jewels they had given her, and Margherita took to bed disheartened: "Questa Principessa di Mantova vistosi levare . . . non solo le gioie donatele dal Signor Duca di Mantova, ma quelle ancora che haveva havute dal cardinal Farnese et altri parenti di lei, si è posta in letto con febre, dandosene la colpa al dispiacere preso." This information is in an "Avviso" from Milan of August 24, 1583, in ASF, MDP 3255, DocID 10760. Gazettes feeding dubious facts and sporting titillating coverage had just become fashionable. On the status of information at the time, see Mario Infelise, "From Merchants' Letters to Handwritten *Avvisi*: Notes on the Origins of Public Information," in *Cultural Exchange in Early Modern Europe: 1400–1700*, ed. Francisco Bethencourt and Florike Edmond (New York: Cambridge University Press, 2006), 33–52.

83. On April 13, 1583, Cavriani informed Vincenzo that Margherita had written the pope because she had no intention of becoming a nun. In ASM, AG, busta 1381, fol. 149r–v.

84. Margherita's entrance in the convent took place on September 23, 1583. See ASM, AG, busta 2012, fols. 380r–384v. For the official vows see ASM, AG, busta. 202, fols. 395r–396v. This would not be the last time the wife of a Gonzaga prince would see her marriage annulled and subsequently be made to enter a convent. For the case of Camilla Faà, secret "wife" of Vincenzo's son, Ferdinando, who had to become a nun under the name of Caterina Camilla once her marriage was deemed invalid because it failed to fulfill some conditions established by the Council of Trent, see Valeria Finucci, "The Italian Memorialist: C. Faà Gonzaga," in *Women Writers of the Seventeenth Century*, ed. Katia Wilson and Frank Warner (Athens: University of Georgia Press, 1989), 121–128; and "Remembering the 'I': Faà Gonzaga's *Storia* (1622)," *Italian Quarterly* 28 (1987): 21–32. This was also not the first time when the marriage of a Gonzaga duke had been left unconsummated. The case of Duke Federico II (1500–1540), whose marriage to Maria Paleologo was first annulled by

Pope Clement VII, then revalidated, but which nevertheless remained unconsummated in both circumstances, took place fifty years earlier. For a recent reconstruction, see Deanna Shemek, "Aretino's *Marescalco:* Marriage Woes and the Duke of Mantua," *Renaissance Studies* 16.3 (2002): 366–380.

85. In the last months before the marriage dissolution, Margherita had turned understandably morose. As Cavriani writes from Parma to Vincenzo in Mantua, she had changed her tastes and often sang or recited stanzas from Ariosto centered on the pains of love, such as "Gravi pene in amor si provan molti" and "Dhe, perché voglio anco di me dolermi?" The letter, dated April 19, 1583, is in ASM, AG, busta 1381, fol. 4, cc. 158–159. Earlier, however, her choices of Ariosto's verses were sunnier, as when on November 21, 1582, Margherita asked Cavriani to compose a melody on the stanza starting with "Mi parea sù una lieta et verde riva." See ASM, AG, busta 201, fol. 224r–v. After the annulment, the Farnese honored the dowry contract and returned the jewels and the money that the Gonzaga had spent on the bride. The Gonzaga were able, however, to keep a good portion of the original dowry, valued at 300,000 scudi, although they restituted the jewels that Margherita had given her husband and his sister. ("Chiedeti il signor duca di Parma [Ottavio Farnese] che fossero restituite alcune gioie che la serenissima principessa haveva donate al serenissimo signor principe, et ha fatto anco domandare che se li ne compensino d'altri che'ella havea donati alla serenissima arciduchessa [Anna Caterina Gonzaga] li quali così sua altezza ha passati sì bene il suo obligo non era d'altro che di restituire li sudetti 100 mila scudi." Letter of Theodoro San Giorgio, Duke Guglielmo's secretary, to the Bishop d'Alba, September 16, 1583, in ASM, AG, busta 1513, fol. 9, cc. 731–732; now in *Le collezioni Gonzaga: Il carteggio tra Venezia e Mantova (1563–1587)*, ed. Daniela Sogliani (Milan: Silvana Editoriale, 2002), at 323.

86. "A tutte finalmente questo libretto farà palese et chiare molte cose . . . : universalmente tutte, ma quelle specialmente che si trovassero mal contente della Religione." In *Trattato della verginità et dello stato verginale: molto à proposito delle vergini che desiderano farsi grate al celeste sposo, et à tutti quelli che vogliono menar vista casta, et viver lieti et contenti nel servitio di Dio* (Rome: Bonfadino et Diani, 1584). The dedication is addressed to "Suor Maura Lucenia Farnese." More generally on the new nun, see Arnaldo Barilli, "Maria [sic] Lucenia Farnese," in his *Studi farnesiani* (Parma: La Bodoniana, 1958), 25–113. Maria Bellonci also mentions a sacred comedy, *La vittoria migliorata*, dedicated to Maura Lucenia by the primadonna actress Antonietta Catella Baiardo in the 1620s. See Bellonci, *Segreti dei Gonzaga*, 82. I have been unable to locate this text.

87. See Ferraro, *Marriage Wars in Late Renaissance Venice;* and Pastore, *Il medico in tribunale.*

88. For the shape that baldness seems to take in syphilitics in popular culture, see Bevacqua, "L'ospedale del Brolo," 34. The connection of loss of hair with syphilis made Gabriele Falloppio's remedial oil very much sought after among the Venetian nobility, as the doctor himself tells it in his *De ulceribus* (Venice: Bertelli, 1563), bk. 2, 1:192.
89. The information is in a letter dated February 18, 1583, from Parma by Zibramonti to Duke Guglielmo, in Giancarlo Malacarne, *Le feste del principe: giochi, divertimenti, spettacoli a corte* (Modena: Il Bulino, 2002), 88. A bit earlier, on January 24, Luigi Olivo had written directly to Guglielmo, telling him that his son had an enormous member (*smisurato*) and therefore that it would be dangerous for Margherita to be with him after surgery. See ASM, AG, busta 202, D II (1583), fol. 22. Thus gossip was feeding on a perceived reality.
90. "Per quella sua fistula gli fu dato un bottone di fuoco, il quale venne a offendere qualche nerbetto o cosa simile. Mediante il quale il stile [penis] sia rimasto alquanto indebolito e sottile, restando la cima grossa al solito, e che da questa nasca il non poter forse talvolta resister gagliardamente allo sforzo che bisogna." This explanation is offered by Orazio Urbani to the Grand Duke of Tuscany in a letter dated February 6, 1583, now in Giancarlo Malacarne, *Splendore e declino da Vincenzo I a Vincenzo II (1587–1627)*, vol. 4 of *I Gonzaga di Mantova: Una stirpe per una capitale europea*. (Modena: Il Bulino, 2007), 55.
91. "Hanno visitato la fistola che S. A. ha, . . . li medici non l'hanno potuta veder bene non l'havendo aperta; et però bisognarebbe che l'aprissero per chiarirsi s'ella vada verso quelle parti che possono impedir il coito; ma havendo io risposto che ciò non si potrebbe fare senza dolore del S.or Principe, et sarebbe fuori di proposito perché non gl'impedendo la detta fistola il 'correse la posta più che da corriere,' molto meno gli può impedire l'atto carnale." Letter of Zibramonti from Reggio to Duke Guglielmo, February 15, 1583, now in Malacarne, *Le feste del principe*, 88. For a study of herbal therapies and surgical interventions on anal fistulae in the period, see F. Sandei et al., "Le fistole dell'ano. Cenni storici," *Rivista italiana di colon-proctologia* 7.1 (1988): 34–41. As I mentioned in the introduction, Vincenzo's fistula could have been a misdiagnosis of bilateral psoas, whose pus-like abscesses are now associated with Pott's disease, afflicting the Gonzaga for generations. See R. Maron et al., "Two Cases of Pott Disease Associated with Bilateral Psoas Abscesses: Case Report," *Spine* 31 (2006): E561. See also Chapter 2.
92. "Ma perché in puoco tempo cessò l'errettione, nella quale era il predetto membro quando esso S.or Principe fece chiamare li medici, non è bastante questa visita. . . . Bisogna ch'il membro sia eretto per far giudicio sicuro si vi sia proportione fra esso et la natura della Ser.ma S.ra Principessa. Nella visita hanno li sopradetti tre medici dimandato a S. A. quanta parte della gianda [penis] ella ha introdotto con essa Ser.ma S.ra et S. A.

ha risposto che non ne ha introdotto niente." Letter of Zibramonti to Guglielmo, February 15, 1583, in ASM, AG, busta 201, cc. 344–347. As Michel de Montaigne was sadly to acknowledge, men are easy hostages to their sexual organ: "I ask you to reflect whether there is one single part of our body which does not often refuse to function when we want it to, yet does so when we want it not to." See Montaigne, "On the Power of the Imagination," in *The Complete Essays*, 115.

93. As Zibramonte tells it, "Alcuni di loro [doctors] reputano la predetta S.ra [Margherita] non haver impedimento che non sia naturale, et che se il Ser.mo Prencipe havesse minor membro et più duro di quello che essi hanno veduto nelle due visite fatte a Reggio, ove non gli lo trovarono ben duro forsi come dicono, perché S. A. o non ebbe occasione che l'incitasse alla lussuria, o non si trovava in termine di perfetta erettione, come molte volte avviene a gli huomini, S. A. haverebbe di già consumato il matrimonio." Letter from Parma to Guglielmo, February 18, 1583, now in Malacarne, *Le feste del principe*, 88.

94. "Dicono anco essersi fatto prova se può reggere peso honesto con il membro ritto, et se pùo aspettare incontro fattoli col palmo delle mani tanto che potesse una cittella. Et di più fatto una misura in forma di natura per veder se il membro suo è tanto disforme che causi l'impotentia. Qual cose pare, che tutte mostrino esser potenti." Avviso of December 22, 1583 (date unclear), in ASF, MDP 3255, DocID 10834.

95. "Il Vescovo di Casale fa iuramenti grandi che esso sa certissimo che il principe ha sverginato due vergini et una di esse ne ha ingravidata." Letter of November 18, 1583, in Nina Glassman, *Lettere proibite: I 'cimenti' del principe Vincenzo Gonzaga* (Ravenna: Longo, 1991), 28.

96. "[Vincenzo] volse provare con una vergine alcuni mesi sono, et si mostrò tanto potente che la trattò male e bisognò medicarla." Cesi's letter to the grand duke is from August 21, 1583, in Glassman, *Lettere proibite*, 22. See also Adalberto Pazzini, "La medicina alla corte dei Gonzaga a Mantova," in *Mantova e i Gonzaga nella civiltà del Rinascimento*, ed. Accademia Nazionale dei Lincei (Mantua: Accademia Virgiliana, 1977), 341. Beato was consulted often by Duke Guglielmo for his ailments and was invited to move to Mantua; he went to Rome instead in 1587. See Barbara Furlotti, "Università, scienza e arte: Uno sguardo generale e alcuni esempi della corrispondenza bolognese," in *Le collezioni Gonzaga: Il carteggio tra Bologna, Parma, Piacenza e Mantova (1563–1634)*, ed. Furlotti (Milan: Silvana Editoriale, 2000–2003), 29.

97. "Et haver' a esser' la favola d'Italia, come è stato Parma, che a me sarebbe doppio smacco." Letter to Ferdinando de' Medici, who was cardinal at the time and resided in Rome, in ASF, MDP 5109, DocId 17625.

98. Joanna died falling from the stairs. She was heavily pregnant and gave birth to a premature son, who died. Recent research by archeologists and physiopathologists has shown, however, that she had suffered a ruptured

uterus (the child entered the birth canal with his arm, as recorded at the time) and that her pelvis was critically deformed by scoliosis. See Gino Fornaciari et al., "The Medici Project: First Anthropological and Paleopathological Results." In http://www.paleopatologia.it/articoli/aticolo.php?recordID=18.

99. "Il fine mio è di rimanere sicuro, che con fanciulla vergine quello amico possa consumare il matrimonio et che però se ne faccia costì la prova, eleggendosi una fanciulla sana della quale si assicurino che la sia vergine." Letter of January 10, 1584, in Glassman, *Lettere proibite*, 46. Alfonso was Vincenzo's brother-in-law, having married his sister, Margherita. The documents relative to the test with Giulia are in Filippo Orlando and Giuseppe Baccini, "Il parentado fra la principessa Eleonora de' Medici e il principe Don Vincenzo Gonzaga ed i cimenti a cui fu costretto il detto principe per attestare come egli fosse abile alla generazione. Documenti inediti tratti dal Regio Archivio di Stato di Firenze," in *Bibliotechina Grassoccia: Capricci e curiosità letterarie inedite o rare*, no. 5 (Florence, 1886). Repr. *Una prova di matrimonio* (Rome, 1961). See also Filippo Orlando, "Altri documenti inediti sul parentado fra la principessa Eleonora de' Medici e il principe Don Vincenzo Gonzaga e i cimenti a cui fu costretto il detto principe per attestare la sua potenza virile," in *Giornale di erudizione: corrispondenza letteraria, artistica e scientifica*, ed. Filippo Orlando (Florence, 1893).

100. "Non potendo io per debito di conoscienza mancare d'affirmare quello ch'io so dell'attitudine del serenissimo Sig. Principe di Mantova, dico et affermo che all'A. S. si rizza il membro come a qual si voglia altro huomo, et che so che S. A. può usare carnalmente con ogni donna vergine o non vergine così prontamente quanto qualunque altro che sia, et in fede del vero ho fatto la presente di mia mano." Letter of Cesare d'Este, December 11, 1583, in Glassman, *Lettere proibite*, 29.

101. Letter of December 28, 1583, in Glassman, *Lettere proibite*, 44–45.

102. Letter of Guglielmo to the Bishop of Alba, November 12, 1583: "Quanto alla chiarezza che dimanda se esso nostro figliolo sia potente a consumare matrimonio con giovane vergine, che considerando esso signore [the Granduke] da chi le sia stato messo avanti questo dubio, può far certo argumento su che sia fondato." In Glassman, *Lettere proibite*, 26.

103. "Il signor Principe mandò a dire al Signor Don Alfonso [d'Este] che non si contentava di farla in una notte sola, ma volerne tre o quattro, et sendoli replicato che quello che non si fa in una notte non riesce anco in dua, il Principe la sera medesima s'andò a licenziare, et la mattina si partì per Mantova senza voler' fare altra prova." Letter of January 21, 1584, to Ferdinando de' Medici, in ASF, MDP 5109, DocId 17646. Vincenzo arrived in Ferrara on January 3, 1584, and the negotiations on the length of the meeting broke on January 20. See Bellonci, *Segreti dei Gonzaga*, 87–90.

104. "Rispetto a certa voce uscita da' Farnese che il Principe era impotente, non volemmo firmare le capitulazioni, se prima non restavamo giustificati della sua potenza, et così convenimmo che in Venezia se ne facessi la prova, dove inviammo una giovane con la quale egli ci rese molto ben chiari et giustificati della vanità della voce sparsa." Letter of April 10, 1584, to the king through Ambassador Bongianni di Piero Gianfigliazzi. Francesco was also asking for the sovereign's formal approval of the marriage. In ASF, MDP 5046, DocId 16148.

105. As Nicholas Terpstra puts it, "It helps us to understand how girls like the Pietà's Giulia were perceived by Florentine patricians: as objects or items of property, worthy of protection and a degree of care, but valued above all for their utility, convenience, and availability. Their sexuality was something to be protected so that it could be used, and the terms and conditions of that use would not be up to the girls to decide." In Terpstra, *Lost Girls: Sex and Death in Renaissance Florence* (Baltimore: Johns Hopkins University Press, 2010), 171. For more on the practice of female guardianship in Florentine convents, see Sharon Strocchia, "Taken into Custody: Girls and Convent Guardianship in Renaissance Florence," *Renaissance Studies* 17.2 (2003): 177–200. Recently "Giulia" has been identified as Giulia Albizi, perhaps an illegitimate daughter of the Albizi (or Albizzi) family. See Malacarne, *Splendore e declino*, 58. But the jury is still out as to her true identity.

106. "Avvertisca quella donna che ammaestri la Giulia, avvertendola che non si facessi forza con qualche instrumento inanzi havesse che far seco." Letter of Pier Cappelli to Belisario Vinta, from Livorno, February 25, 1584, now in the "Appendice documentaria" of Costantino Cipolla and Giancarlo Malacarne, *El più soave et dolce et dilectevole et gratioso bochone: Amore e sesso al tempo dei Gonzaga* (Milan: Franco Angeli, 2006), 432.

107. "Quando l'Altezza Sua non si sente habile a poter dar la sodisfattione di sé che ricerca il Signor Granduca di Toscana, . . . in niun modo entri nella pratica dell'altro matrimonio di Lorena col Signor Ambasciatore Christianissimo come l'Altezza Sua mostra haver pensiero di fare, perché esso Signor Nostro Serenissimo stima esser troppo disconveniente l'entrare in nuove pratiche, che prima non si sia certo di quello che l'Altezza Sua può." Letter of Theodoro San Giorgio, March 12, 1584, giving Guglielmo's instructions to Camillo Capilupi, who was going to Venice. In ASM, AG, busta 203, fol. 381. See also Coniglio, *I Gonzaga*, 349–350.

108. "L'Altezza Sua s'essamini le forze proprie et quando sente d'haverle tali che il mancamento sia stato per il dolor di stomaco et non per impotenza, ch'ella reiteri la prova." Letter of March 12, 1584, in ASM, AG, busta 203, fol. 381.

109. There was some urgency in having the *prova* concluded before Holy Week, so the encounter was scheduled after sundown on Wednesday, March 14, 1584.

110. "Et la condussi [the hand] fra l'uno e l'altro pettiglione, sino che con essa tocai la pube et urtai nel membro duro che la fanciulla haveva in corpo." Letter of Belisario Vinta to the Grand Duke of Tuscany, from Venice, March 16, 1584, in Cipolla and Malacarne, *El più soave et dolce et dilectevole et gratioso bochone,* 434.

111. "When I saw that he [Callimaco, the lover] was healthy, I [Nicia, the husband] dragged him along behind me and in the dark I took him into the bedroom and put him to bed. And before I left, I decided I should feel to make sure everything was going as it should. . . . After I had touched and felt everything, I left the room and locked the door. Then I returned to my mother-in-law by the fire, and we chatted and waited all night." See *The Mandrake Root* [*La Mandragola*], in *Five Comedies from the Italian Renaissance,* ed. and trans. Laura Giannetti and Guido Ruggiero (Baltimore: Johns Hopkins University Press, 2009), 5.2.111–112. Earlier, in a letter of February 25, Vinta had told the grand duke that he would try to touch the organ in order not to be deceived ("m'ingegnerò anche di toccar con la mano se poterò").

112. As in this letter of March 19, 1583, by Antonio Serguidi, secretary of the Medici, to Pietro di Francesco Usimbardi in Rome: "Il principe di Mantova riuscì felicemente, poichè non solo sverginò la fanciulla, ma la chiavò tre volte in sei hore che stette seco. Et non contento di questo, volse tornar la seconda notte et fece il medesimo, oltre all'haver lassato toccare il membro al Vinta mentre l'haveva dentro, talché in questo atto si è havuto ogni satisfattione." In ASF, MDP 5109, DocId 17660.

113. Alfred Kinsey's pathbreaking *Sexual Behavior in the Human Female* (Philadelphia: Saunders 1953) is based on research he conducted in 1936 in the classroom of Indiana University. Kinsey and MacMillen have recently been the subject of a biographical film, *Kinsey* (2004), which reenacts their initial sexual difficulties. In the equally pathbreaking *Human Sexual Response* (Toronto: Bantam, 1966), Virginia Johnson and William Masters recorded through direct observation in a laboratory at Washington University the anatomy and physiology of human sexual responses.

114. The text of the interview is now in the section "Interrogatori fatti alla fanciulla il dì 15 marzo 1583" of Cipolla and Malacarne, *El più soave et dolce et dilectevole et gratioso bochone,* 435–436; and most recently in Terpstra, *Lost Girls,* 187–189.

115. The Galenic theory of female seed as corresponding to male semen and thus predicating that women also experience heat, warm pneuma, and ejaculate—contributing potentially to generation—was put to rest first by William Harvey, when he argued in 1651 that he could see no seed in mammals. Harvey proceeded to criticize Fabrici's view of semen as "the agent or efficient cause of generation" expressed in *De formation foetu* in 1604. See his *Exercitationes de generatione animalium. Quibus accedunt quaedum de partu: de membranis ac humoribus uteri et de conceptione* (London:

Typis Du Gardinis, 1651. Yet as Clara Pinto-Correia points out, Harvey still believed "that the semen activates the egg by 'contagion' rather than by providing the 'efficient cause.'" See Pinto-Correia, *The Ovary of Eve: Egg and Sperm and Preformation* (Chicago: University of Chicago Press, 1997), 111.

116. Little mention was made at the time of female secretions and discharges. Mondino de' Luzzi had likened women's vaginal dampness to saliva. See Jacquart and Thomasset, *Sexuality and Medicine in the Middle Ages*, 37. Vesalius simply acknowledged "a thin and very scant and watery semen" coming from the ovaries to the womb. See Vesalius, *The Epitome of Andreas Vesalius*, trans. L. R. Lind (New York: Macmillan, 1949), 85.

117. As Albertus Magnus wrote in *De animalibus*, quantitatively, women have greater pleasure, but men have greater intensity. See Cadden, *Meanings of Sex Difference*, 157.

118. Although official documents in the Medici archives no longer talk of her, the lore went that she indeed had a boy and was married to a certain "Giuliano," a Roman musician. This Giuliano has been confused with Giulio Caccini (1551–1618), a composer and singer at the Medici court who later moved to Rome. According to Timothy McGee, the boy, Pompeo, became a famous singer as well as a sexual profligate. See McGee, "Pompeo Caccini and *Euridice:* New Biographical Notes," *Renaissance and Reformation* 26.2 (1990): 81–99. This hypothesis, however, is far-fetched, not least because the woman who raised Pompeo is named "Lucia" in the documents. See Terpstra, *Lost Girls*, 190.

119. "E V. S. [Belisario Vinta] sta vedere e considerer molto bene . . . se il membro è ben formato e se gli manca cosa alcuna; se i testicoli sono grandi a proportione et se gli ha tutti e due. E potendo chiarirsi V. S. coll'occhio in sul fatto, finirebbe questo negotio perfettamente." Letter of Pier Cappelli to Belisario Vinta, from Livorno, February 25, 1584, in Cipolla and Malacarne, *El più soave et dolce et dilectevole et gratioso bochone*, 432.

120. "Et tocchai et parvemi il membro in quello stato, che era chinato, membro ordinario ma ben fatto, et così i due testicoli in ogni lor parte, et messa la mano sotto d'ogni lato dei testicoli, non vi trovai male né impedimento nessuno." Letter of Piero Galletti to the Grand Duke of Tuscany, March 16, 1584, in Cipolla and Malacarne, *El più soave et dolce et dilectevole et gratioso bochone*, 436.

121. "Questa mattina andatomene di sua volontà nell'anticamera del Sig. Principe, mi fece chiamar ben presto drento che diaceva in letto, et mostrommi il membro ritto et sodo come un fuso, appuntato et proportionatissimo, et lo maneggiai et lo scalpellai con la mia mano, et così maneggiai li testicoli et rimasi contentissimo, parendomi la grossezza et la lunghezza del membro assai grande, ma non però fuor di natura, et le forme della fanciulla che l'hanno ricevuto non hanno patito lesione." Letter of Piero Galletti to

the Grand Duke of Tuscany, from Venice, March 16, 1584, in Cipolla and Malacarne, *El più soave et dolce et dilectevole et gratioso bochone*, 436.
122. See Giovanni Marinello, *Le medicine partenenti alle infermità delle donne* (Venice: Valgrisio, 1574), 53v, 63v.
123. The wedding took place in the church of Santa Barbara in Mantua. See ASM, AG, busta 168, fols. 1r–72v. Eleonora was given a dowry of 300,000 scudi, which included numerous jewels. As for illegitimate children, there is no official counting, but Vincenzo had at least four.
124. The movie, with Vittorio Gassman as Vincenzo, was directed by Pasquale Festa Campanile in 1965.
125. Vesalius, *De humani corporis fabrica*, bk. 5.
126. See Jacquart and Thomasset, *Sexuality and Medicine*, 47. In his teaching Peter of Abano (1257–1316) followed Avicenna and the Arabic school of thought.
127. For example, Henri de Monteville (1260–1316) in *La chiurgie* wrote that "the uses of this membrane are twofold: first, that urine could issue through it so that it does not spill into the uterus through the vulva; and second, it is able to alter the air that enters the womb though the vulva." He states that the clitoris (*tentigo*) has the same function that the uvula has in the throat. See Jacquart and Thomasset, *Sexuality and Medicine*, 45. I am indebted to Marzio Barbagli for my more in-depth look at the medieval understanding of this organ. Among Barbagli's copious writings on sexuality and the legal history of families in Italy, see his most recent *Storia di Caterina che per ott'anni vestì abiti da uomo* (Bologna: Il Mulino, 2014).
128. Falloppio, *Observationes anatomicae*, 2:369.
129. Costanzo Varoli, *Anatomiae, sive de resolutione corporis umani libri IIII* (Frankfurt: Wechel and Fischer, 1591), 99. But the Hippocratics had already mentioned it. See Thomas Laqueur, "Amor Veneris, Vel Dulcedo Appelletur," in *Zone: Fragments for a History of the Human Body*, part 3, ed. Michael Feher (New York: Zone, 1989), 90–131; Katharine Park, "The Rediscovery of the Clitoris," in *The Body in Parts: Fantasies of Corporeality in Early Modern Europe*, ed. David Hillman and Carla Mazzio (New York: Routledge, 1997), 171–193; and Valerie Traub, "The Psychomorphology of the Clitoris or, the Reemergence of the *Tribade* in English Culture," in *Generation and Degeneration: Tropes of Reproduction in Literature and History from Antiquity to Early Modern Europe*, ed. Valeria Finucci and Kevin Brownlee (Durham: Duke University Press, 2001), 153–186. Recently Karma Lochrie has cogently argued that in the medieval period there was more knowledge of this organ than it has been acknowledged by early modern historians and "what differentiates Falloppia's or Colombo's clitoris from Avicenna's is not a new pleasure principle or normalizing effect, but the argument for militant empiricism itself and the case for a new anatomical

science." See her *Heterosyncrasies* (Minneapolis: University of Minnesota Press, 2005), 74.
130. See Mathes, "As Long as a Swan's Neck?," 123.
131. Andreas Vesalius, *Anatomicarum Gabrielis Falloppii observationum examen* (Venice: Francesco de' Franceschi da Siena, 1564), 143.
132. Colombo, *De re anatomica*, 447–448.
133. Thomas Bartholin (1616–1680), *Bartolinus Anatomy, Made from the Precepts of His Father, and from Observations of All Modern Anatomists, Together with His Own* (London: John Streater, 1668), 72.
134. "E affine a questo altro intervento, che si compie sulle donne, quando la ninfa o coda come chiamano va asportata. Infatti talvolta la ninfa cresce tanto smisuratamente che porta con sé molta molestia o turpidine. Per cui fatta adagiare all'indietro la donna, con una pinzetta si prende ciò che è superfluo della ninfa e si toglie con lo scalpello. . . . Bisogna togliere anche il clitoride come le ninfe." In Gaspare Tagliacozzi, *La chirurgia plastica per innesto di Gaspare Tagliacozzi*, ed. and trans. Werner Vallieri (Bologna: Montaguti, 1964), 173.
135. The wax models have been housed in the University of Cagliari since 1806 and are available in the beautifully illustrated text by Riva, *Flesh and Wax* (see the two figures at 74–75). I thank Professor Riva for having alerted me to these detailed, life-size ceroplastic creations.
136. Susan Williamson and Rachel Novak, "The Truth about Women," *New Scientist*, August 1, 1998, 1–5. See also Elizabeth Harvey, "Anatomies of Rapture: Clitoral Politics/Medical Blazons," *Signs* 27 (2001): 315–346, at 320. Williams and Novak did not know, unfortunately, of Susini's accurate anatomical waxes.
137. Fabrici, "Rari 117.23," in Biblioteca Nazionale Marciana, Venice. Also in Rippa Bonati and Pardo-Tomás, eds., *Il teatro dei corpi*, 330.
138. Plenty of ink has been spread in the last few years following Thomas Laqueur's famous statement that the male and female bodies were considered homologous ("one sex/one flesh model") in the early modern period, following Galen's insights, and that the difference between the two bodies were "of degree and not of kind." This difference became "incommensurate" only in the late eighteenth century. See Laqueur, *Making Sex: Body and Gender from the Greeks to Freud* (Cambridge: Harvard University Press, 1990), 25. Laqueur's study has been extremely influential in cultural studies, but his statements on the topic have often been revised with arguments regarding the limited number of authors mentioning homology in their texts in the sixteenth century (such as Alessandro Benedetti's *Anatomice* in 1502 and Berengario da Carpi's *Isagogae brevis* in 1522). See Katharine Park and Robert Nye, "Destiny Is Anatomy," *New Republic* 204 (February 18, 1991): 53–57; Katharine Park, "Cadden, Laqueur, and the One-Sex Body," *Medieval Feminist Forum* 46.1 (2010): 96–100; Janet Adelman,

"Making Defect Perfection: Shakespeare and the One-Sex Model," in *Enacting Gender on the English Renaissance Stage*, ed. Viviana Comensoli and Anne Russell (Urbana: University of Illinois Press, 1999), 23–52; Michael Stolberg, "A Woman Down to Her Bones: The Anatomy of Sexual Difference in the Sixteenth and Early Seventeenth Centuries," *Isis* 94.2 (2003): 274–299; Monica H. Green, "Bodies, Gender, Health, Disease: Recent Work on Medieval Women's Medicine," *Studies in Medieval and Renaissance History* 3rd ser., 2 (2005): 6–12; and Patricia Simons, *The Sex of Men in Premodern Europe: A Cultural History* (Cambridge: Cambridge University Press, 2011), 121–156. Thomas Laqueur's response is in "Sex in the Flesh," *Isis* 94.2 (2003): 300–306.

139. André Du Laurens, *Historia anatomica* (Frankfurt: Rhodius, 1600), 359–360. The translation comes from Stolberg, "A Woman Down to Her Bones," 287. On the debates taking place already by the late sixteenth century on the difference between male and female bodies, see Ian Maclean, *The Renaissance Notion of Woman: A Study in the Fortunes of Scholasticism and Medical Science in European Intellectual Life* (Cambridge: Cambridge University Press, 1980), 28–46.

140. Caspar Bartholin, *Anatomicae institutiones corporis humani* (Oxford: Turner, 1633), 98.

141. Sigmund Freud, "The Taboo of Virginity," in *The Standard Edition of the Complete Psychological Works of Sigmund Freud*, ed. and trans. by James Strachey, vol. 11 (London: Hogarth Press, 1957), 193–208, at 193.

142. Bellonci, *Segreti dei Gonzaga*, 343.

143. Freud, "The Taboo of Virginity," 188–189.

144. Bellonci, *Segreti dei Gonzaga*, 343.

145. "Si va credendo che Sua Altezza sia finalmente per ammogliarsi, per viver fuori del peccato." Letter of February 2, 1612, in ASF, *Urbino*, fol. 241, c. 955v.

146. See Bellonci, *Segreti dei Gonzaga*, 341–344.

147. For a reconstruction and an assessment of that very complicated event, "one which was to shape the politics of Europe for the next three decades," see David Parrott, "The Mantuan Succession, 1627–31: A Sovereignty Dispute in Early Modern Europe," *English Historical Review* 112 (1997): 20–65, at 20.

148. See Nina Treadwell, "'Simil combattimento fatto da Dame:' The Musico-Theatrical Entertainments of Margherita Gonzaga's *Balletto delle donne* and the Female Warrior in Ferrarese Cultural History." In *Gender, Sexuality and Early Music*, ed. Todd Borgerding (New York: Routledge, 2002), 27–40. Letters commenting on Margherita's love for dancing and singing are present everywhere in the correspondence of chief entertainer Cesare Cavriani. See ASM, AG, busta 201, fol. 41, fol. 61, and fols. 74r–75v.

2. The Aesthetic Cure

1. On Vincenzo's military collection, see Dario Franchini et al., *La scienza a corte. Collezionismo eclettico, natura e immagine a Mantova fra Rinascimento e Manierismo* (Rome: Bulzoni, 1979), 122.
2. Margherita Paleologo, who belonged to a cadet branch of the family, had married Vincenzo's grandfather, Federico II, in 1531.
3. As in the second crusade: "Partì lunedì passato il sig.r Duca mio per la volta d'Ongaria, et porto seco la cassetta de' medicamenti mandatami da V.A. [Ferdinando] la quale egli serba per testimonio del zelo che l'A.V. ha della sua salute." Letter of August 1, 1597, in ASF, MDP 2942, DocID 16315.
4. An anonymous contemporary chronicle of this crusade, entitled "Relatione del primo viaggio che il serenissimo signor duca Vincenzo di Mantova fece alla guerra d'Ongheria l'anno 1595 et di tutto quello che successe mentre S. A. si fermò in corte Cesarea et in Campo," is in ASM, AG, busta 388, now in Giancarlo Malacarne, *Splendore e declino: da Vincenzo I a Vincenzo II (1587–1627)*, vol. 4 of *I Gonzaga di Mantova: Una stirpe per una capitale europea* (Modena: Il Bulino, 2007), 339–343. Vincenzo's second crusade of two years later, 1597, in which he completed a successful sortie at Giavarrino (Raab), Hungary, also ended earlier than expected because of disagreements with the new imperial commander. As to why the third crusade of 1601 ended earlier as well, see Chapter 3.
5. "Restituitosi pertanto il nostro Duca al campo, si ammalò anch'egli . . . a cagione d'essersi tenuto tre giornate intiere sempre armato a cavallo, con poco e disagiato riposo, per essere pronto alle scorrerie de' Turchi fin sotto de' suoi alloggiamenti." In Federigo Amadei, *Cronaca universale della città di Mantova* (Mantua: CITEM, 1956), 3:147; also in Malacarne, *Splendore e declino*, 122. Vincenzo's letters from the field are in ASM, AG, busta 2155. See also Leonardo Mazzoldi, Renato Giusti, and Rinaldo Salvatori, eds., *Mantova: La storia, le lettere, le arti* (Mantua: Istituto Carlo d'Arco per la Storia di Mantova, 1963), vol. 3.
6. "Quivi si fermò S. A. alcuni dì alloggiando in un comodo palagio a spese sue. . . . In questo tempo che S. A. stette in Possonia pigliando essa molto miglioramento per conto di detta Crisipilla et trovandosene quasi libera, si risolse di tirar innanti alla volta di Vienna." In "Relatione del primo viaggio che il serenissimo signor duca Vincenzo di Mantova fece alla guerra d'Ongheria l'anno 1595," ASM, AG, busta 388, fol. 321r, now in Malacarne, *Splendore e declino*, 342.
7. See Giuseppe Coniglio, *I Gonzaga* (Milan: Dall'Oglio, 1967), 367.
8. Ulisse Aldrovandi, *Ornithologiae, hoc est de avibus historiae . . . libri XII* (Bologna: Fraciscum de Franciscis, 1599), vol. 1, bk. 1, at 27. Tagliacozzi was also the doctor of Duke Ranuccio Farnese in Parma and of Virginio Orsini, the nephew of Ferdinando de' Medici.

9. Letter of Tullio Petrozzani to Federico Pendasio, February 10, 1596. In Martha Teach Gnudi and Jerome Pierce Webster, *The Life and Times of Gaspare Tagliacozzi, Surgeon of Bologna (1545–1599)* (New York: Reichner, 1950), 168. See also Alfonso Silvestri, "Gaspare Tagliacozzi a Mantova," *Archiginnasio* 32 (1937): 89–100.
10. Letter of Tullio Petrozzani to Federico Pendasio, February 23, 1596, in Gnudi and Webster, *The Life and Times of Gaspare Tagliacozzi*, 169.
11. Letter of Tullio Petrozzani to Federico Pendasio, February 10, 1596, in Gnudi and Webster, *The Life and Times of Gaspare Tagliacozzi*, 168. We know the identity of another doctor who participated to the consult, Gerolamo Conforti, from nearby Brescia. He had cured Vincenzo in the past for unspecified problems.
12. He was consulted on March 14 in Bologna on how to get rid of a catarrh by Francesco dall'Armi, a noble working for the Gonzaga family. Tagliacozzi also wrote a letter justifying Dall'Armi's absence from Mantua, since he had recommended him to remain in bed and eat light for at least eight days. The relative letters are in Gnudi and Webster, *The Life and Times of Gaspare Tagliacozzi*, 421–422.
13. The rumor that "vi sono principi c'hanno gran mira di levar cotesto soggetto da Bologna con prometterli dupplicato partito di quello che li vien dato dal Publico" comes from a letter of Camillo Gozzadino, the Bolognese ambassador in Rome, July 24, 1596. In Gnudi and Webster, *The Life and Times of Gaspare Tagliacozzi*, 422. In a letter a few days earlier of July 16, 1596, Tagliacozzi had asked the Bolognese authorities for an increase to his income, since not only, he wrote, people younger than him were making more money but he had received no monetary recognition when he was last promoted. The petition was denied for lack of funds ("lo stato di quelle entrate . . . è ridotto in tanta strettezza") on July 20, 1596. See Gnudi and Webster, *The Life and Times of Gaspare Tagliacozzi*, 423.
14. Letter of Vincenzo to Francesco dall'Armi, in Gnudi and Webster, *The Life and Times of Gaspare Tagliacozzi*, 177; and Silvestri, "Gaspare Tagliacozzi a Mantova," 96, for the Italian version. In a letter sent to the Duchess of Mantua ten years earlier, on July 13, 1586, by the Bolognese physician Gabriello Beato, we know that Tagliacozzi was curing the cardinal, but since the patient was not showing any apparent benefit, Beato recommended the services of another doctor, Bonifacio Granata. The Gonzaga still preferred Tagliacozzi. See Gnudi and Webster, *The Life and Times of Gaspare Tagliacozzi*, 96–97.
15. Letter of Francesco Dall'Armi to Guido Caffini of August 22, 1596, in Gnudi and Webster, *The Life and Times of Gaspare Tagliacozzi*, 177; and Silvestri, "Gaspare Tagliacozzi a Mantova," 96.
16. "Se n'ongerà la sera, come andrà in letto dove è l'escoriatione nelle nari, et la mattina si laverà con un puoco d'acqua della villa tepida." In Gnudi and Webster, *The Life and Times of Gaspare Tagliacozzi*, 424.

17. We know of this visit from a letter that the alchemist Giovanni Antonio Magini wrote from Bologna to Vincenzo asking that Tagliacozzi, who was going to Mantua, carry home to Bologna on his return trip a drawing of the map of the Mantuan territory: "Con l'occasione del signor Tagliacozzi, ho voluto con questa mia far riverenza all'A. V. Ser.ma." In ASM, AG, busta 1166, fol. 1, cc. 32–33; also in Gnudi and Webster, *The Life and Times of Gaspare Tagliacozzi*, 424.
18. Gaspare Tagliacozzi, *De curtorum chirurgia per insitionem*, trans. Joan H. Thomas, with an introduction by Robert M. Goldwyn (New York: Gryphon Editions, 1996), vii–viii.
19. On Vincenzo's brand-new provisions (for the times) to cure the sick and wounded in war—he was preceding by two centuries what Napoleon's doctors would set up during military campaigns—see Adalberto Pazzini, "La medicina alla corte dei Gonzaga a Mantova," in *Mantova e i Gonzaga nella civiltà del Rinascimento*, ed. Accademia Nazionale dei Lincei (Mantova: Accademia Virgiliana, 1977), 291–351, at 336.
20. "La natura della infermità non è precisata, ma tutto ci fa pensare che fosse sifilide, benché i dati siano troppo scarsi per poterlo affermare con certezza." In Jerome Pierce Webster and Martha Teach Gnudi, "Documenti inediti intorno alla vita di Gaspare Tagliacozzi," in *Studi e memorie per la storia dell'Università di Bologna* 13 (Bologna: Istituto per la Storia dell'Università, 1935), 41. The claim is omitted in their later book, 179.
21. "Et perché da lei sono avvisato del pigliare ch'ella fa del decotto del legno, forza è che per la incredibile mia affitione per la serenissima sua persona, le scriva che mi dispiace d'udire che l'altezza vostra erudita di scientia singolare, usi medicamenti volgari ripieni di molte imperfettioni sottoponendosi a astinenze e strettezze insopportabili." In ASM, AG, busta 1534, fol. 3, cc. 433–434, now in *Le collezioni Gonzaga: Il carteggio tra Venezia e Mantova (1588–1612)*, ed. Michaela Sermidi (Milan: Silvana Editoriale, 2003), 300. There is also a reference to Vincenzo's undergoing the "cura del legno" in Maria Bellonci, *I segreti dei Gonzaga* (Milan: Mondadori, 1947). The "wood therapy" was used for an array of problems. In fact, Eleonora de' Medici underwent the treatment in the final months of her life, as in this letter from Vincenzo to Ferdinando de' Medici, apprising him of his wife's ongoing recuperation: "Sono alquanti giorni ch'ella piglia l'acqua del legno con molta toleranza et con qualche segno di profitto, a che cooperando la stagione et il continuo aginto d'altri rimedij che si porgerà alla natura, ne vado sperando ogn'hora meglio." Letter of April 1, 1611, in ASF, MDP 2646, DocID 5204. We have a recipe of a decoction of holy wood made in Mantua and consisting of "libbr. 1 di legno santo limato infuso in 8 librr. d'acqua, onc. 4 di acqua di rose, bolito alla consumazione di un terzo." This common recipe appears in a list of drugs ordered at the Gonzaga court in a specific month, December 1587, entitled "Robbe vive per servitio di S. A. Ser.ma et della Ser.ma Sig.a Duchesse et altre ocorente

con bolete." Some of the concoctions and elixirs in this list may have been used not only by Vincenzo and his wife and sister, but also by various residents at court. See Cristoforo Masino and Giuseppe Ostino, "Le forniture di medicinali e 'robbe vive' alla corte di Mantova nel mese di dicembre del 1587," in *Mantova e i Gonzaga nella civiltà del Rinascimento,* 375–379, at 377. Affected by syphilis in any case were many men in the Gonzaga line, including Vincenzo's grandfather, Federico II, and his great-grandfather, Francesco.

22. Adalberto Pazzini, "La medicina alla corte dei Gonzaga a Mantova," in *Mantova e i Gonzaga nella civiltà del Rinascimento,* 291–351, at 319. Also Achille Neri thought that syphilis could be a reason for Vincenzo's bath therapy in Sampierdarena. See Neri, "Il duca di Mantova a San Pier D'Arena," *Giornale ligustico* 13 (1886): 160–164, at 160.

23. I have seen only one drawing of Vincenzo with an exaggerated, longish, depressed nose, in a book of portraits of rulers at the Marciana Library in Venice by Giacomo Franco, *Effigie naturali dei maggior principi et più valorosi capitani di questa età con l'arme loro. Raccolte et con diligenza intagliate da Giacomo Franco* (Venice: Apud Iacobum Francum, 1596). The book is composed of thirty-five images, including all European princes as well as Turks, Persians, and Tartars. Vincenzo is at plate 23. He has blondish hair, a young looking figure, curly mustaches, and a pointed beard; is fully armed; and wears the collar of the Redeemer. None of the other figures in the book has such a remarkably low, almost caricaturesque nose as Vincenzo. It is possible of course that because the drawing was not made from a live model but from a medal, some features may have been less true to life.

24. See Gnudi and Webster, *The Life and Times of Gaspare Tagliacozzi,* 221–222. In any case, Tagliacozzi kept corresponding with the Gonzaga during the year, as testified in a letter he sent to Eleonora de' Medici on October 15, 1597, recommending her patronage for his student Francesco Bruschi. See Gnudi and Webster, *The Life and Times of Gaspare Tagliacozzi,* 219. Tagliacozzi died on November 7, 1599. The duke had been informed in advance of the physician's impending death and was notified by Tagliacozzi's son two days following the event.

25. Giorgio Vasari (1511–1574), "Preface III," in *The Lives of the Most Excellent Painters, Sculptors and Architects,* ed. George Bull (Baltimore: Penguin, 1965 and 1971), 35.

26. Marsilio Ficino (1433–1499), *Commentary on Plato's Symposium on Love,* trans. Sears Jayne (Dallas: Spring Publications, 1985); and Baldesar Castiglione, *The Book of the Courtier,* trans. George Bull (New York: Penguin, 1967).

27. Francesco Petrarca, *De remediis utriusque fortunae libri II,* in *In Our Image and Likeness: Humanity and Divinity in Italian Humanist Thought,* ed. Charles Trinkaus (Notre Dame: University of Notre Dame Press, 1955), at 451.

28. See Gabriele Falloppio, *Secreti diversi e miracolosi* (Venice: Imberti, 1640) and "De decoratione" in *Opera genuina omnia, tam practica quam theorica* (Venice: De Franciscis, 1606); Girolamo Mercuriale, *De decoratione* (Venice: Apud Paolum Meietum, 1585); Giovanni Tommaso Minadoi, *De humani corporis turpitudinibus cognoscendis et curandis libri tres* (Padua: Bolzetta, 1600).
29. Mariacarla Gadebush Bondio, "I pericoli della bellezza 'mangonica.' Aspetti del dibattito su protesi, trucchi e chirurgia estetica tra '500 e '600," *Micrologus: natura, scienza e società medievali* 15 (2007): 425–449, at 441. See also Sabrina Veneziani, "Le lezioni dermatologiche di Girolamo Mercuriale," in *Girolamo Mercuriale: Medicina e cultura nell'Europa del Cinquecento*, ed. Alessandro Arcangeli and Vivian Nutton (Florence: Olschki, 2008), 203–215.
30. To get a sense of the intensity of this correspondence, see Elena Venturini, ed., *Le collezioni Gonzaga: Il carteggio tra la Corte Cesarea e Mantova (1559–1636)* (Milan: Silvana Editoriale, 2002).
31. It is no surprise, then, that Vincenzo thought it proper to pay a rumored 7,000 scudi to have a painting by Raphael in his palace. In fact, since the Canossa family, which owned the painting, was making the sale difficult, he threw into the bargain "the title of Marquis of Cagliano and the territory of Monferrato that came with it," just to make sure the sale would go through. See Barbara Furlotti and Guido Rebecchini, *The Art and Architecture of Mantua: Eight Centuries of Patronage and Collecting* (New York: Thames and Hudson, 2008), 220.
32. The authorization came on September 8, 1610. It was then left to his son Ferdinando to implement his father's wish, officially chart it, and further the infrastructure. See Paul Grendler, *The University of Mantua, the Gonzaga and the Jesuits, 1584–1630* (Baltimore: Johns Hopkins University Press, 2009), 53ff.
33. A good part of the collection was sold to King James I in 1628; much of what was left was stolen or destroyed by German mercenaries during the sack of Mantua. A sample of the collection was reassembled in Mantua in 2002, and it took millions of euros just to insure it. The reassembled works of art are now printed in Raffaella Morselli, ed., *Gonzaga, La Celeste Galeria: Le raccolte* (Milan: Skira, 2002). See also Roberta Piccinelli, "Le facies del collezionismo artistico di Vincenzo Gonzaga," in Raffaella Morselli, ed., *Gonzaga, La Celeste Galeria: L'esercizio del collezionismo* (Milan: Skira, 2002), 341–347; and Furlotti and Rebecchini, *The Art and Architecture of Mantua*, 220.
34. Adriano Valerini, *La celeste galeria di Minerva* (Verona: Appresso Girolamo Discepolo, 1588).
35. The famous botanist Zenobio Bocchi was invited from Pisa to create a "giardino dei semplici" in Mantua. See also Dario Franchini et al., *La scienza a corte*, 30–62.

36. Tagliacozzi, *De curtorum chirurgia per insitionem*, 10.
37. "In fact, the main purpose of this procedure is not the restoration of the original beauty of the face but rather the rehabilitation of the part in question. Its beauty lies in the faultless performance of the functions decreed it by Nature. . . . These are the reasons for placing my procedure in the realm of the curative and no other. I would not disagree, however, with the claim that this operation does, in fact, restore the beauty of the face." In Tagliacozzi, *De curtorum chirurgia per insitionem*, 59.
38. See Alfonso Corradi, "Dell'antica autoplastica italiana," in *Memorie del Regio Istituto Lombardo di Scienze e Lettere. Classe di scienze matematiche e naturali*, ser. 3, vol. 13 (Milan, 1883), 225–275, at 244; and Gadebush Bondio, "I pericoli della bellezza 'mangonica,'" 443. More generally on rhinoplasty I am indebted to the study of Luigi Monga, "Odeporica e medicina: I viaggiatori del Cinquecento e la rinoplastica," *Italica* 69 (1992): 378–393.
39. J. C. Lascaratos et al., "From the Roots of Rhinology: The Reconstruction of Nasal Injuries in Hippocrates," *Annals of Otology, Rhinology, and Laryngology* 112.2 (2003): 159–162.
40. Aulus Cornelius Celsus (25 B.C.–50 B.C.), *De medicina*, trans. G. W. Spencer (Cambridge: Harvard University Press, 1935–1938). Celsus's work was rediscovered by Pope Nicholas V and published in 1478.
41. Johann Caspar Lavater, *Essays on Physiognomy: For the Promotion of the Knowledge and the Love of Mankind* (Boston: Spotswood and West, 1794).
42. Lanfranco of Milan (d. 1315), who writes about the nose in chapter 2 of his *Cyrurgia parva*, did not believe that it was possible to repair a detached nose. This treatise is inserted in Guy de Chauliac (1300–1368), *Cyrurgia Guidonis de Cauliaco* (Venice, Octaviani Scoti, 1498). De Chauliac had the same opinion as did his student Pietro d'Argellata, a surgeon in Bologna around 1400. Theodoric, Bishop of Cervia (1205–1298) and son of Ugo Borgognoni, the founder of the Bolognese surgical school, described how to treat a partially severed nose but did not mention grafting. See also Rolando Capelluti (b. ca. 1430), *La chirurgia di Mo. Rolando da Parma detto dei Capezzuti. Riproduzione del Codice Latino n. 1382 della R. Biblioteca Casanatense di Roma* (Rome: Istituto Nazionale Medico Farmacologico Serono, 1927); and Henri de Mondeville (14th cent.), *Chirurgie de Maitre Henri de Mondeville, chirurgien de Philippe Le Bel, roi de France, composée de 1306 à 1320*, ed. E. Nicaise (Paris: Baillière et Cie, 1893), 346. More generally on the inroads surgery made in the Middle Ages thanks to these academically minded medical practitioners, see the impressive study by Michael McVaugh, *The Rational Surgery of the Middle Ages* (Florence: Edizioni del Galluzzo, 2006).
43. Sushruta, who practiced around the fifth century B.C., is the most celebrated Indian physician and surgeon, recognized as the father of ophthalmology for his pioneering work on cataracts.

44. The surgery is described in detail and with admiration by Bartolomeo Facio (d. 1457) in his *De viris illustribus liber* (Florence: Giovanelli, 1745). See also Domenico Tripodi, "Sull'arte di acconciare i nasi: i Vianeo e la 'Magia Tropaensium,'" *Valsalva* 44 (1968): 54–56.
45. Alessandro Benedetti (1460–1525), *Anatomice, sive Historia corporis humanis*, ed. and trans. Giovanna Ferrari (Florence: Giunti, 1998). Benedetti also gave suggestions on what he considered the appropriate time for surgery and how to prepare for it.
46. Ambroise Paré, *Opera chirugica*, bk. 22, ch. 2, "Qua arte exacta naris portio reparari" (Frankfurt: Apud Johannen Feyrabend, 1594).
47. Camillo Porzio (1526?–1580?), *L'istoria d'Italia nell'anno 1547 e la descrizione del regno di Napoli* (Naples: Tramater, 1839), 14.
48. "Fu dispartita la zuffa e il povero gentiluomo restò senza naso; e io che lo avea in mano tutto pieno di arena, li pisciai suso e lavato col piscio gli lo attaccai e lo cuscì benissimo e lo medicai col balsamo e lo infasciai e lo feci stare così otto giorni, credendo che si dovesse marcire; nondimeno, quando lo sligai, trovai che era ritaccato benissimo e lo tornai a medicare solamente un'altra volta e fu sano e libero, che tutto Napoli ne restò maravigliato; e questo fu pur la verità e il Sig. Andrés lo può raccontare perché è ancora vivo e sano." In Leonardo Fioravanti (1518–1588), *Il tesoro della vita humana. Dell'Eccellente dottore e cavaliere M. Leonardo Fioravanti Bolognese. Diviso in quattro libri* (Venice: Sessa, 1570), c. 64r; cited in Piero Camporesi, *Camminare il mondo: Vita e avventure di Leonardo Fioravanti medico del Cinquecento* (Milan: Garzanti, 1997), 115.
49. On this pseudo-Vesalius work, *Chirurgia magna* (Venice: Valgrisi, 1568), see Gnudi and Webster, *The Life and Times of Gaspare Tagliacozzi*, 122.
50. Gabriele Falloppio, "De decoratione," ch. 10, in *Opera genuina*, 3.1, 19v.
51. Ambroise Paré, *Les Oevvres d'Ambroise Paré* (Paris: Gabriel Buon, 1585). See also Thomas Gibson, "The Prostheses of Ambroise Paré," *British Journal of Plastic Surgery* 8 (1955–1956): 3–8.
52. See Gnudi and Webster, *The Life and Times of Gaspare Tagliacozzi*, 282.
53. Paolo Zacchia (1584–1659), *Quaestiones medico-legales*, 7 vols. (Rome: Brugiotti, 1621–1635). Zacchia was the personal physician of Pope Innocent X.
54. The letter of February 22, 1586, is now published as an appendix to chapter 18 of the second edition of Girolamo Mercuriale's *De decoratione*. English translation from Gnudi and Webster, *The Life and Times of Gaspare Tagliacozzi*, 138.
55. "There have been several gentlemen—among whom Messer Sigismundus Barianus, a noble, Messer Alexander Vinstinus, also a noble, both of Piacenza, whose noses were cut off while they were duelling, Octavius Facinus, also of Piacenza, and a Fleming, Messer Henricus van Banesghem of Antwerp—for all of whom we restored noses so resembling

nature's pattern, so perfect in every respect that it was their considered opinion that they liked these better than the original ones which they had received from nature." In Gnudi and Webster, *The Life and Times of Gaspare Tagliacozzi*, 139.

56. The difference between the two techniques is explained by Ocsko (1537–1599), who had studied at the University of Bologna before returning to his native Poland in 1569. He judged the Vesalius method very difficult and recommended instead the one used by his professor, Giulio Cesare Aranzi: "Si serviva della pelle del bracci, e questo lembo di pelle si attecchiva al moncone del naso senza grandi dolori, come se fosse la pelle del naso stesso, lasciando non solo intatti i muscoli del braccio, ma formando anche un naso bello . . . Miracolosa davvero questa operazione, ma non occorre dirlo, richiede un paziente adatto, con buona complessione, perché negli individui col corpo guasto, non solo non atteschino (i lembi), ma producono spesso piaghe e il naso nuovo cadrà." See Eugenio Dall'Osso, "Giulio Cesare Aranzio e la rinoplastica," *Annali di medicina navale e tropicale* 61 (1956): 617–627, at 622. See also Arpad Fischer, "Rapporti tecnico-chirurgici in rinoplastica tra i Branca-Vianeo e Giulio Cesare Aranzio," *Coll. Pag. Storia Med.* 22 (1969): 79–90. I mentioned Aranzi (or Aranzio) in Chapter 1, when he was called to the Farnese court for a consult over princess Margherita's sexual anatomy.

57. "If trees of different types can be joined by means of a graft, albeit only after a long interval, and if one can take on the other's characteristics, then it should be a much simpler and swifter process to restore amputated parts to soundness with the help of suitable material. The skin of the upper arm (from which the graft is taken) is, after all, very similar in nature to the skin of the parts for which restoration is possible. Moreover, if the bark of one tree can coalesce with the bark of another, as in the case of inoculation, there is no reason to believe that skin, which is analogous to bark, cannot be firmly and safely conjoined to other parts of the same body." In Tagliacozzi, *De curtorum chirurgia per insitionem*, 61. For a detailed study of Tagliacozzi's technique, besides the work of Gnudi and Webster previously cited, see Corradi, "Dell'antica autoplastica italiana"; and Silvia Marinozzi, "The Vianeo and Gaspare Tagliacozzi: The Development of Rhinoplasty in the XV Century," *Medicina nei secoli* 11.3 (1999): 603–610.

58. See, respectively, chapters 17, 22, and 24 of Tagliacozzi's *De curtorum chirurgia per insitionem*.

59. For the identification of Tagliacozzi's arm flap as "the Italian method," see I. Eisenberg, "A History of Rhinoplasty," *South African Medical Journal* 62 (August 21, 1982): 286–292, at 288.

60. The soporific sponge was first used in the Middle Ages by the School of Salerno. To wake up the patient after surgery, a sponge imbibed in vinegar would usually be sufficient. For other techniques used for sedation

before surgery, see Blair O. Rogers, "Nasal Reconstruction 150 Years Ago: Aesthetic and Other Problems," *Aesthetic Plastic Surgery* 5 (1981): 283–327, at 287–288.

61. "Because the true nature of infection was unknown at that time and hygiene was neither prized nor practiced, it was estimated that up to the end of the eighteenth century, the mortality rate from all operations ranged from 50 to 80%, depending upon the type of operation performed." In Rogers, "Nasal Reconstruction 150 Years Ago," 291.
62. Tagliacozzi, *De curtorum chirurgia per insitionem*, 105.
63. Giovanni Marinello, *Gli ornamenti delle donne scritti per M. Giovanni Marinello. Et divisi in Quattro Libri* (Venice: Valgrisio, 1574), bk. 3, pt. 3, 149–150, "Nella quale si parla del Naso": "Il Naso è una di quelle parti del viso, che chi non la ha perfetta, non può apparere bello in profilo. Egli deve essere piccolo e affilato, e nel suo principio e base, che è sopra la bocca, e su la sua punta, e vuole con un segno di rivoltura mostrar quella distinta con un poco quasi di soprasalto, colorito, ma non rosso. . . . Ma, se un pochetto di rilevato, non aquilino: percioche in bella donna non sta bene. . . . Convengosi le nari asciutte, e nette. Non è bello il naso arricciato: percioche guasta il profilo."
64. Franco Rollo, M. Mascetti, and R. Cameriere, "Titian's Secret: Comparison of Eleonora Gonzaga della Rovere's Skull with the Uffizi Portrait," *Journal of Forensic Sciences* 50.3 (May 2005): 602–607.
65. See Paul Barosky, *Michelangelo's Nose: A Myth and Its Maker* (University Park: Penn State University Press, 1990).
66. "Quindi il naso per mezzo il viso scende, / che non trova l'invidia ove l'emende." In Ludovico Ariosto, *Orlando furioso*, ed. Marcello Turchi (Milan: Garzanti, 1974), 7.12. Amedeo Quondam canvasses the entire Petrarchist tradition to see why Laura's nose was not mentioned in "Il naso di Laura: considerazioni sul ritratto poetico e la comunicazione lirica," in his *Il naso di Laura. Lingua e poesia lirica nella tradizione del classicismo* (Modena: Panini, 1991).
67. As Stefano Guazzo (1530–1593) writes, "Par quasi ch'egli [the nose] sia più tosto soggetto da romanzi e da capitoli berneschi, dove piacevolmente si ragiona degli uomini nasuti." See *La civil conversatione del signor Stefano Guazzo* (Venice: Salicato, 1575), 304r.
68. Thomas Aquinas, *Summa theologica* (Paris: Blot, 1926), IV, sententiarum, 22, 25. For the case of eunuchs and castrati, see Valeria Finucci, *The Manly Masquerade: Masculinity, Paternity, and Castration in the Italian Renaissance* (Durham: Duke University Press, 2003), 256.
69. Otto Hildebrand, *Die Entwicklung der plastischen Chirurgie* (Berlin: Hirschwald, 1909), 9.
70. Cosimo de' Medici to Pedro Afán Ribera (Duque de Alcala), May 15, 1561: "Et quanto alli dua schiavi turchi ripresi approviamo che per exempio delli altri si faccia lor tagliare ambidue gli orecchi affatto e il naso, ma

non già che si cavi loro l'occhio, et ci piace che a chi gli ha trovati si faccia pagar il premio promesso a spese delle guardie," in ASF, MDP 211, DocID 8868.

71. As in this list of slaves at starboard of the ducal galley, "Toscana," of April 13, 1555: "Amor d'Affrica, d'anni 35, taglato la punta del naso venne d'Affrica [Medhia] col signor Giordano." In ASF, MDP 627, DocID 10868.
72. See, for example, Vincenzo Giusti, *Irene* (Venice: Gio. Battista Somasco, 1588).
73. Italo Calvino, "The Silver Nose," in *Italian Folktales* (London: Penguin, 2000).
74. See Klaus Van Eickels, "Gendered Violence: Castration and Binding as Punishment for Treason in Normandy and Anglo-Norman England," *Gender and History* 16.3 (2004): 588–602.
75. Margherita Costa, *Li buffoni* (1641), now in *Commedie dell'Arte* 2, ed. Siro Ferrone (Milan: Mursia, 1986).
76. Virgil, *Aeneid*, trans. Robert Fagues (London: Penguin, 2006), 6.493–496.
77. This was the punishment, for example, for Simeone. His sentence was later commuted to twenty-five lashes and banishment from Venice for five years. See Guido Ruggiero, *The Boundaries of Eros: Sex Crime and Sexuality in Renaissance Venice* (New York: Oxford University Press, 1985), 122. For a similar case in Florence, in which both the active and the passive partner were condemned to have their noses and ears cut off, see Michael Rocke, *Forbidden Friendships: Homosexuality and Male Culture in Renaissance Florence* (New York: Oxford University Press, 1996), 78. As Rocke notices, the two were also given the choice of paying fines instead, with the larger amount paid by the active partner. For cases of homosexuals whose noses were cut off in Nuremberg, see Valentin Groeber, *Defaced: The Visual Culture of Violence in the Late Middle Ages* (New York: Zone, 2004), 80. As he eloquently puts it: "Cutting off the nose, like similar ignominious punishments, functioned by pointing downward, or by defining a below" for men as well as women (82).
78. Jane Tibbetts Schulenburg, "The Heroics of Virginity: Brides of Christ and Sacrificial Mutilation," in *Women in the Middle Ages and the Renaissance: Literary and Historical Perspectives*, ed. Mary Beth Rose (Syracuse: Syracuse University Press, 1986), 29–72.
79. "This mutilation," he continues, "not a shameful one, but rather a proper and virtuous one, ensured that each woman's chastity, which she had promised to God, would remain intact." In Tagliacozzi, *De curtorum chirurgia per insitionem*, 25.
80. Giulio Mancini, *Del Disonore*, Biblioteca Apostolica Vaticana, Barb. Lat. 4314, 151v–152r.
81. Girolamo Fracastoro, *De contagionibus, morbisque contagiosis et eorum curatione. Libri tres*, in *Hieronymous Fracastorius and His Poetical and Prose Works*

on Syphilis, ed. and trans. William Riddell (Toronto: Canadian Social Hygiene Council, 1928), 8–25, at 9.

82. William Shakespeare, *Timon of Athens*, ed. Anthony Dawson and Gretchen Minton (London: Arden Shakespeare, 2008), 4.3.
83. The first documented repair of a saddle nose through a bone rather than a skin graft is dated 1896. The surgeon was James Israel in Berlin. See Sander Gilman, *Making the Body Beautiful: A Cultural History of Aesthetic Surgery* (Princeton: Princeton University Press, 1999), 57.
84. Giovanni Marinello provides a cure for a smelly nose in a chapter entitled "Il fiato puzzolente, che esce dal naso, con quali medicine curare si debba," of his *Gli ornamenti delle donne*, bk. 3, pt. 3, 150.
85. Giovanni della Casa (1503–1556), *Galateo, a Renaissance Treatise on Manners*, ed. and trans. Konrad Eisenbicher and Kenneth B. Bartlett (Toronto: CMRS, 1994).
86. Tycho Brahe's (1546–1601) astronomic observations were fully developed after his death by his student Johannes Kepler.
87. "Nel quale assalto fu tagliato il naso a Ricoverino de' Cerchi da uno masnadiere de' Donati . . . Il quale colpo fu la distruzione della nostra città, perché crebbe molto odio tra i cittadini." In Dino Compagni (1255–1324), *Cronica*, ed. Davide Cappi (Rome: Istituto Palazzo Borromini, 2000), 37. An English version is in *Dino Compagni's Chronicle of Florence*, trans. Daniel Bornstein (Philadelphia: University of Pennsylvania Press 1986), 25.
88. Annibal Caro (1507–1566), *La nasea*, in *Commento di ser Agresto da Ficaruolo sopra la prima ficata del padre Siceo* (Bologna: Romagnoli, 1961).
89. "Il naso risponde alla verga: ché avendolo alcuno lungo e grosso, overo acuto e grosso, o breve, il medesimo si giudica di quella; così le nari rispondono ai testicoli. Nasuti appresso Lampridio si dicono quelli che più maschi sono. Onde è il proverbio del naso assai volgare, dalla grandezza del naso conoscersi la sua grandezza." In Giambattista della Porta, *Della fisionomia dell'uomo*, ed. Mario Cicognani (Milan: Longanesi, 1971), ch. 7, "Del naso," 251. On Della Porta's treatise, see also Alfred David, "An Iconography of Noses: Directions in the History of a Physical Stereotype," in *Mapping the Cosmos*, ed. Jane Chance and R. O. Wells Jr. (Houston: Rice University Press, 1985); and Juliana Schiesari, "The Face of Domestication: Physiognomy, Gender Politics and Humanism's Others," in *Women, Race, and Writing in the Early Modern Period*, ed. Margot Hendricks and Patricia Parker (New York: Routledge, 1994), 55–70. Tagliacozzi too provides a list of the physiognomists' take on the shape of the nose to signify character in *De curtorum chirurgia per insitionem*, 27.
90. "Desiderarei che la Ser.ma mi honorassi di solecitare il Bronzino del mio ritratto aciò che questa [questi] altri imparirano a fare i nasi, poiché quello che fanno a me qua è per tre volte quello che fanno a San Carlo [Borromeo]." January 16, 1617, in ASF, MDP 2951.

91. Laurent Joubert, *Popular Errors*, trans. Gregory David de Rocher (Tuscaloosa: University of Alabama Press, 1989), 215. The Latin phrase is also used by Francois Rabelais in *Gargantua and Pantagruel*, in *Oeuvres complètes* (Paris: Editions du Seuil, 1995), XI.
92. "Il naso è parte spermatica, e però, se intieramente staccata, né cresce, né si conglutina quando sia rimessa." In Giovanni Andrea Della Croce (1514–1575), *Della cirurgia libri sette* (Venice: Ziletti, 1574), sec. 2, bk. 2, ch. 3. Croce, however, felt that a partially detached nose could be readjusted.
93. "Nel seicento . . . le operazioni più gravi, o che esigevano particolare maestria, non si facevano od erano lasciate ai norcini; ed i rinoplasti andavano uguagliati ai *castratori* dell'Umbria." In Corradi, "Dell'antica autoplastica italiana," 252.
94. Freud describes the gastric spot in relation to Dora's nose in "Fragment of an Analysis of a Case of Hysteria," in *The Standard Edition of the Complete Psychological Works of Sigmund Freud*, ed. and trans. James Strachey, vol. 7 (London: Hogarth Press, 1953), 3–122, at 78. For the correspondence between Freud and Fliess regarding reflex nasal neuroses, see *The Complete Letters of Sigmund Freud to Wilhelm Fliess, 1887–1904*, ed. and trans. Jeffrey Moussaieff (Cambridge: Harvard University Press, 1985), 45–48. See also Dianne Hunter, *Seduction and Theory: Readings of Gender, Representation, and Rhetoric* (Urbana: University of Illinois Press, 1989), 102.
95. Sander Gilman, "The Jewish Nose: Are Jews White? Or, the History of the Nose Job," in *Encountering the Other(s): Studies in Literature, History and Culture*, ed. Gisela Brinker-Gabler (New York: SUNY Press, 1995), 149–182.
96. J. C. (Joseph Constantine) Carpue (1664–1746), *An Account of Two Successful Operations for Restoring a Lost Nose from the Integuments of the Forehead* (London: Longman, Hurst, Rees, Orme, and Brown, 1816). See also Marinozzi, "I Vianeo e Gaspare Tagliacozzi," 607. The first account of such an Indian method was described in 1794 in a report of *The Gentlemen's Magazine* and involved a patient, named Cowasjee, who was operated on by Indian brickmakers. See Frank McDowell, *The Source Book of Plastic Surgery, Compiled and Edited by Frank McDowell* (Baltimore: Williams and Wilkins Company, 1977). Not many patients were surviving the procedure, according to the French doctor Baron Larrey, who vehemently opposed nasal surgeries. Writing in 1831 and citing no statistical support, he claims that in India, 99 out of 100 patients would die following the procedure out of pain or tetanus. See Rogers, "Nasal Reconstruction 150 Years Ago," 290.
97. Carl Ferdinand von Graefe (1787–1840), *Rhinoplastik* (Berlin: Reimer, 1818). See also Maxwell Maltz, *Evolution of Plastic Surgery* (New York: Froben Press, 1946), 223–225.
98. Johann Friedrich Dieffenbach (1782–1847), *Surgical Observations on the Restoration of the Nose and on the Removal of Polypi and Other Tumours from the*

Nostrils (London: Highley, 1833). Many plates illustrating Dieffenbach's method are in Rogers, "Nasal Reconstruction 150 Years Ago," 298–306.

99. Philippe Frédéric Blandin (1798–1849) and Johann Friedrich Dieffenbach (1792–1847) were contemporary surgeons. For the term "autoplasty," see Corradi, "Dell'antica autoplastica italiana."

100. Warren describes the procedure in "Rhinoplastic Operation," *Boston Medical and Surgical Journal* 16 (1837): 69. See also Rogers, "Nasal Reconstruction 150 Years Ago," 314–315.

101. "Essendo stato sepellito Gasparo Tagliacozzo Dottore di Medicina nella Chiesa delle Monache di S. Gio. Battista fù d'indi alcune settimane udita una voce in quel Monastero notificando la sua dannatione, per il che fù il suo corpo d'indi disoterrato, et portato alle mura, per la quale voce s'inspiritarono alcune Monache." This information is in Valerio Rinieri, *Diario*, vol. 4, c. 2v (1600), now in Gnudi and Webster, *The Life and Times of Gaspare Tagliacozzi*, 437.

102. Sbaraglia (1641–1693), also known for his polemic against Marcello Malpigli, participated in the debate on the uselessness of anatomy in 1689. He felt that the data doctors had on the body were therapeutically insufficient, and thus the humoral Galenic theory offered real value. Sbaraglia was specifically against microscopic anatomy. According to Webster and Gnudi, he was thus against Tagliacozzi. See their *Documenti inediti intorno alla vita di Gaspare Tagliacozzi*, 46, n. 2.

103. "After the malevolent actions of some persons envious of the fame of Tagliacozzi, who was accused of magic, had been discovered, his body was restored to its first place of burial with all the rightful solemnities and with the complete re-establishment of his fame, name and official dignity, and he was completely exonerated of the charges. Every act in paper against him was destroyed and a verdict of full absolution was given with, furthermore, the condemnation of the accusers and the persons declared guilty who, in addition to being obliged to deny their accusations, were also required to have themselves absolved of the judgment incurred. Thus it is annotated marginally in the chronicles of those times under the fifteenth of July 1600." See Gnudi and Webster, *The Life and Times of Gaspare Tagliacozzi*, 235–236. Further research from Pietro Capparoni has uncovered nothing new. See his "Le vicende della tomba di Gaspare Tagliacozzi" (Rome: Istituto Nazionale Medico Farmacologico Serono, 1933), 1–11; repr. from *Bollettino dell'Istituto Storico Italiano dell'Arte Sanitaria* 32.4 (July–August 1933).

104. "If the physician attempted to take the graft from a person other than that patient, the outcome would surely be imperiled. The skin flap must be firmly sutured to the mutilated nose or lips until the parts coalesce; moreover, we must restrict its motion as much as possible lest the delicate union be weakened. Would two people ever consent to being bound together so intimately and for so long? I certainly cannot imagine it. How

could the physician ensure the survival of the graft? . . . It is best, then, to leave this method unattempted. . . . It must be clear to everyone by now that the graft should be taken from the patient himself, because this method alone provides reliable results. Using another person's body as the source of the graft cannot produce anything but despair." In Tagliacozzi, *De curtorum chirurgia per insitionem*, 77.

105. Tommaso Campanella (1568–1639), *De sensu rerum et magia. Libri quatuor* (Frankfurt: Apud Emmelium, 1620), bk. 4, ch. 2, at 308.
106. Samuel Butler (1612–1680), *Hudibras*, ed. John Wilders (London: Clarendon Press, 1967), pt. 1, canto 1, lines 281–286.
107. "Juste à la mort du préteur, / tombait le nez de l'emprunteur, / et souvent dans la meme bière, / par justice et par bon accord / en remettait au gré du mort / le nez auprès de son derrière." In Voltaire (1694–1778), *Oeuvres completes* (Paris: Imprimerie de la Société Littéraire Typographique, 1785), 42: 413–414.
108. For a modern history, see Elizabeth Haiken, *Venus Envy: A History of Cosmetic Surgery* (Baltimore: Johns Hopkins University Press, 1999); Gabriella Glaser, *The Nose: A Profile of Sex, Beauty, and Survival* (New York: Simon and Schuster, 2002); Gilman, *Making the Body Beautiful*; and Virginia Bloom, *Flesh Wounds: The Culture of Cosmetic Surgery* (Los Angeles: University of California Press, 2003).

3. The Comfort Cure

1. Vincenzo's second crusade of 1597 did not bring any remarkable victory (the decisive attack on the fortress of Giavarrino—that is, Raab, the key to Hungary—on September 30 saw also the death in the field of the commander general, John of Prinistein) and did not come any closer to offering a resolution to the problem of the Ottomans' steady expansion to the West.
2. On April 12, 1601, Vincenzo had written a letter from Gratz to his personal physician, Paolo Caraccio (nicknamed il Contorti), asking him to solicit one of the alchemists at his court, a man named Pedrocca, to work on a chemical compound that could destroy, or at least sufficiently drug, the enemy so that he could take Canissa. The duke's order was put in motion, and a letter of August 28, 1600, by Cesare della Riviera communicated that the poison was ready and that if deemed not too deadly, more arsenic would need to be added. See Roberto Navarrini, "La guerra chimica di Vincenzo Gonzaga," *Civiltà mantovana* 4 (1969): 43–47.
3. Vincenzo had been given by the pope the title of general lieutenant to Generalissimo Gian Francesco Aldobrandini, the pope's nephew, but this title was not recognized by Aldobrandini or any of the other Italian commanders.

4. An anonymous contemporary chronicle of this crusade, titled "Relatione delle cose di Canissa," is in ASM, AG, busta 975, now in Giancarlo Malacarne, *Splendore e declino: da Vincenzo I a Vincenzo II (1587–1627)*, vol. 4 of *I Gonzaga di Mantova: Una stirpe per una capitale europea* (Modena: Il Bulino, 2007), 343–346.
5. For more on Vincenzo's third crusade, see Vincenzo Errante, "'Forse che sì forse che no': La terza spedizione del duca Vincenzo Gonzaga in Ungheria alla guerra contro il turco (1601) studiata su documenti inediti," *Archivio storico lombardo* 42.1 (1915): 15–114.
6. "Nel tempo più opportuno di travagliare et di proseguire a codesta impresa così ben disposta, mi trovo alcuni giorni oppresso da febbri, chè la quartana s'è fatta quasi quotidiana, con l'aggiunta della solita enfiaggine al ginocchio." In Errante, "'Forse che sì forse che no,'" 53. The *quartana* is an intermittent fever that comes every fourth day, to distinguish it from the *terzana*, which comes every third day. See Carlo Cipolla, *Miasmi e umori* (Bologna: Il Mulino, 1989), 117. We also know that Vincenzo was suffering from a not-too-indisposing *terzana* ("un poco di terzanella") on August 2, 1602, as his wife reports. See ASF, MDP 2943, DocId 5014. In time, the *terzana* and the *quartana* came to stand for all recurring fevers.
7. Letter by Striggio to Eleonora from Canissa, September 29, 1601, in Errante, "'Forse che si forse che no,'" 55.
8. For example, when he was sixteen, his secretary Marcello Donati felt that it was unhealthy for him to swim in a pool in Innsbruck, where he was visiting his sister, as noted in this letter of August 17, 1578, by Teodoro Sangiorgio to Vincenzo's father, Guglielmo: "L'altro hieri s'era posto in voler andar a nuotare in certo bagno, il che lo vietai co' qualche fatica, aitato dal S.r Marcello che disse ch'hera cosa mal sana." In ASM, AG, busta 546, 3/1.
9. The Roman doctor Andrea Bacci (1524–1600) lamented in his *De thermis* that for the people of his time, going to church had somehow substituted for going to the baths, as had been customary in Roman times. See *De thermis* (Venice: Valgrisi, 1571). Bacci's erudite commentary on therapeutic waters, especially those near Rome, made his book popular, and it was reprinted often. Pope Sixtus V later named him his archiater.
10. See Camillo Brunori (da Meldola) (1681–1756), *Il medico poeta, ovvero la medicina esposta in versi, e prose italiane* (Fabriano: Gregorio Marriotti, 1726), 292, 450.
11. "Qual dal Bulicame esce ruscello / che parton poi tra lor le peccatrici, / tal per la rena giù sen giva quello." (As issues from the Bulicame [a bubbling thermal place] a rivulet which then the sinful women share among themselves, so this ran down across the sand.) In Dante Alighieri, *Inferno*, ed. and trans. Charles Singleton (Princeton: Princeton University Press, 1970), 14:79–81.

12. Roy Porter, "The Patient's View: Doing Medical History from Below," *Theory and Society* 14 (1985): 175–198, at 186.
13. The inflammation of the bursa over the kneecap bone had already been recognized at the time as an occupational disease in various categories of workers, such as women and men doing repetitive joint movements, as in spinning. See Leonardo Botallo (1519–1588), *I doveri del medico e del malato,* ed. Leonardo Carerj and Anita Bogetti Fassone (Turin: UTET, 1981), 46.
14. Incidents while jousting were common. We know, for example, that Vincenzo suffered a serious hand injury in 1606 in a court tournament (the Giostra della Quintana). See ASF, MDP 4796, DocId 2945.
15. Adalberto Pazzini writes convincingly about rickets and also identifies a pathology affecting the Gonzaga line that comes from congenital malformations in the womb: obesity, a metabolic disease, which involved many members of the extended Gonzaga family. See Pazzini, "La medicina alla corte dei Gonzaga a Mantova," in *Mantova e i Gonzaga nella civiltà del Rinascimento,* ed. Accademia Nazionale dei Lincei (Mantua: Accademia Virgiliana, 1977), 291–351, at 306–310. The first important book on infantile rickets, Francis Glisson's (1599?–1677) *De rachitide, sive morbo puerili* (London: Sadler and Beaumont, 1650), classified the disease as a moist distemper caused by unequal bone growth. The role of vitamins in rickets was understood only in the nineteenth century.
16. Tuberculosis of the knee constitutes 28 percent of all kinds of tuberculosis in infancy and is secondary only to tuberculosis of the spine. See Giuseppe Canepa, *Osteopatologia infantile: manuale-atlante di ortopedia per pediatri* (Padua: Piccin, 1996), 348; and Halfdan Sundt, "The Diagnosis and Frequency of Tuberculous Disease of the Knee," *Journal of Bone and Joint Surgery* 13 (1931): 740–758, which also addresses cases of knee pathologies in syphilitic patients.
17. Today this abscess is easily cured with antibiotics.
18. After reading the report on the fistula, Cardinal Carlo Borromeo counseled Vincenzo to keep it more under control: "Il S.or Principe non dovrebbe curar così puoco come fa la ditta fistola." The information is in a letter by Aurelio Zibramonte to Duke Guglielmo Gonzaga of February 15, 1583, now in Giancarlo Malacarne, *Le feste del principe: giochi, divertimenti, spettacoli a corte* (Modena: Il Bulino, 2002), 88. The fistula was examined again following Vincenzo's "victorious" sexual tournament with Giulia at Francesco de' Medici's request (see Chapter 1).
19. See, for example, Thomas Benedek, "The History of Gold Therapy for Tuberculosis," *Journal of the History of Medicine and Allied Sciences* 59.1 (2004): 50–89; Philip Ellman and J. Stewart Lawrence, "Gold Therapy in Rheumatoid Arthritis," *British Medical Journal* 2 (1940): 314–316; and Chiara Crisciani, "Oro potabile fra alchimia e medicina: due testi in tempo di peste," in *Convegno nazionale di storia e fondamenti della chimica: L'Aquila,*

8–11 Ottobre 1987, ed. Franco Calascibetta (Rome: Accademia Nazionale delle Scienze, 1997), 83–93.

20. Vincenzo's correspondence with Giacomo Alvise Cornaro is illustrative of the duke's increasingly compelling desire to obtain potable gold not only, as it has been assumed, to find a solution to his debts but also for health reasons, as in the cited correspondence in which Cornaro declares that he has found a secure and easy method to make gold a most healthy medicament in a day ("trovato modo facile et sicuro di ridurre l'oro in medicamento salubrissimo in un giorno"). The letter to Vincenzo of August 6, 1607, is in Paola Goretti, "Limatura della luna argentea: La scienza dei magnifici apparati, tra malinconia, vestiario e vaghezze d'antico," in *Gonzaga: La Celeste Galeria. L'esercizio del collezionismo,* ed. Raffaella Morselli (Milan: Skira, 2002), 185–211, at 203.

21. Before undertaking a potable-gold cure offered to him in 1514, Duke Francesco asked that somebody else affected by the disease try it out first to confirm its value: "Uno che vol far aurum potabile per liberar il Sig. farassi experientia in uno affranciosato prima che il Sig. il pilia." In Pazzini, "La medicina alla corte dei Gonzaga," 317–318. Liquid gold was also used to coat pills to eliminate their foul taste, a custom that actually rendered the medicine useless, since gold is not absorbed by the body. The common Italian expression *indorare la pillola* (sweeten the pill) comes from this context. On the understanding that if something is costly it must be more beneficial, a number of expensive gelatinous facial creams and masks containing gold particles are once again being touted as having anti-aging, anti-inflammatory properties, and as being able to give the skin a plumped glow while also controlling pigmentation. Colloidal gold at $580 an ounce is indeed becoming the new facial elixir. See "Gold Face Cream: A Costly Leap of Faith," *New York Times,* May 27, 2010, E3. More generally, see Ernst Darmstaedter, "Per la storia dell'*aurum potabile,*" *Archivio di Storia della Scienza* 5.3 (1924): 251–271.

22. Tobacco was used not only in pills but also in lotions and in syrups; infusions of leaves were good in warm baths for syphilitics. For the use of tobacco to address a variety of health issues at the time, see Peter C. Mancall, "Tales Tobacco Told in Sixteenth-Century Europe," *Environmental History* 9.4 (2004): 648–678; and Alberico Benedicenti, *Malati, medici e farmacisti: storia dei rimedi traverso i secoli e delle teorie che ne spiegano l' azione sull'organismo* (Milan: Hoepli, 1924), 1:732, 1:741–742.

23. Marcello Donati, *De variolis et morbillis tractatus. . . . Eiusdem De radice purgante quam Mechioacan vocant* (Mantua: Philoterpsem et Philoponos, 1569). The book was even translated into French in 1572. See Attilio Zanca and Adriano Galassi, "Saggio di bibliografia medica mantovana rinascimentale," in *Mantova e i Gonzaga nella civiltà del Rinascimento,* ed. Accademia Nazionale dei Lincei (Mantua: Accademia Virgiliana, 1977), 399–421, at 407.

24. As in this letter to Vincenzo by his counselor Marcello Donati in 1589: "Mi spiace che ella sia inchodata dalla gotta." In ASM, AG, busta 2645, cited in Malacarne, *Splendore e declino: da Vincenzo I a Vincenzo II*, 85.
25. See Francesco Puccinotti, "Della rachitide," in *Opere complete edite ed inedite* (Naples: Pellerano, 1858), 1:117ff., cited in Pazzini, "La medicina alla corte dei Gonzaga a Mantova," 314. Rickets in the Gonzaga line was of course not determined by a bad diet.
26. See Thomas Benedek and Gerald Rodnan, "Petrarch on Medicine and the Gout," *Bulletin of the History of Medicine* 37 (1963): 397–416, esp. 408–409. In his old age, Petrarch moved permanently from Venice to the nearby town of Arquà, south of Padua, perhaps because of the proximity of the *stufe* of Abano and Montegrotto, where he could cure his ailments. We know he was in Montegrotto in 1365, probably to resolve a skin disease. See Paolo Ghedino, " 'Dilettose venete fonti': Le terme di Abano, Montegrotto, Battaglia, Galzignano e Teolo," in *Alle fonti del piacere: la civiltà termale e balneare fra cura e svago*, ed. Nelli-Elena Vanzan Marchini (Milan: Leonardo Arte, 1999), 102–117, at 105. For more on the distinction between gout and other joint diseases, such as rheumatoid arthritis, osteoarthritis, and ankylosing spondylitis, see Roy Porter and G. S. Rousseau, *Gout: The Patrician Malady* (New Haven: Yale University Press, 1998), 7–10.
27. The diagnosis by rheumatologist Frank Arnett at the University of Texas Medical School in Houston was made at a historical clinicopathological conference sponsored by the University of Maryland School of Medicine in 2005. See http://www.umm.edu/news/releases/columbus.htm.
28. Thomas Sydenham (1624–1689), *Methodus curandi febres, propriis observationibus superstructa* (London: Crook, 1666), cited in Porter and Rousseau, *Gout: The Patrician Malady*, 8.
29. "Non havendo potuto continovare nell'uso d'altri medicamenti giudicati a proposito per rimediare alle indispositioni che mi vengono cagionate da questo mio catarro, son consigliato da medici a ritornarmene quest'anno ancora a pigliar l'acque delli Bagni di Spa per dove ritrovandomi quasi di partita, ho voluto darne parte a V. Alt.zza. . . . Resta qui al gioverno la Duchessa mia." In ASF, MDP 2943, DocID 5011.
30. "Il Duca di Mantova Vincenzo Gonzaga è venuto qua per farsi alla marina alcuni bagni per un ginocchio che l'ha offeso di catarri." In Anon., "Racconto delle cose successe in Genova dall'anno 1600 fino al 1610," Ms. Seventeenth century, fol. 1373, July 6, 1607, in Archivio del Comune, Genoa, Fondo Brignole Sale, 109. D. 4. Vincenzo had already been in Genoa for an official visit in 1592, when he was magnificently hosted. See Achille Neri, "Il duca di Mantova a Genova nel 1592," *Archivio storico lombardo* 13 (1886): 113–126.
31. "Mentre sua eccellenza è stata oppressa dal catarro dicono c'habbi fatto voto d'andar alla santa casa di Loreto con la signora duchessa sua mo-

glie." In ASM, AG, busta 1735, now in Roberta Piccinelli, ed., *Le collezioni Gonzaga: Il carteggio tra Milano e Mantova (1563–1634)* (Milan: Silvana Editoriale, 2003), 432. Vincenzo went back to Loreto at least one additional time, in 1605, stopping in Assisi as well, and then went incognito to Rome in order to further the canonization of his relative Luigi Gonzaga. See Federigo Amadei, *Cronaca universale della città di Mantova* (Mantua: CITEM, 1956), 3:215.

32. See Amadei, *Cronaca universale della città di Mantova*, 3:279.
33. Shigehisa Kuriyama, "The Forgotten Fear of Excrement," *Journal of Medieval and Early Modern Studies* 38 (2008): 413–442, at 422–423.
34. Giovanni Tommaso Minadoi, *De arthritide* (Padua: Bolzetta, 1602). See also Lucia Samaden, "Giovanni Tommaso Minadoi (1548–1615): da medico della 'nazione' veneziana in Siria a professore universitario a Padova," *Quaderni per la storia dell'università di Padova* 31 (1998): 91–164, at 159–160.
35. Richard Lower (1631–1691), *De catarrhis*, ed. Richard Hunter and Ida Macalpine (London: Dawsons of Pall Mall, 1963), 10.
36. Ibid., 11. On the importance of managing perspiration for Santorio Santorio, a professor of medical theory in Padua who monitored his daily solid and liquid intake and discharge in *De statica medicina* (1614), see Lucia Dacome, "Balancing Acts: Picturing Perspiration in the Long Eighteenth Century," in *Studies in History and Philosophy of Biological and Biomedical Science* 43 (2012): 379–391.
37. Katharine Park, "Natural Particulars: Medical Epistemology, Practice, and the Literature of Healing Springs," in *Natural Particulars: Nature and the Disciplines in Renaissance Europe*, ed. Anthony Grafton and Nancy Siraisi (Cambridge: MIT Press, 1999), 347–367, at 348.
38. "Io parlai iersera a parecchi medici: l'uno dice che io vadia a San Filippo, l'altro alla Porretta, e l'altro alla Villa; e' mi parvono parecchi uccellacci, e a dirti il vero, questi dottori di medicina non sanno quello che si pescono." In Niccolò Machiavelli, *Mandragola*, ed. Nino Borsellino (Rome: Newton and Compton, 1996), 35–36. English version from *Five Comedies from the Italian Renaissance*, ed. and trans. Laura Giannetti and Guido Ruggiero (Baltimore: Johns Hopkins University Press, 2003), 78.
39. Ventura Minardo, *De balneis Calderii in agro veronensi* and *Compendio delle regole contenute ne gli Eccellentissimi Autori, che de' bagni di Caldiero nel territorio veronese hanno scritto del modo di usar dette acque e fango* (Venice: Ad instantiam Alexandri F. Thomae de Salodiis, 1571). The list occupies five pages in the treatise, 9v–11v.
40. Antonio Filarete, *Treatise on Architecture*, ed. and trans. John R. Spencer (New Haven: Yale University Press, 1965), 1:294.
41. Lampridio Anguillara, *Vaticinio et avertimenti per conservare la sanità, et prolongar la vita humana* (Ferrara: Vittorio Baldini, 1589), 18–19.
42. David S. Chambers, "Federico Gonzaga ai bagni di Caldiero," *Civiltà mantovana*, n.s. 4 (1984): 45–61, at 48–49.

43. Ibid., 50.
44. Bathhouses too provided bloodletting, cupping, and massage to their clientele, both male and female. See Mary Fissell, "Introduction: Women, Health, and Healing in Early Modern Europe," *Bulletin of the History of Medicine* 82 (2008): 1–17, at 12.
45. Paola Malatesta was in Petriolo from February 20 to September 3, and spent a considerable amount of money. See Giuseppe Coniglio, *I Gonzaga* (Milan: Dall'Oglio, 1967), 50; Attilio Portioli, *I Gonzaga ai bagni di Petriolo presso Siena nel 1460–61* (Mantua: Eredi Segna, 1870); and Pazzini, "La medicina alla corte dei Gonzaga a Mantova," 310.
46. "Smontati et intrati in camera, esso sig. Bonifacio prese licentia et lo Ill. mo S.mio [Ludovico II Gonzaga], spogliatosi et postassi una turca in dosso, s'è posto a zugar a scacchi, et nel vero, fino qui non gli è alcuno se sia meglio mantenuto." Letter of Francesco Secco to Barbara Hohenzollern, April 30, 1475, in ASM, AG, busta 745. On May 9, 1460, Ludovico asked for books: "Per lo primo corriere vi accaderà mandare in qua, vedite mandarmi el Lucano nostro e Quinto Curtio . . . et mandarne ancora quello Augustino *De civitate Dei*." In ASM, AG, busta 2096, c. 126r. Now both in Malacarne, *Le feste del principe,* 173, 176.
47. Gabriele Falloppio, "De medicatis aquis," in *Opera genuina omnia* (Venice: De Franciscis, 1606). A student of his, Andrea Marcolini—*ipsius discipulo amantissimo,* as he presents himself in the title (we encountered him in Chapter 1)—published posthumously a cycle of lectures by Falloppio on thermal waters, *De thermalibus aquis atque de fossilibus* (Venice: Ziletti, 1564). I thank Maurizio Rippa Bonati for this reference. Falloppio's booklet was also translated into English by Robert Leese as "A Brief View of All Baths." The manuscript is in the Folger Shakespeare Library's collection. See Jean Dietz Moss, "The Promotion of Bath Waters by Physicians in the Renaissance," in *Rhetoric and Medicine in Early Modern Europe,* ed. Stephen Spender and Nancy Struever (Aldershot: Ashgate, 2012), 61–82.
48. Michel de Montaigne, *Journal de voyage de Michel de Montaigne . . . en Italie . . . en 1580 et 1581* (Rome and Paris: Le Jay, 1774).
49. For Vincenzo's case, see Martha Tech Gnudi and Jerome Pierce Webster, *The Life and Times of Gaspare Tagliacozzi* (New York: Reichner, 1950), 178n. For Francesco's case, see Pazzini, "La medicina alla corte dei Gonzaga."
50. The information is in a letter of Guidobono Guidoboni to the ducal counselor Tullio Petrozzani of July 30, 1591, from Prague: "Il signor ambasciatore di Spagna [Guillén de San Clemente], al quale ho fatto sapere la benigna cura presa da sua altezza nostro signore [Vincenzo Gonzaga] in ordinare al signor medico Salamonio la relatione sopra li bagni d'Acqui conforme a quello che vostra signoria mi scrisse, ne rende dovute grazie all'altezza sua et starà aspettando detta relatione." In ASM, AG, busta 465, fol. 1, cc. 260–261, now in *Le collezioni Gonzaga: Il carteggio tra la Corte*

Cesarea e Mantova (1559–1636), ed. Elena Venturini (Milan: Silvana Editoriale, 2002), 338.

51. "Consigliato da questi miei Medici, et da altri ancora son sforzato ad esseguire hora quello che per confermarmi in buona salute pensai di fare sin' l'anno passato, cioè di transferirmi in Fiandra a pigliar l'acque delli Bagni di Spa, le quali mi vengono sopramodo commendate per singolar rimedio della mia indispositione. Credo che la partita mia di qua sarà verso il fine di questo mese." In ASF, MDP 2942, DocID 4991.
52. "Havendo io havuto ultimamente avviso dal S. Duca et da' suoi che S. Alt. si ritrovava verso il fine del pigliar quell'acqua della fonte di Spa, et che ne sentiva già notabile giovamento, ho voluto darne la nova a V. S. acciocchè la participi al Ser.mo Gran Duca mio Zio." In ASF, MDP 2942, DocID 4996.
53. To Ferdinando de' Medici he wrote: "Sapendo io che l'A.V. sentirà quell contento del mio ritorno di Fiandra, Dio gratia, con buona salute, et con molto miglioramento dell'indispositione per la quale mi trasferij colà . . . vengo con questa a darlene parte." In ASF, MDP 2942, DocId 4998. To Christine de Lorraine he gave the same news: "Non volendo io lassar passare occasione alcuna con la quale io possa ragguagliare V. A. dello stato mio, vengo con questa a darle parte del mio ritorno di Fiandra, Dio lodato con prospera salute, et con molto miglioramento dell'indispositione per la quale me ne passai a pigliare l'acque dei bagni di Spa." In ASF, MDP 2945, DocID 4788.
54. "Sono cinque giorni che S. A. si beve, et adesso si piglia cent' once ogni mattina, suda molto et anco la passa per l'orina; non si può se non sperarsi buono effetto, che piaccia a Dio concedergli." In ASM, AG, E. XI.3, busta 574.
55. Letter of Hercole Achilli from Spa to Annibale Chieppio in Mantua, August 5, 1599. By August 12, Vincenzo was in Liège. In ASM, AG, E. XI.3, busta 574.
56. For Henri III's visit to Spa, see L. W. B. Brockliss, "The Development of the Spa in Seventeenth-Century France," *Medical History*, Supplement 10 (1990): 23–47, at 25.
57. Ferrante II Gonzaga di Guastalla wrote from Lièges to Fabio Gonzaga in July 3, 1590: "Son venuto a Spa et o pigliata quest'acqua venti giorni de la quali mi ritrovo benissimo gratia a Dio." In ASF, MDP 2941, DocID 4837.
58. As in this letter of Antonio Costantini from Nancy to Andrea Cioli in Florence, May 17, 1619, regarding Vincenzo's II visit of 1619: "Il S.r Principe Don Vincenzo è per inviarsi a questa volta fra pochi giorni andandosene alli bagni di Spa per consiglio de' medici per rimediare ad un certo suo ordinario dolor di testa." In ASF, MDP 2951, DocID 5542.
59. Spa "giova ad infiniti mali, come S. A. potrà notare dal qui alligato libretto, ch'io li mando in lingua francese." The letter of July 26, 1599, is in ASM, AG, E. XI.3, busta 574.

60. Letter of Ferdinando Persia to Annibale Chieppio, July 26, 1599, in ASM, AG, E. XI.3, busta 574.
61. Although we are led to assume by contemporary commentators that women were often taking the baths half-naked, this was not necessarily the case. When Queen Elizabeth went to take the hot waters of Charing Cross upon the recommendation of her doctors to address her crippling rheumatism, we are told that she immersed herself fully clothed, gloves and ruffle collar included. See Doretta Davanzo Poli, "La moda ai bagni di moda," in *Alle fonti del piacere,* ed. Nelli-Elena Vanzan Marchini, 77–99, at 78.
62. "Tutto è venuto a notitia di questa corte con poca sua riputatione, se pur sono vere le dette cose." The letter, which has no sender and addressee, is in ASF, MDP 4255, DocID 25843.
63. "Alli 8 di giugno 1602, in sabato, il serenissimo nostro signor duca Vincenzo partì da Mantova con una nobilissima compagnia de cavaglieri mantovani per andare in Fiandra et, per quanto ho inteso, al bagno nell villaggio di Spa, dove andò anco l'altra volta come di sopra, havendo il giorno istesso disinato cone le serenissime moglie et sorella duchessa di Ferrara et anco tutti gli figliuoli al pallazzo di Porto, nel giardino del quale doppo il detto pranso, fu ricetato una bellissima comedia." In Giovanni Battista Vigilio, *La insalata. Cronaca mantovana dal 1561 al 1602,* ed. Daniela Ferrari and Cesare Mozzarelli (Mantua: Gianluigi Arcari Editore, 1992), ch. 133, 63v, at 119.
64. Letter of May 17, 1602, in ASF, MDP 2943, DocID 5011.
65. She wrote to her uncle in June 21, 1602, that she was sending him some men condemned to the galleys to serve in the Tuscan fleet, in the absence of her husband, gone to the baths at Spa: "Trovandosi qui gli infrascritti destinati al remo, ho dato ordine in assenza del Sig.r Duca mio, che come sa V.A. è andato alli bagni di Spa, che sieno consignati secondo 'l solito all'Ambasciatore suo in Modona perche venghino a servire nelle galere della A.V." In ASF, MDP 2943, DocID 16223.
66. "Dopo havere comminciato a ripigliar forze il Sig.re Duca mio è passato in Bressana [Bresciana] e alla volta del Lago d'Ise [Iseo], paese di molte delitie per mutar aria, conforme al riccordo datole da Vostra Alt.za così anco persuaso da medici, sperandosi che per la buona stagione che passa et per la perfettione dell'aria di quei luoghi sia per riaversi affatto della sua pristina sanità." In ASF, MDP 2943, DocId 5019.
67. "Il medico incaricato di difendere la salute del principe bisogna che adotti prudenza ed un atteggiamento di ricerca dovendo arrivare non solo a conoscere la natura dell'aria che egli respira, ma anche ad armonizzarla al suo temperamento ed a procurargli una giusta traspirazione in relazione alla caratteristica del suo organismo che può essere robusto o gracile." In Bernardino Ramazzini, *La salute dei principi ovvero come difendersi dalle malattie e dai medici,* ed. Francesco Carnevale (Florence: Tosca, 1992), 45.

68. Among the health tourists who visited the place in later years was the poet and novelist Alessandro Manzoni (1785–1873), who attempted to address his liver problems.
69. In Naples Vincenzo brought along a retinue of eight ministers, eleven or twelve gentlemen of the Chamber, his secretarial staff, servants for any possible need, as well as his son Francesco and his own court. Upon arrival he was received by the viceroy and was offered an array of entertainments and banquets, including a tournament: "All'incontro il Duca proseguì a Napoli, ove da quel Vice-Re fu ricevuto con grandi onori e servito di vari divertimenti, ed in ispecie d'un nobilissimo torneo, di armoniose serenate e lauti banchetti nel dilizioso Posillipo ed in altri luoghi ameni." In Amadei, *Cronaca universale della città di Mantova*, 3:201.
70. There were a number of booklets circulating at the time on the bath culture of the era, such as Scipione Mazzella, *Opusculum de Balneis Puteolanum Baiarum et Pithecusarum* (Naples: Ex typographia Stelliolae, 1593). See also Sean Cocco, *Watching Vesuvius: A History of Science and Culture in Early Modern Italy* (Chicago: University of Chicago Press, 2012).
71. Agnano itself lies in a volcano crater, which after an eruption in 1198 became filled with water. This created a four-mile-long lake, which was eventually drained in the nineteenth century to clear it of malaria.
72. A long list of emperors, from Nero to Hadrian, had visited the area regularly or had built their villas there. Cicero called the place "a little Rome" (*pusilla Roma*), and Cornelius Celsus and Galen praised its water as miraculous. Gnaeus Cornelius had already found relief in the Cumane springs for his arthritis by the 2nd century B.C.
73. Pozzuoli was the most important port in Italy under the Romans and was connected to Baiae by a pontoon bridge built by Caligula.
74. C. M. Kauffmann, *The Baths of Pozzuoli: A Study of the Medieval Illuminations of Peter of Eboli's Poem* (Oxford: Bruno Cassirer, 1959), 19.
75. "I soliti rimedi delli fumaroli che si dicono di Agnano . . . e domenica prossima giorno della Pentecoste fu l'ultima volta a prendere ditti fumaroli." These steam vents induced "sudori in molta copia che si spera possano col tempo apportarle molto di giovamento." In Anon. "Narrativa di tutto il viaggio di S.A. nel regno di Napoli de l'anno 1603," Archivio Generale di Sinancas, Estado Napoles, leg. 1099, fol. 44, April 30, 1603, in ASM, AG, busta 388, cc. 418–438. See also Coniglio, *I Gonzaga*, 376.
76. Giovanni Boccaccio, *L'elegia di Madonna Fiammetta* (Florence: Moutier, 1829), 91–92.
77. See Amadei, *Cronaca universale della città di Mantova*, 3:258, 3:283. Vincenzo names this son in his last will as being circa nine years of age at the time ("filium Illegitimum nomine Franciscus etatis annorum nove circuiter"). See ASM, AG, busta 330, fols. 297r–298r.
78. Pourbus completed two portraits but was unable to send the duke his most desired painting, that of a noblewoman named Spinelli, which only arrived

in Mantua later that year. After Pourbus left, a second Flemish painter was left in charge of finishing the commissioned portraits, which were sent to Mantua in January 1608. See Roberta Piccinelli, "Le *facies* del collezionismo artistico di Vincenzo Gonzaga," in *Gonzaga: La Celeste Galeria, L'esercizio del collezionismo,* ed. Raffaella Morselli, 342. In the same book, see also Italo Iasiello, "Vincenzo I e il Regno di Napoli," 357–362.

79. "Correva l'anno 1607 e il duca Vincenzo sui primi di maggio si era condotto a diporto sul lago di Garda, donde si restituì a Mantova 'molto risentito del dolore al ginocchio.'" In Achille Neri, "Il Duca di Mantova a San Pier D'Arena," *Giornale ligustico,* 160.

80. See Amadei, *Cronaca universale della città di Mantova,* 3:60.

81. Letter of June 23, 1607, from Van Manin [last name illegible], in which he declares himself delighted of the charge. In ASM, AG, E. XXI.3, busta 777, cc. 709r–710v). He also states the reason clearly: "Sendo ritornato [di Corsica] due giorni sono, ho trovato una lettera del Mons. Iberti, che mi avvisa la risoluzione fatta da V. A. d'andar alli bagni di Spa" (711r).

82. The letter of Annibale Iberti, stating that Vincenzo gave the order to bring him water from Spa, is dated July 7, 1607: "Pigliar et condursi in Italia del'acqua di Bagni di Spa in Fiandra." In ASM, AG, E. XXI.3, busta 777, c. 520r.

83. Letter of Iberti from Sampierdarena to the Gonzaga court, August 1, 1607, in ASM, AG, E. XXI.3, busta 777, c. 552r. As for containers, we know from a letter that when the weather was not conducive to a personal visit to the spring, the hot water was brought in *zucche* to keep it at a warm temperature for a while. See Chambers, "Federico Gonzaga ai Bagni di Caldiero," 47.

84. Cornaro to Vincenzo, May, 11, 1602: "Intendendo che ella è per andare in Fiandra, per fare l'acqua di Spa . . . posso affermare che portate in Italia non perdono di virtù, ancorché si riscaldino co'l fuoco, potendosi anco riscaldare in vaso d'argento coperto in modo che non possa essalare vapore alcuno." In ASM, AG, busta 1534, fol. 3, cc. 492–493, now in Michaela Sermidi, ed., *Le collezioni Gonzaga: Il carteggio tra Venezia e Mantova (1588–1612)* (Milan: Silvana Editoriale, 2003), 304. In the same letter, Cornaro wrote that he used water from Spa to make a medicinal drink as healthy as that of Spa, but better tasting. The issue of whether mineral waters lost their property when taken away from the original spring had been addressed at the time by a number of doctors with uneven recommendations. For Michele Savonarola, it was better to use water *in loco*. See Savonarola, *De balneis et thermis naturalibus omnibus Italiae,* in *De balneis omnia quae extant apud Graecos, Latinos, et Arabas,* ed. Tomaso Giunta (Venice: Giunta, 1553), 2.3, fol. 16v.

85. Letter of Annibale Iberti from Sampierdarena to Vincenzo's son, Francesco, July 8, 1607, in ASM, AG, E. XXI.3, busta 777, cc. 522r–523r.

86. "Coi bagni dell'acqua di mare che piglia in casa." In ASM, AG, E. XXI.3, busta 777, 533r.
87. Writing in 1602, Bartolomeo Paschetti (fl. 1578–1616) judged these waters better than those of Lombardy for drinking too, for they were "very light and good." See his *Del conservare la sanità, et del vivere de' Genovesi,* in *Del conservare la sanità di Bartolomeo Pascetti,* ed. Gino Fravega (Pisa: Tip. Giradini, 1964). See also Stephanie Hanke, "Bathing 'all'antica': Bathrooms in Genoese Villas and Palaces in the Sixteenth Century," *Renaissance Studies* 20.5 (2006): 674–700; and Maria Rosa Moretti, *Musica e costume a Genova: Tra Cinquecento e Seicento* (Genoa: Pirella, 1990), 56, 58.
88. "Hora che mi trovo alcuni di sono in questa villa di San Pietro d'Arena fuori di Genova per usar certi bagni." In ASF, MDP 2444, DocID 5074. The use of wooden tubs to keep mineral water extended to a good number of resorts. Galileo, for example, was in the habit of getting them brought from Abano to Padua when he was living there. In Tomaso Giunta, ed., *De balneis omnia quae extant apud Graecos, Latinos, et Arabas* (Venice: Giunta, 1553)—a collection of approximately seventy short treatises on baths from Roman times up to the date of publication in Venice—the Paduan doctor Ludovico Pasini remarks that this was usually done by the nobility, as in the case of Duke Alfonso I of Este. Among the sixteenth century writers in *De balneis* we find well-known doctors: Girolamo Cardano, Nicolò Massa, and Bernardino Tomitano. Representing the fifteenth century is Michele Savonarola, as already mentioned.
89. "Il Duca di Mantova Vincenzo Gonzaga è venuto qua per farsi alla marina alcuni bagni per un ginocchio che l'ha offeso di catarri." In Anon., "Racconto delle cose successe in Genova dall'anno 1600 fino al 1610."
90. Letter of Iberti from Sampierdarena to the Gonzaga court, July 21, 1607, in ASM, AG, E. XXI.3, busta 777, c. 537r.
91. "Et si gli sli è enfiata la gamba . . . dalli dolori." Letter of Iberti from Sampierdarena, August 21, 1607, in ASM, AG, E. XXI.3, busta 777, c. 570r.
92. See Moretti, *Musica e costume a Genova,* 58–59.
93. "La sera [Vincenzo] si gode la riviera dove han cominciato a concorrere molte dame per vedere et per essere vedute, sebben ancor non si è venuto a stringere conversatione con loro." In Achille Neri, "Il duca di Mantova a San Pier d'Arena," 161.
94. See Moretti, *Musica e costume a Genova.*
95. "Era aspettato in Mantova hieri sera il Signor Duca con non poca mala satisfattione di quei del suo sangue e de' suoi sudditi, havendo egli in questo suo viaggio di Genova fatto per semplice inclinatione di questi ct di giovu consumato presso a cento mille scudi che haveriano potuto servire a miglior uso per i bisogni della sua casa che non sono pochi." In Vincenzo Errante, "'Forse che sì forse che no,'" 25–26.

96. Letter of June 20, 1608, from Eleonora to her uncle, who had sent the medicinal gift of a porcupine stone for Vincenzo. She wrote that her husband had left two days earlier. ASF, MDP 2944, DocID 5099.
97. Fabrici sent the box right away: "Mando a V.A. Ser.ma un scatolino de pillole, et mi piace ch'ella seguiti di usarle, perché con queste, piacendo al S.re, viverà longo tempo et sana." In ASM, AG, E, XLV.3, busta 1540. See also Giuseppe Favaro, "Girolamo Fabrici d'Acquapendente e la medicina pratica," *Bollettino dell'Istituto Storico Italiano dell'Arte Sanitaria* 7.1 (1927): 1–10, at 8.
98. See ASF, MDP 4256, DocId 23079. Roberta Piccinelli puts the departure date for the Catholic Flanders at September 5, 1608; see "Le *facies* del collezionismo artistico di Vincenzo Gonzaga," in *Gonzaga*, ed. Morselli, 47.
99. The letter from Fra' Gregorio is addressed to Vincenzo's son, Ferdinando Gonzaga: "Il Ser. Sig. Duca è tuttavia travagliato della gamba ma spera liberarsene presto." In ASM, AG, Serie F. fasc. 2. See also Leonardo Mazzoldi, "Vita cittadina del primo '600: Lettere inedite dell'Archivio Gonzaga," *Bollettino Storico Mantovano* 3 (1956): 200–213, at 204.
100. Letter of Giovanni Pietro Tornatore to the ducal conselor Annibale Iberti, March 16, 1611, from Milan: "Mentre sua eccellenza è stata oppressa dal catarro dicono c'habbi fatto voto d'andar alla santa casa di Loreto con la signora duchessa sua moglie, et che dopo Pasqua partirà alla volta di Parma per tener a battesimo quel principe. Per pigliar qualche sollevamento par che dissegni sua eccellenza d'andar a Sesto a goder delle delitie d'un giardino, fontane e palazzo del signor Benedetto Pieno, qual fa preparamenti per ricevere l'eccellenza sua." In ASM, AG, busta 1735, now in Roberta Piccinelli, ed., *Le collezioni Gonzaga: Il carteggio tra Milano e Mantova (1563–1634)* (Milan: Silvana Editoriale, 2003), 432.
101. Gonzalo Fernández de Oviedo (1478–1557), *Historia General y Natural de las Indias* (Madrid: Nabu Press, 2010); Antonio de Herrera y Tordesillas (1559–1625), *Historia general de los hechos de los castellanos en las islas y tierra firme de el mar Oceano* (Madrid: Emplenta Real, 1601–1615). In the fourth installment of the recent film saga *Pirates of the Caribbean,* subtitled *On Stranger Tides,* Captain Sparrow's journey is meant to locate the fountain of youth.

4. The Sexual Cure

1. Dante Alighieri, *Il Convivio,* trans. Richard Lansing (New York: Garland, 1990), 4:24.
2. Until 1776 not only Cuzco in Peru but also La Paz, Quito, and Potosí in Bolivia, as well as Panama, belonged to the viceroyalty of Peru.
3. "Il signor cavaliere Emanuel Cimenes, . . . è quello che ha quel verme che con vostra altezza trattai, et oltre a quello credo che habbia molti segreti." In ASM, AG, busta 1126, fol. 5, c. 185, now in Roberta Piccinelli, ed., *Le*

collezioni Gonzaga: Il carteggio tra Firenze e Mantova (1554–1626) (Milan: Silvana Editoriale, 2002), 219.

4. "Serenissimo Signore, stante l'ordine da V.A. m'informai et trovo che nel Isola de Carga, per legue trenta discosto da la Città di Ozmus su la bocqa del Eufrates, si trova un genero di rane [grane?] da Portuguesi chiamato Carangolo de Carga, quale tenuto [sentito?] in mano facci l'effetto acennatomi V. A. Ser.ma. Però questi debbono essere rarissimi poi che uno portoguese altro che ha servito là per soldato, mi afferma non ne avere maj visto si bene sentitolo dire. Onde per la incertitudine esorterei piuttosto V.A. Ser.ma al fare l'essencia o olio di Perle per qualche mese che se fuora de ogni pericolo, et in pochi mesi fa notabile effetto et la estrattione di satyrione, di che V.A. sé degnata prendere un vasetto qui, fa similemente efetto grande." In ASM, AG, E. XI.3, busta 575, c. 865.

5. Raffaello Putelli, *Il duca Vincenzo I Gonzaga e l'interdetto di Paolo V a Venezia* (Venice: Istituto Veneto di Arti Grafiche, 1911).

6. During Vincenzo's life, this portrait and similar others were displayed prominently in the ducal palace. For more on the activity of Pourbus in Mantua, see Donatella Mattioli, "Fiamminghi a Mantova tra Cinque e Seicento," in Mulazzani et al., *Rubens a Mantova* (Milan: Electa, 1977), 68–86. For more in general about portraits of Vincenzo, mostly now belonging to private collections, see Paolo Bertelli, "Appunti sulla ritrattistica di Vincenzo I Gonzaga," in *Scritti per Chiara Tellini Perina*, ed. Daniela Ferrari and Sergio Marinelli (Mantua: Arcari, 2011), 229–249. I borrow the description of the duke as alert and erect from Patricia Simons, "Alert and Erect: Masculinity in Some Italian Renaissance Portraits of Fathers and Sons," in *Gender Rhetorics: Postures of Dominance and Submission in History*, ed. Richard C. Trexler (Binghampton: MRTS, 1994), 162–186.

7. Morosini's comment is in *Relazioni degli ambasciatori veneti al senato*, ed. Arnaldo Segarizzi (Bari: Laterza, 1912), 1:87–111, at 91. See also Giuseppe Coniglio, *I Gonzaga* (Milan: Dall'Oglio, 1867), 391.

8. The missive from 1547 in which Aretino, boasting of his "quaranta volte il mese," sets himself apart from those who luxuriate only once a year, is in his *Lettere*, ed. Paolo Procaccioli (Rome: Salerno, 1997–2002), 4:188–190.

9. Letter of March 6, 1608, in ASM, AG, busta 2712, fasc. 23, n. 41, now in Leonardo Mazzoldi, "Vita cittadina del primo '600: Lettere inedite dell'Archivio Gonzaga," *Bollettino Storico Mantovano* 3 (1956): 202–213, at 206.

10. Giuseppe Verdi, *Rigoletto* (New York: Riverrun, 1982), 1.1: "Questa o quella per me pari sono. La costanza, tiranna del core, detesto qual morbo crudele."

11. Or, as the old *Diccionario de autoridades* of the Real Academia Española, which also explains old words, puts it, "Qualquier insecto largo y delgado, de varios colores y figuras, que se cria en la tierra, en el agua, en los cuerpos vivos y en los muertos." Today there are more than 4,400 named

species of worms on the planet, making it difficult to identify precisely this *gusano*.
12. Bellonci, *Segreti dei Gonzaga*, 289.
13. The cantharis, the Venetian doctor Giovanni Marinello writes, was particularly helpful when pulverized with the penis of a bull and that of a deer, mixed with black pepper, ginger, cardamom, borax, pine nuts, pistachios, satyrion, birds' tongues, arugula seed, sugar, and a few other ingredients. See Marinello, *Le medicine partenenti alle infermità delle donne* (Venice: Valgrisio, 1574), 29r. Writing in 1565 on the duties of doctors and patients, Leonardo Botallo warned, however, that it could bring on convulsions and even death on lovers too eager to perform: "So di un altro [uomo] che, avendo sentito dire che la cantaride potenzia la virilità, per meglio amare l'amica, ingerì in abbondanza polvere di cantaride e preso da convulsioni morì in tre giorni." In Botallo, *I doveri del medico e del malato*, ed. Leonardo Carerj and Anita Bogetti Fassone (Turin: UTET, 1981), 109–110. Botallo's original Latin treatise, *Commentarioli duo, Alter de medici, alter de Aegroti munere*, was published in Lyon by Antonium Gryphium in 1565. Pulverized Spanish fly was also notoriously used to abort for many centuries. The lore of the cantharis still attracts interest today. One has only to check through the many Internet sites selling cantharidin. Still, its only reliable medical use is for wart removal.
14. Giuseppe Marcobruno was a Mantuan pharmacist who directed the Pharmacy of the Coral and then the Pharmacy of the King around 1588. He was still directing it in 1599, when the pharmacy first disappeared from the *Libro degli statuti e paratici degli speziali di Mantova;* see ASM, AG, busta 3106, fols. 348r–349r. See also Attilio Zanca and Adriano Galassi, "Saggio di bibliografia medica mantovana rinascimentale," in Attilio Zanca et al., *Mantova e i Gonzaga nella civiltà del Rinascimento* (Mantua: Accademia Virgiliana, 1977), 399–421, at 408.
15. As Bonatti writes to Duke Vincenzo on July 5, 1609: "Ho fatto ogni diligenza per sapere se le cosse desiderate da V.A. che gli siano portate da Evangelista spetiale si ritrovino nele Indie Orientali o Occidentali ma sin hora non si è ritrovato persona che ne sappia dar notizia." In ASM, AG, busta 609, fol. 322r.
16. "Mi par mille anni esser colà. Il signor mi conceda la sanità, acciò possi felicemente pervenire al suo desiderio." In ASM, AG, busta 609, fol. 321r.
17. "Hebbi la notta per informatione delli animaletti che desidera sua altezza dalle Indie; ma dovendosi procurare del Perù che è provincia delle Indie occidentali, non potrà servire questo nostro huomo qual va in India e non passerà Ormus [Hormuz]. Ma con tutto ciò ogni servitio che occorrerà a sua altezza et a vostra signoria illustrissima [Chieppio] si trova anche a Goa il signor Giovan Battista Chiut nostro qual da vostra eccellenza è conosciuto, complirà con molto amore tutto quello che gli sarà comandato. Et quando pur fosse tale la curiosità di sua altezza di voler a tutti i

modi gli animaletti significatemi, darò ordine a nostri di famiglia che scrivino a loro corrispondenti a Mexico Città di America che selli facino venire con li Perulieri che ivi capitano, ma avanti di poterli havere di qua, passarà almeno due anni per essere il viagio lontano." In ASM, AG, busta 1540, fol. 2, cc. 307–308, now in Michaela Sermidi, ed., *Le collezioni Gonzaga: Il carteggio tra Venezia e Mantova (1588–1612)* (Milan: Silvana Editoriale, 2003), 465–466. There are previous letters, of April 12, 1609, and April 20, 1609, that confirm that Vincenzo was looking for imports from the East Indies.

18. "Sig. re. Tanto si è ricercato in questa corte, che finalm.e si è ritrovato un prete indiano, che ne ha datto cognitione dell'animaletto ad erectione virge, dice che no è più longo che l'ungia d'un detto della mano, è peloso, di varij colori, la testa ha come di moscone, che passato sopra il membro opera meraviglios.e, ovvero posto nell'olio hore 24 et onto fa l'istesso effetto, si ritrova nel Perù nella valle di Chiuchiago, da questo allora si è inteso alcune pietre, et gomme di grandiss.a virtù. Sto aspettando con desid. di giungere, se ci sia passaggio per l'Indie Occ.li, che colà ha scritto il S. Bonatti qual procura la licenza, et subitamente espedito colà m'inviarò non perdonando a fatica alcuna per adempir il comandam'di V.A.S. e per fine con ogni umiltà faccio reverenza a V.A.S. Di Madrid gli 14 luglio 1609." In ASM, AG, busta 609, fol. 323r. Most of Marcobruno's correspondence is now printed in Giuseppe Ostino, "L'avventuroso viaggio al Perú di Evangelista Marcobruno, speziale mantovano nei primi anni del '600 alla ricerca di una curiosa droga," *La farmacia nuova* 24.8–9 (1968): 3–22; and in Stefano Scansani, *L'amor morto* (Milan: Mondadori, 1991). The same day Marcobruno also wrote to Ferdinando Gonzaga, a budding alchemist and botanist, to tell him that he had found in Madrid some plants and was planning to bring them to him on his way back. See ASM, AG, busta 609, fol. 325r.

19. Galileo presented his spyglass to the Venetian Senate that August 1609, and by October or November he directed it toward the heavens. Vincenzo Gonzaga invited Galileo to come to his court from the University of Padua, perhaps as a military architect, but there was a disagreement regarding the stipend.

20. "Tra molti Indiani che qui sono alla Corte ho ritrovato un pré di S. Franc.o che m'ha accertato detto gusano ritrovarsi nella Montagnas dellos Andes, et li Indiani li portano essicati nella cità di Chiuchiago e di Potosì; detto verme è longo poco meno ch'il detto della mano, di color velluto vario, et che con esso toccandosi solo il membro fa così valorosam. e erregere, che non ritrovandosi a quel punto appresso a qualche dona, sente così acerbo dolore, che quasi muore, ne ho potuto intendere se vi è il maschio e la femina, questo si è inteso da questo prè, qual è statto guardiano in quella cità et sopra esso gusano ha predicato, acciò quelli se ne astenessero. Si ritrovano dentro il Perù 400 leghe per terra, et a questo

Novembre parte l'armata di Siviglia per il Perù." In ASM, AG, busta 609, fol. 333r. Marcobruno here revises some information he sent Vincenzo one month earlier: then the *gusano* was as long as a finger's nail; now it is just short of a finger.

21. "Sereniss.mo mio Signore, Sono venuti in questa flotta alcuni padri di S. Franc.o dall'Indie de quali uno è Genovese, che per ani 28 è che se ne sta nel Perù, et conferma l'istesso della virtù di detto Gusano, et che si ritrova nella montagna de los Andes et si porta in Chiuchiago, conferma esser lungo come el detto picciolo della mano, non men grosso; tutto peludo, et che con esso solo toccandosi fa l'effetto miracoloso, che già scrissi a V.A. Ser.ma di Sagovia, overo lo pongono in olio, et di quello si onta, et che per remedio di questo hano la contra hierva altrimente morirebbono, la quale non ho potuta sapere, ma che colà si ritrova." In ASM, AG, busta 609, fol. 335r.

22. "Da questi padri ancora ho inteso alcuni semplici medicam.si di grandiss. ma virtù e questi come altri cosa non restarò per fatica di conseguirli. Medesimamente qui da uno moro schiavo mi ho d.o cognitione di un altro gusano dell'istessa virtù, che si ritrova in Nuova Spagna chamato dandastica et se è il vero che ci sia lo pigliarò. Della partita che sarà in breve sto aspetando con grandiss.o desid.o già che io so ove ho io andare, et informatomi beniss.o di detto viaggio, come anco per li libri che tengo. Sono stato avvertito che in questo viaggio si spende molto e che li 500 scudi che mi pagararo nell'Indie non ponno supplire." In ASM, AG, busta 609, fol. 335r.

23. "Scriverò tutto quello che in viaggio mi si rappresenterà." Letter of July 14, 1609, to Annibale Iberti, in which Marcobruno conferma from Madrid that he will keep a travel diary. In ASM, AG, busta 609, fol. 327r.

24. Letter of Marcobruno, from Segovia, to the ducal counselor, Annibale Iberti, August 29, 1609, in ASM, AG, busta 609, fol. 333r. Marcobruno gloats when he finds out that because of a difference in shape, the "gusano" sent from Seville was not the right one, as he writes in a letter of October 20: "Da questo ha potuto comprendere il s.r. Bonatti, quello che mandò a V.A.S. di Siviglia non è il vero." In ASM, AG, busta 609, fol. 335r. Then again in another letter of November 18, "come molti m'hanno testim.o che hora con questa flotta sono venuti dall'Indie, et tutti vengono a confrontarsi in una istessa relazione, si che vediamo che il scaravaggio ['cockroach'] mandato dal Bonatti non è il legittimo per esser molto diverso si di forma come per applicarlo." In ASM, AG, busta 609, f. 337.

25. "Ai miei Presidente e giudici ufficiali della Casa de Contratación della città di Siviglia ordino di lasciar passare alle provincie del Perù Evangelista Marcobruno di 28 anni di età, di statura media, bianco, grosso di viso e di corpo, senza chiedere alcuna notizia per quanto riguarda ad affari relativi all'Illustrissimo Duca di Mantova, il mio molto caro Cugino,

ciò che adempirete benché egli sia straniero e per quanto si riferisce ad altro do esenzione, restando per il resto in forza e valido. Fatto in Madrid addì 17 novembre 1609. Io il re." This royal decree was added to Marcobruno's travel documentation by Pedro de Contreras of the Casa de Contratación of Seville, who issued the permit on January 4, 1610; in Archivio General de Indias, Contratación 5, 317, n. 1. r. 9. I cite from Scansani's translation in *L'amor morto,* 181. For the importance of the Casa de la Contratación in fostering scientific knowledge in the New World, see Clarence Henry Haring, *Trade and Navigation between Spain and the Indies* (Cambridge: Harvard University Press, 1918); and Antonio Barrera-Osorio, *Experiencing Nature: The Spanish American Empire and the Early Scientific Revolution* (Austin: University of Texas Press, 2006), 29–48.

26. See Mario Cermenati, "Ulisse Aldrovandi e l'America," *Annali di Botanica* 4 (1906): 313–366, at 362–363. On the relationship between Aldrovandi and Mantuan naturalists, see Dario Franchini, "Ulisse Aldrovandi ed i naturalisti mantovani," in Dario Franchini et al., *La scienza a corte: Collezionismo eclettico, natura e immagine a Mantova fra Rinascimento e Manierismo* (Rome: Bulzoni, 1979), 10–19.

27. "Se io narrassi a V.A.S. el travaglio che ho passato per terra del Pirù che in sei mesi ho caminato 673 leghe, tanto despoblado donde non hai memoria di paro camino (?) de quindesi giorni el passar tanti presipitij de montagne donde en tutto el ano continuamente stano tanti fiumi grandiss.mi da passare et altri accidenti che passeno li poveri passageri." In ASM, AG, busta 610, fols. 603r–604r. Contemporary narratives abound of Peruvian harshness within the forbidding Andean inland. José de Acosta called Potosí terribly cold, barren, dry, and bleak. See his *Natural and Moral History of the Indies,* ed. Jane Mangan (Durham, NC: Duke University Press, 2002), bk. 4, ch. 6, "Of the Mountain of Potosí and Its Discovery," 172–174.

28. Niccolò Machiavelli, *Mandragola/Clizia* (Milan: Feltrinelli, 1995), 4.2: "Io pigliarò prima una presa d'uno lattovaro che si chiama satirione . . . che farebbe, quanto a quella faccenda, ringiovanire un uomo di novanta anni non che di settanta, come ho io." Earlier I mentioned that Vincenzo too was advised to use satyrion as a recreational drug by Emanuel Ximenes.

29. Enrico Malizia, *Ricettario delle streghe: Incantesimi, prodigi sessuali e veleni* (Rome: Edizioni Mediterranee, 1992), 141. I give other recipes throughout *The Manly Masquerade: Masculinity, Paternity, and Castration in the Italian Renaissance* (Durham: Duke University Press, 2003), 28–107.

30. Charles Thompson, *The Mystic Mandrake* (New York: University Books, 1968), details the use of the mandrake through the centuries to increase male sexual drive as well as to address women's infertility.

31. Malizia, *Ricettario delle streghe,* 130–133.

32. Likewise, Marinello writes, the dried and pulverized genital member of a bull spread over an egg yolk worked "marvelously." In Marinello, *Le medicine partenenti alle infermità delle donne*, 27r.
33. Caterina Sforza (da Forlì), *Esperimenti de la Ex.ma S.ra Caterina da Furlj matre de lo Inlux.mo Signor Giovanni de Medici*, ed. Desiderio Pasolini (1525; Imola: Tip. D'Ignazio Galeati e figli, 1894), 229: "Cum predicto unguento omni die enim magnificabitur virga mirabiliter."
34. Giambattista della Porta, *Phytognomonica seu methodus nova facillimaque qua plantarum ac rerum omnium vires ex solo faciei inspection assignatur* (Naples: 1583). The reference is in Alberico Benedicenti, *Malati, medici e farmacisti* (Milan: Hoepli, 1924), 1:525.
35. Malizia, *Ricettario delle streghe*, 172.
36. Isabella Cortese, *I secreti della signora Isabella Cortese ne' quali si contengono cose minerali, medicinali, arteficiose, e alchemiche* (Milan: La vita felice, 1995), 94.
37. Castore Durante, *Il tesoro della sanità: nel quale si da il modo da conservar la sanità, et prolungar la vita, et si tratta della natura de' cibi ed de' rimedij de' nocumenti loro* (Mantua, 1590). I quote from the English translation, *A Treasure of Health* (London: William Crook, 1685), 168–169.
38. "Era veramente mirabile, per eccitare gli appetiti venerei, un'erba, la quale aveva portata un indiano; imperocché non solamente mangiata, ma toccata, tanto incitava gli uomini al coito, ch'essa li faceva potenti ad esercitarlo quante volte lor fosse piaciuto. Di modo che dicevano, che coloro che l'avevano usata, l'avevano fatto più di dodici volte, come che più fosse stato udito dire quell'indiano, il quale era grave di corpo e robusto, averlo fatto tal giorno settanta volte; ma però con spargimento di poche gocciole di seme per volta." In Pietro Andrea Mattioli, *Discorsi . . . ne' sei libri di Pedacio Dioscoride Anazarbeo della materia medicinale* (Venice: Pezzano, 1744), 513. Mattioli was probably referring to the East Indies. See also Piero Camporesi, *I balsami di Venere* (Milan: Garzanti, 1989), 31.
39. "In questa terra si trova una specie d'arboro, ch'è di legno tenero. Li Indiani piuttosto si lasceriano ammazzare, che andar al suo lume; perche dicono, che mettendo l'indiano alla luce di questo arboro, o dandole il suo fumo; resta impotente con donne." The citation comes from a letter from Lima, Peru, of December 26, 1568, by the soldier Pietro di Osma to Nicolás Monardes. In Monardes, *Delle cose che vengono portate dall'Indie Occidentali, pertinenti all'uso della medicina* (Venice: Ziletti, 1575), 69–82, at 78.
40. Leo Africanus (Leone Africano), "Della descrittione dell'Africa et delle cose notabili che ivi sono," in Giovanni Battista Ramusio, *Navigationi et viaggi* (Venice: Giunti, 1565), 1:95e.
41. See Daniela Sogliani, ed., *Le collezioni Gonzaga: Il carteggio Venezia-Mantova (1563–87)* (Milan: Silvana Editoriale, 2002), 60–61.
42. The story of Nicola is in Antonello Gerbi, *La natura delle Indie Nove: Da Cristoforo Colombo a Gonzalo Fernandez de Oviedo* (Milan: Ricciardi, 1975), 263.

43. Mattioli, *Discorsi . . . ne' sei libri di Pedacio Dioscoride;* Caspar Bauhin, *Pinax theatri botanici* (Basel: Ludovici Regi, 1623).
44. See Giuseppe Olmi, *L'inventario del mondo: Catalogazione della natura e luoghi del sapere nella prima età moderna* (Bologna: Il Mulino, 1992), 242; Benedicenti, *Malati, medici e farmacisti,* 716–732; Guenter Risse, "Transcending Cultural Barriers: The European Reception of Medicinal Plants from the Americas," in *Botanical Drugs of the Americas in the Old and New Worlds,* ed. Wolfgang-Hagen Hein (Stuttgart: Wissenschaftliche Verlagsgesellschaft, 1984), 31–42; J. Worth Estes, "The Reception of American Drugs in Europe, 1500–1650," in *Searching for the Secrets of Nature: The Life and Works of Dr. Francisco Hernandez,* ed. Simon Varey, Rafael Chabrán, and Dora Weiner (Stanford: Stanford University Press, 2000), 111–121; and Maria Luz López Terrada and José Pardo-Tomás, *La primeras noticias sobre plantas americanas en las relaciones de viajes y crónicas de Indias (1493–1553)* (Valencia: Instituto de Estudios Documentales, 1993). The most imported therapies from the New World, beyond the guaiacum, the sarsaparilla, and the maca, were tobacco, sassafras, jalap, and *tacamahácha.*
45. "Gelsomini di Catalogna, fichi d'India, aloe, et altri fiori d'Italia." See Elena Venturini, "Il vestibolo dell'imperatore: Vicende di collezionismo artistico nelle relazioni tra Gonzaga e Asburgo," in *Le collezioni Gonzaga: Il carteggio tra la Corte Cesarea e Mantova (1559–1636),* ed. Elena Venturini (Milano: Silvana Editoriale, 2002), 15–134, at 31. The list of naturalists, apothecaries, doctors, herbalists, and "speziari" who operated in Mantua at the time of Vincenzo's reign is a long one, with men such as Filippo Costa, Ippolito Genifroti, Antonio Bertioli, Paolo Carazzi, Marcello Donati, Giovanni Battista Luchini, and Giovanni Battista Cavallara. For a study of these men and their similar interests in herbal material and medicine, as well as for a list of what was contained in the cabinets of Filippo Costa, see Dario Franchini et al., *La scienza a corte,* 30–62, especially 48–55.
46. "Nel passaggio di qua del signor conte Marcello [Donati], li diedi un poco di ragguaglio nel particolar del segreto di questi nostri concittadini intorno alla multiplicazione dell'oro, che dicono di haver trovato." Letter from Bologna of Ulisse Bentivoglio to Vincenzo Gonzaga of March 13, 1590, in ASM, AG, busta 1164, fol. 3, cc. 372.
47. "Hora avrei potuto sperare di dare a vostra altezza qualche nova della riuscita che si spera di trarre oro dall'argento, se no s'interponevano queste feste di Pasqua con li giorni santi trascorsi senza lavoro temporale." Letter from Bologna of Gregorio Capilluti to Vincenzo Gonzaga of April 24, 1590, in ASM, AG, busta. 1164, fol. 3, cc. 396–397.
48. The information is in Kate Simon, *I Gonzaga: Storia e segreti* (Milan: Newton Compton, 2004), 316.
49. "Volendo Sua Signoria Illustris. e Reverendis. provedere opportunamente a questo abuso [people selling vipers to make money] . . . ordina a comanda

che niuno (dalli Speciali, che essercitano il medicinale in poi) debba, né possa comprare alcuna quantità di Vipere vive o morte, sotto pena di L. 25 per ciascuna di loro." This *Bando sopra le vipere* of April 20, 1606, is in Piero Camporesi, "Speziali e ciarlatani," in *Cultura popolare nell'Emilia Romagna: Medicina, erbe e magia,* ed. Giuseppe Adani and Gastone Tavagnini (Milan: Silvana, 1981).

50. See the report of the Venetian ambassador Pietro Gritti of 1612, in *Relazioni degli ambasciatori veneti,* ed. Segarizzi, 1:118. See also Antonino Bertolotti, *Le arti minori alla corte di Mantova nei secoli XV, XVI e XVII* (Milan, 1889; repr. Bologna: Forni, 1974), 91–96.

51. The citation from Giovan Battista Cavallara is in Paula Findlen, *Possessing Nature: Museums, Collecting, and Scientific Culture in Early Modern Italy* (Berkeley: University of California Press, 1994), 105. On cabinets of curiosities, see Oliver Impy and Arthur MacGregor, eds., *The Origins of Museums: The Cabinets of Curiosities in Sixteenth- and Seventeenth-Century Europe* (Oxford: Oxford University Press, 1986).

52. The corpse was that of Passerino Bonacolsi, which gave the gallery the name of "Passerino," still used today.

53. In 1607, for example, the jaw and the shinbone of a unicorn arrived from Bologna for Vincenzo, because it was known that a drink containing shavings of these bones "worked marvelously" and cured a number of diseases. See ASM, AG, busta 1168, fol. 3, c. 464. In 1609 Vincenzo sent Grand Duke Cosimo II de' Medici two leopards, a male and a female, presumably for breeding purposes, from his well-stocked menagerie of exotic animals. See the letter of April 25, 1609, in ASF, MDP 2944, DocID 5114. See also *Le collezioni Gonzaga: Il Carteggio tra Bologna, Parma, Piacenza e Mantova (1563–1634),* ed. Barbara Furlotti, 124ff. for this and similar letters.

54. Christopher Columbus, *Textos y documentos completos: Relaciones de viajes, cartas, y memoriales,* ed. Consuelo Varala (Madrid: Allianza, 1982), 143: "Esta es para desear, e vista, es para nunca dexar." See also Roland Greene, "Petrarchism among the Discourses of Imperialism," in *America in European Consciousness, 1493–1750,* ed. Karen Ordhal Kupperman (Chapel Hill: University of North Carolina Press, 1995), 130–165.

55. See Agnes Arber, "A Chronological List of the Principal Herbals and Related Botanical Works Published between 1470 and 1670," in Arber, *Herbals: Their Origin and Evolution; A Chapter in the History of Botany, 1470–1670* (Cambridge: Cambridge University Press, 1912), 227–237.

56. Maca was recommended to overcome frigidity in women too, to regulate menstruation and menopausal symptoms, to increase sperm activity in livestock, to cure arthritis and joint pain, to restore cognitive functions, and to address respiratory disorders. Maca was used by the locals before battle to make them strong and courageous, but it was forbidden to use it

afterward, for fear that the increased libido would unleash itself on the conquered enemy women.

57. Mixing local medicine and European techniques, Augustín Farfan published *Tractato brebe de Anatomia y Chirurgia* in 1579, in which he recommended about sixty local remedies. See Guenter Risse, "Medicine in New Spain," in *Medicine in the New World: New Spain, New France, and New England*, ed. Ronald Numbers (Knoxville: University of Tennessee Press, 1987), 12–63, at 49. For a thorough study of curative imports, see Charles Talbot, "America and the European Drug Trade," in *First Images of America: The Impact of the New World on the Old*, ed. Fredi Chiappelli (Berkeley: University of California Press, 1976), 833–844.

58. See Bernardino de Sahagún, *Florentine Codex: A General History of the Things of New Spain*, ed. and trans. Arthur Anderson and Charles Dibble (Santa Fe and Salt Lake City: School of American Research and University of Utah, 1982), 12:67, 12:75, 12:79. See also Miguel De Asua and Roger French, *A New World of Animals: Early Modern Europeans on the Creatures of Iberian America* (Aldershot: Ashgate, 2005).

59. Thus, there were descriptions of trees that bore oysters and of opossums with human feet. The flower *granadiglia* (*fior messicano*) even displayed the five wounds of Christ's passion.

60. As many as 4,000 books mentioning the New World and its riches had been published by the end of the sixteenth century. See John Alden, ed., *European Americana: A Chronological Guide to Works Printed in Europe Relating to the Americas, 1493–1776*, vol. 1 (New York: Readex, 1980).

61. On the richness of the Gonzaga library, see Irma Pagliari, "'Una libreria che in Italia non v'era una simile ne' anco a Roma': La biblioteca dei Gonzaga," in *Gonzaga: La Celeste Galeria, L'esercizio del collezionismo*, ed. Raffaella Morselli (Milan: Skira, 2002), 111–125; and C. H. Clough, "The Library of the Gonzaga of Mantua," *Librarium* 15 (1972): 50–63. On books and cosmographic treatises about America available in the nearby Veneto libraries at the time, see Federica Ambrosini, *Paesi e mari ignoti: America e colonialismo europeo nella cultura veneziana (secoli XVI–XVII)* (Venice: Deputazione Editrice, 1982).

62. Francisco Hernández, *Rerum medicarum Novae Hispaniae thesaurus* (Rome: Mascardi, 1651). The full herbal in facsimile is now available in *Historia natural de Nueva España*, 2 vols. (México: Universidad Nacional de México, 1959). See José López Piñero and José Pardo, "The Contribution of Hernández to European Botany and *Materia Medica*," in *Searching for the Secrets of Nature: The Life and Works of Dr. Francisco Hernández*, ed. Simon Varey (Stanford: Stanford University Press, 2000), 122–137. In 1580 Nardo Antonio Recchi, an Italian scientist named to the post of royal botanist in Madrid, was given the task of making a selection from Hernández's still-unpublished manuscript by Philip II of Spain. The interest in Recchi's

selection of 400 plants among scientists and herbalists was high from the start, even though only a few copies of his work were ever printed (in 1628 by the Accademia dei Lincei in Rome). See Risse, "Transcending Cultural Barriers," 36; and José Pardo-Tomás, *Oviedo, Monardes, Hernández: El tesoro natural de America; Colonialismo y ciencia en el siglo XVI* (Madrid: Nivola, 2002).

63. Fabio Colonna, *Phytobasanos sive plantarum aliquot historia: in qua describuntur diversi generis plantae veriores* (Naples: Carlinum et Pacem, 1592). Also, Marcobruno did not know of the Badianus manuscript, which contained 184 local plants and trees, written in 1552 by an Indian doctor in Nahuatl and translated into Latin by Juan Badiano. It soon disappeared from view until it was found in the Vatican Library in 1929. See Martín de la Cruz, *The Badianus Manuscript (Codex Barberini, Latin 241), Vatican Library: An Aztec Herbal of 1552,* trans. Emily Walcott Emmart (Baltimore: Johns Hopkins University Press, 1940). Nor did Marcobruno know book 11, *Of Earthly Things,* on medicaments in Bernardino de Sahagún's *Historia general de las cosas de Nueva España,* which found its home in the Biblioteca Medicea Laurenziana in Florence and became known as the *Florentine Codex* (1577–1580). See also Debra Hassig, "Transplanted Medicine: Colonial Mexican Herbals of the Sixteenth Century," *Res: Anthropology and Aesthetics* 17/18 (1989): 30–53.

64. Juan Fragoso, *Discursos de las cosas aromaticas* (Madrid: Yuañez, 1572); José de Acosta, *Historia natural y moral de las Indias* (Seville: de Leon, 1590), *Historia naturale, e morale delle Indie* (Venice: Basa, 1596). Acosta was sent to Peru in 1571, visiting Cuzco, La Paz, Charcas, Potosí, and Chuquisaca. The text appeared in Italian almost immediately. See also Martín Martín and Valverde, *La farmacia en la América colonial;* René Taton, ed., "Las Ciencias in la America Colonial," in his *Historia general de las ciencias,* trans. Manuel Sacristán, vol. 2, *La ciencia moderna* (Barcelona: Ediciones Destino, 1972), 791–822.

65. Nicolás Monardes, *Delle cose, che vengono portate dall'Indie Occidentali pertinenti all'uso della medicina* (Venice: Ziletti, 1575 and 1597). Carolus Clusius (Charles de l'Ecluse) soon translated a widely circulated edition of Monardes, to which he added a commentary, *Rariorum aliquot stirpium per Hispanias observatarum historia* (Antwerp: Piantini, 1576). See also his *Exoticorum libri decem* (Leiden: Raphelenghi, 1605), in which he puts together information gathered from Monardes, da Orta, Acosta, and other Spanish herbalists. For more on European medical imports, see Daniela Bleichmar, "Books, Bodies, and Fields: Sixteenth-Century Transatlantic Encounters with the New World *Materia Medica,*" in *Colonial Botany: Science, Commerce, and Politics in the Early Modern World,* ed. Londa Schiebinger and Claudia Swan (Philadelphia: University of Pennsylvania Press, 2005), 83–99.

66. See the letter that Alfonso Pancio wrote to Aldrovandi in Bologna on April 15, 1570, now in Biblioteca Universitaria di Bologna, Fondo Aldrovandi, MS 38, 156r, cited in Franchini et al., *La scienza a corte*, 59. In his own "giardino dei semplici" in Mantua, Donati, moreover, cultivated the mechiocan root (or jalap), used as a purgative, about which he wrote a book, *De variolis et morbillis tractatus . . . Eiusdem De radice purgante qua mechiocan vocant* (Mantua: Philoterpsem et Philoponos, 1565).
67. Gonzalo Fernández de Oviedo, *Libro secondo delle Indie Occidentali. . . . Summario della naturale et generale historia dell'Indie occidentali, composta da Gonzalo Ferdinando del Oviedo* (1534), reproduced in Giambattista Ramusio, *Terzo volume delle Navigationi et viaggi* (Venice: Giunti, 1556) and in all later editions. The *Sommario* is now in vol. 5 of the new edition of Ramusio's *Navigazioni*, ed. Marica Milanesi, 6 vols. (Turin: Einaudi, 1978–1988). Oviedo corresponded with a number of Italian intellectuals, such as Pietro Bembo and Gerolamo Fracastoro. See the brief introduction by Marica Milanesi to Oviedo's text, 5:210.
68. Castore Durante (1529–1590), *Herbario Nuovo . . . con figure che rappresentano le vive piante che nascono in tutta Europa, et nelle indie orientali et occidentali* (Rome: Bonfadino and Diani, 1585). Durante mentions a number of New World herbs, like the American aloe, effective against viper's poison (18–19); the "guacatan," recommended for wounds (219); the "lentisco del Perù," a purgative (219); and the "mecciocan," prescribed to regulate humors. The index also includes herbs necessary to heal the male organ, such as those for the "verga e i suoi ardori" (172) and the "verga infiammata" (188), and provides remedies to help women in childbirth (319). See also Frank Anderson, *An Illustrated History of the Herbals* (New York: Columbia University Press, 1977), 187–192. For a sense of the herbals available in Mantua, often illustrated by anonymous painters, see Franchini, "L'illustrazione scientifica a Mantova," in Franchini et al., *La scienza a corte*, 64–77.
69. These may have included Girolamo Ruscelli's *Secreti del reverendo donno Alessio Piemontese* (1555), which enjoyed eighteen editions by the end of the century; Timotheo Rossello's *Della summa de' secreti universali in ogni materia* (1561), with five editions; pseudo-Gabriele Falloppio's *Secreti diversi e miracolosi* (1563), with nine editions; Leonardo Fioravanti's *Del compendio de i secreti rationali* (1564), also with nine editions; Isabella Cortese's *I secreti* (1561), with seven; and finally, the blockbuster, Giambattista della Porta's *Magia naturalis* (1560), with three editions in Italian and a whopping fifteen in Latin. For more on books of secrets, see William Eamon, "Science and Popular Culture in Sixteenth-Century Italy: The Professors of Secrets and Their Books," *Sixteenth Century Studies* 16 (1985): 471–485.
70. In Venice, according to Richard Palmer, "No one was to open a pharmacy (*bottega medicinale*) unless he had been an apprentice (*garzone*) for five

years, and had served a further three in dispensing and composing medicines." See Palmer, "Pharmacy in the Republic of Venice in the Sixteenth Century," in *The Medical Renaissance in the Sixteenth Century,* ed. A. Wear, R. K. French, and I. M. Lonie (Cambridge: Cambridge University Press, 1985), 99–117, at 103.

71. Given the time of Marcobruno's trip, it is debatable whether he knew of Giuseppe Quercetanus (Joseph Du Chesne) and his extremely influential *Pharmacopoea dogmatorum restituta,* published in Latin in 1607 (Paris: Morellus) and in Italian in 1609 as *Le ricchezze della riformata pharmacopea del Sig. Giuseppe Quercetano, medico e consigliere regio,* although of course given Vincenzo's (and his chemists') interests, the text may have reached Mantua right away. For distilling techniques, another popular text, Pietro Mattioli's *Del modo di distillare le acque da tutte le piante* (Venice: Valgrisi, 1581), could also have been in Marcobruno's shop.

72. On these travel books, see Tomás, "Obras Españolas," 59–61.

73. Giovanni Lorenzo d'Anania, *L'universale fabrica del mondo, overo Cosmografia* (Venice: Muschio, 1596); the section on Peru is at 399–402. In *Il mondo e le sue parti cioe Europa, Africa, Asia, et America* (Florence: Tosi, 1595), Gioseppe Rosaccio describes the inhabitants of Peru as ugly, fearful, and stupid. More generally, see Silvana Serafin, *La natura del Perù nei cronisti dei secoli XVI e XVII* (Rome: Bulzoni, 1988); and Carmelo Samonà, "La letteratura dell'esperienza vissuta: I cronisti delle 'Indie,'" in *La letteratura spagnola dei secoli d'oro,* ed. Carmelo Samonà et al. (Florence: Sansoni, 1973), 100–134. For an understanding, on the other hand, of what the conquest meant to the people of Peru, see Nathan Wachtel, *The Vision of the Vanquished: The Spanish Conquest of Peru through Indian Eyes, 1530–1570* (New York: Barnes and Noble, 1977).

74. See, for example, *Avisi particolari delle Indie di Portugallo* (Rome: Dorico and Bressani, 1552); *Nuovi avisi dell'Indie di Portogallo* (Venice: Tramezzino, 1562); *Diversi avisi particolari dall'Indie di Portogallo, ricevuti dall'anno 1551 sino al 1558 dalli reverendi padri della Compagnia di Giesù* (Venice: Tramezzino, 1565).

75. This *gusano* was not, in any case, the maggot of a Spanish fly, since this emerald-green beetle is not present in the New World.

76. "Hanno anche le femine un'altra usanza crudele, e lontana da ogni humano vivere esse (percioche sono sopra modo lussuriose) per sodisfare al lor dishonesto piacere, usano questa crudeltà, che danno a bere a gli huomini il sugo d'una certa herba, il qual beuto si gonfia loro il membro, et cresce grandemente e se quello non giova, accostano al membro certi animali venenosi, che lo mordano in sin che si gonfia, onde aviene che appresso di loro molti perdono i testicoli e diventano eunuchi." In "Sommario di Amerigo Vespucci Fiorentino di due sue navigationi al Magnifico M. Piero Soderini Gonfalonier della Magnifica Republica di Firenze," in Giovanni Battista Ramusio, *Navigationi et viaggi,* ed. with an introduction

by F. R. A. Skelton and George Parks (Amsterdam: Theatrum Orbis Terrarum, 1967–1970), 1:131r. See also Adalberto Pazzini, "La medicina alla corte dei Gonzaga a Mantova," in *Mantova e i Gonzaga nella civiltà del Rinascimento,* ed. Accademia Nazionale dei Lincei (Mantua: Accademia Virgiliana), 291–344, at 298.

77. "Mentre potevano haver copia de christiani, è cosa maravigliosa da dire quanto dishonestamente porgessero i lor corpi, e invero che sono lussuriose oltra il creder di ognuno." In Ramusio, *Navigationi et viaggi,* 132v.

78. The geographer Alberto Magnaghi was the first to demonstrate that out of the four trips he claims to have made to South America—two for the Spanish crown (1497–1498 and 1499–1500) and two for the Portuguese crown (1501–1502 and 1503–1504)—Vespucci never made the first and the last. See his *Amerigo Vespucci* (Rome: Treves, 1926).

79. And indeed, in some contemporary accounts, women are held responsible even for cannibalism in the New World. As Antonio Pigafetta explains, the custom of eating human flesh started when a woman threw herself onto one of the men responsible for killing her only son and started to bite his shoulder. Thus, men later inaugurated the habit of eating their enemy's flesh. See *Viaggio atorno il mondo fatto e descritto per messer Antonio Pigafetta vicentino,* in Ramusio, *Navigazioni,* ed. Milanesi, 2:874.

80. "Ancora in questo proposito desiderato dalle donne, scrive Amerigo Vespucci, che discoperse il Brasil, in una sua lettera a Piero Soderini, che le donne di quel paese, lusoriosissime, davano da bere certo sugo d'erbe agli uomini per farli crescere il loro membro, et che se quel sugo non giovava glie lo facevano mordere o pungere da animali velenosi." The diary of Francesco Carletti (1573?–1636) was not printed until 1701. I cite from the modern critical edition, *Ragionamenti del mio viaggio intorno al mondo,* ed. Gianfranco Silvestro (Turin: Einaudi, 1958), 196. See also Daria Perocco, *Viaggiare e raccontare: Narrazione di viaggio ed esperienze di racconto tra Cinque e Seicento* (Alessandria: Edizioni dell'Orso, 1997), 62–72.

81. "Costumano alcuni Indi, et per valentia et per farsi crescere el capo della verga; di darsi tre o quattro tagli sopra esso, di modo l'aprono come dita della mano, cioè in 4 o 5 parte; di poi vi spremono su certe herbe che guariscono subito, cioè in poco tempo, facendo enfiare quella carne con certa callosità di modo che dicono le Indie ne hanno gran piacere." In Galeotto Cey, *Viaggio e relazione delle Indie, 1539–1553,* ed. Francesco Surdich (Rome: Bulzoni, 1992), 94.

82. Anne McClintock, *Imperial Leather: Race, Gender, and Sexuality in the Colonial Conquest* (New York: Routledge, 1995), 22.

83. At the time it was not known of course that this infection was caused by a wormlike, microscopic organism called spirochete, which tunnels into the mucous membrane of the genitalia, but everybody could see that the chancres and wart-like lesions that appeared on the penis in men afflicted by the disease gave the organ the appearance of being worm eaten.

Also gumma appearing on the face, scalp, and legs gave the visual impression of being infested with worms.

84. "The natural Conjunction of a leprous Man with a monstrous Woman; or from the unnatural or Sodomitical, of another with a diseased Beast; from poisoned Wine; the influence of some malevolent Star; the venomous Bite of a Serpent. Which were the opinions of Paracelsus, Van Helmont, Coesalpinus, Fracastorius, and our Lister." In Daniel Turner, *Syphilis: A Practical Dissertation on the Venereal Disease* (London: Walthoe et al., 1732), 1–2. Although Monardes too writes extensively about the diffusion of syphilis, whose origin he traces back to the return of Christopher Columbus in Europe, he limits himself to saying that the disease spreads sexually and makes no mention of women's lasciviousness. See Monardes, *Delle cose che vengono portate dall'Indie Occidentali*, part 1, 24–27.

85. Simeon Zuccolo (Zuccolo da Cologna), *La pazzia del ballo* (Bologna: Forni, 1969), 27.

86. See Gabriele Mina, "Una costruzione melanconica: Il primo dibattito sul tarantismo," in *Il morso della differenza: Antologia del dibattito sul tarantismo fra il XIV e il XVI secolo*, ed. Gabriele Mina (Nardò: Besa, 2000), 9–68, at 16. For the sexual fever at the center of this dance, see Finucci, *Manly Masquerade*, 100–101; and, more generally, Ernesto De Martino, *La terra del rimorso: Contributo a una storia religiosa del sud* (Milan: Saggiatore, 1961).

87. Piero Camporesi, *The Anatomy of the Senses: Natural Symbols in Medieval and Early Modern Italy,* trans. Allan Cameron (Cambridge: Polity Press, 1995), 111.

88. Francesco Redi, *Esperienze intorno alla generazione degli insetti,* in *Scienziati del Seicento,* ed. Maria Luisa Altieri Biagi and Bruno Basile (Milan: Ricciardi, 1980), 314–463. See also Finucci, *Manly Masquerade*, 68–78.

89. Oviedo, *Naturale e generale historia dell'Indie,* in Ramusio, *Navigazioni,* ed. Milanesi, 5:675.

90. Piero Camporesi, *Bread of Dreams: Food and Fantasy in Early Modern Europe,* trans. David Gentilcore (Chicago: University of Chicago Press, 1989), 155.

91. Giovan Battista Codronchi, *De morbis qui Imolae* (Bologna: Battista Bellagamba, 1603).

92. "Gl'indiani si spulciano l'un l'altro, e quelli massime che fanno questo essercizio sono le femmine, e tutto quel che pigliano in questa sua caccia si mangiano, e sono tanto avezzi a questo che con difficoltà grande possiamo noi cristiani far che gl'Indiani che ci servono in casa non faccino il medesimo." In *Sommario della naturale e generale istoria dell'Indie occidentali,* in Ramusio, *Navigazioni e viaggi,* ed. Milanesi, 5:319. The story of the lice is also told by Hernández, who finds the custom disgusting. See Hernández, "The Antiquities of New Spain," in *The Mexican Treasury: The Writings of Dr. Francisco Hernández,* ed. Simon Varey (Stanford: Stanford University Press, 2000), 75.

93. *Sommario,* in Ramusio, *Navigazioni,* ed. Milanesi, 5:319, 5:285. For other detailed descriptions of New World insects in Oviedo, bk. 15, see Ramusio, *Navigazioni,* ed. Milanesi, 5:718–735.
94. Acosta, *Historia natural y moral,* bk. 5, ch. 26; *Natural and Moral History,* ed. Mangan, 309.
95. Tobacco was used in pills, lotions, and syrups; infusions of leaves were good for warm baths for syphilitics.
96. Paolo Boccone, *Osservazioni naturali,* 78–79; in Piero Camporesi, *The Incorruptible Flesh: Bodily Mutation and Mortification in Religion and Folklore,* trans. Tania Croft-Murray (New York: Cambridge University Press, 1988), 211. Dr. Johnson, for example, who later in life had asthma, dropsy, gout, rheumatoid arthritis, and a malignant tumor in his left testicle, "consumed a vast quantity of medicines: opium, oil of terebinth, valerian, ipecacuanha, . . . musk, dried squills, and Spanish fly." See Henry Hitchings, *Defining the World: The Extraordinary Story of Dr. Johnson's Dictionary* (New York: Farrar, Straus and Giroux, 2005), 119.
97. The recipe is in Enrico Benassi, *I consulti medici di Giambattista Morgagni* (Bologna: Cappelli, 1934), 203. See also Camporesi, *Incorruptible Flesh,* 102.
98. Monardes, *Delle cose, che vengono portate dall'Indie Occidentali,* pt. 2, ch. 10, 102–103.
99. Antonio Bertioli, *Delle considerazioni . . . sopra l'olio di scorpioni dell'eccellentissimo Matthioli* (Mantua: Francesco Osanna, 1585). See also Loren MacKinney, "Animal Substances in *Materia Medica:* A Study in the Persistence of the Primitive," *Journal of the History of Medicine and Allied Sciences* 1 (1946): 149–170, at 157.
100. He had said so in his letter to Vincenzo of August 29, 1609, and repeated it in the letter with the same date addressed to the ducal counselor, Iberti: "Hora che mi è palese ritrovarsi quello commessomi dal Ser.mo S.r N.ro dentro al Perù per terra 400 leghe." In ASM, AG, busta 609, fol. 329r.
101. Letter of June 10, 1609, from Barcelona to Cardinal Ferdinando Gonzaga, in ASM, AG, busta 609, fol. 319. Friars and priests were often considered possessions easy to monetize because they were usually ransomed by their order or confraternity.
102. Portobelo had a better harbor and was used after 1598 when Nombre de Dios on the isthmus itself was abandoned. According to José de Acosta, the eighteen leagues in the inhospitable land between Nombre de Dios and Panama were more difficult to pass than 2,300 leagues of ocean. See Acosta, *Historia natural y moral,* bk. 3, ch. 10.
103. This scheme had been followed more or less since 1564, when two annual convoys would leave each year between March and September to account for the winds and the hurricane season. A *flota* was composed of thirty-five to seventy ships and was accompanied by warships for protection, especially when coming from the southern route, with its huge amounts of silver and gold. The trip back started around the middle of

March by way of Cuba, Bermuda, and the Azores to Seville. Because of the winds, the trip west from Seville to Panama (Nombre de Dios) usually lasted 75 days; the entire return trip could take as many as 130 days. See Carla Rahn Phillips, "The Growth and Composition of Trade in the Iberian Empires, 1450–1750," in *The Rise of Merchant Empires: Long-Distance Trade in the Early Modern World, 1350–1750*, ed. James Tracy (New York: Cambridge University Press, 1990), 34–101, esp. 77–78; and Roy MacLeod, "Spain and America: The Atlantic Trade, 1492–1720," in *Cambridge History of Latin America*, vol. 1 (New York: Cambridge University Press, 1984). Acosta described the trip and the stopovers in somewhat more exact terms than did Marcobruno, in *Historia natural y moral*, bk. 3, ch. 4, fol. 38r–38v; *Natural and Moral History*, ed. Mangan, 106–108.

104. "Li negri che qui servono alli spagnoli per esclavi, che è quantità grandissima vano tutti nudi cobrendosi solo le parti vergognose di huomini come donne. Diferente è la fruta di costì così passa di souavità e di delicatezza a quante ha il Mundo, de' quali uno è il Platano [banana], l'altro la Pigna [ananas] et altre diverse sorti de Meloni che già sono nel fine soavissimi." Letter of April 6, 1610, from Cartagena to Duke Vincenzo Gonzaga, in ASM, AG, busta 610, fol. 231r.

105. "Partissimo del porto [Cartagena] in un grandiss.o galione en el mar del Zur [the Pacific ocean] et in un mese dassimo fondo en el porto de Manta costa del Perù per cargar aqua et manalotage el general de quella mar desembargo sino 50 pasageri en a quel porto tra quali io fui uno et caminai per terra sino a Lima città donde resiede il virei, de alì partij per el Cusco, donde conseguì sette gusanos che chiamano li Indiani pullo pullos et con grandiss.o fatica potessimo tener questi per non esser la staggione di raccoglierli, et questi già erano del altro anno en poter de un teniente de los Andes del Cusco. Passai sino a Chiuchiago et per molta diligensa et de amici giamai potessimo ritrovar niguno per non essere il tiempo che vengano che è per pasqua, de alì passai a Potosì dove me fu dada enformatione che l'indiani li portino de terra callente ne meno li ritrovai. Partei de Potosi per Arica dove me imbarcai sino a Lima deove giongessimo in otto giorni en el Cusco, et in Chiuchiago lasiai pagati li gusani acciò l'inviasino in Lima a mercanti conisciuti li quali enviavano con el primo naviglio che parta per queste parte grandiss.e quantità. . . . Quando gionsi a Cartagena de Indias ritrovai carta del Sig.r Bonati con la nota di quello che me mandava S.A.Ser.ma et de algune cose che se comandavano non ho potuto portarle per non haver tenuto le letere en el Pirù." Letter of Marcobruno to Vincenzo Gonzaga, October 25, 1611, in ASM, AG, busta 610, fols. 603–604.

106. The *dorstenia* was used to forestall epidemics in England at the time of the plague. See Nathaniel Hodges, *Loimologia; or, An Historical Account of the Plague in London in 1665* (London: Bell and Osborn, 1720).

107. Monardes, *Delle cose, che vengono portate dall'Indie Occidentali*, pt. 2, ch. 10, 103. Acosta also mentions *contrayerba* and refers his readers to the work of

Hernández in the version of Recchi and to the work of Monardes in *Historia natural y moral*, bk. 4, ch. 29, fol. 85r.; *Natural and Moral History*, ed. Mangan, 222–223.

108. See Carmen Martín Martín and José Luis Valverde, *La farmacia en la América colonial: El arte de preparar medicamentos* (Granada: Universidad de Granada, 1995), 454. Or the *contrayerba* could be the passionflower (*passiflora normalis*), of which Hernández wrote, which is used to depress the central nervous system and thus sedates spasms and lowers blood pressure.

109. The toxic effects of the Spanish fly are evident, for example, in the account of Prioress Angelica della Macchia recounting how Sister Domenica da Paradiso "took certain syrups prescribed to her by the doctors. In one (and it is not known if it was there by mistake or for some other reason) was a poison, Spanish fly, and as soon as she took it she had many attacks of vomiting, bloody discharge, inflammation, and filming over her eyes, so that she collapsed and almost died." In Giulia Calvi, "A Metaphor for Social Exchange: The Florentine Plague of 1630," *Representations* 13 (1986): 139–163, 158.

110. "Levo de Potosí quatro Aletti che qui me li hanno stimati in grandiss.o pretio i dal virei de nova Spagna et dal general de questi galioni se han morto più de la metà en el camino, a mi se me hano morti due pauxi de pedra che tienen en la fronte che sono come pavoni, due altri tengo de plumas, una guacamaya se ne volo en la mar, tengo trei catalincas e papagalo altri animali se me han morto. Levo altre cose curiose e cose medicinale si di predre come de gume et resine et olji et conserve e qui stan cargando doi navigli per Genova ne gli me imbarcarò credo che saliranno dentro de 15 giorni." Letter of October 25, 1611, in ASM, AG, busta 610, fol. 604. The identification of these animals is offered by Ostino, "Il viaggio," 19. Marcobruno wrote Vincenzo that he would try to collect these items before leaving the New World; he had been given 500 scudi for his expenses. See ASM, AG, busta 609, fol. 335r.

111. "Ando comperando duoi barili picioli de olive di queste così grosse credo sarà gusto di V.A." Letter of Marcobruno to Vincenzo, October 25, 1611, in ASM, AG, busta 610, fol. 604r. Olives and vines were introduced by the Spaniards and thrived in Peru to the point that they were also sent to Mexico, according to Francesco Carletti, who visited the area around 1594–1596. From the context it seems more likely, however, that Marcobruno got the olives just before leaving Spain.

112. "Mi rincresce a dirli che questa settimana si è inteso che la nave dove se imbarcò detto Marcobruno fu presa da corsari et condotta in Algieri, et seben vi ho qualche interesso, più mi duole la captività della persona di esso Marcobruno, che seben ha buon signore che con ogni brevità procurerà sua libertà, non lassa di stare in miserabil statto, et forse lo haveran privatto delle curiosità che portava a Sua Altezza, che non serà poco

suo disgusto a presso al resto. So non essere bisogno importunare a vostra signoria per darne aviso et adoprarsi in sua libertà, che per la affectione li porto ne restarò a vostra signoria obbligatissimo per mia parte, et se di qua vi fosse qualche tratto con Algieri, ne farei pratica con le opere, perciò mi serà gratto sapere a suo loco il negociato et con suo commodo dirmi della receputa di quella, et per fine basio le mani di vostra signoria et nostro Signore la feliciti. Di Sevilla 21 febraro 1612, Filippo Soles." In ASM, AG, busta 611, fol. 270. On the often horrible living conditions reserved for Christian slaves in seventeenth-century Algiers (as the lore went, they could be sold for one onion), see Robert Davis, *Christian Slaves, Muslim Masters: White Slavery in the Mediterranean, the Barbary Coast, and Italy, 1500–1800* (New York: Palgrave Macmillan, 2003).

113. In his letter to Ferdinando from Madrid of July 14, 1609, for example, Marcobruno promised the then cardinal that he would bring back some "noble plants." See ASM, AG, busta 609, fol. 325r. Earlier, when still in Spain, he had sent back to Mantua a pound and seven ounces of *mumia* (dried human flesh), a popular cure of early modern medicine. See the letter of July 14, 1609, from Madrid to Annibale Iberti, in ASM, AG, busta 609, fol. 327r.

114. "Promitto in fede di Principi che liberandosi Evangelista Marcobruno captivo in Algieri per opera del padre fra Felice Beninisi dell'ordine della Trinità e del Padre Ministro del Monasterio di Genova mi contenti di farli pagare trecento ducatoni per il suo riscatto e ricuperando li robbe ch'esso Evangelista portava dall'India gli farò sborsare quello che spendarà per essi. In fede di che ho fatto scrivere e sigillar la presente che sarà firmata di mia mano. Di Mantova li 11 giugno 1613. Ferdinando etc. duca di Mantova." In ASM, AG, Mandati, vol. 98, busta 47. Ferdinando himself was a budding scientist and lover of learning, and worked hard at establishing the reputation of the short-lived but well staffed "Peaceful University" in Mantua: the Pacifico Gymnasio Mantuano (1624–1629). See Paul Grendler, *The University of Mantua, the Gonzaga and the Jesuits, 1584–1630* (Baltimore: Johns Hopkins University Press, 2009).

115. On the various procedures available at the time to ransom Christian slaves from their Muslim captors, see, for example, Andrea Pelizza, *Riammessi a respirare l'aria tranquilla: Venezia e il riscatto degli schiavi in età moderna* (Venice: Istituto Veneto di Lettere, Scienze ed Arti, 2012) and Davis, *Christian Slaves, Muslim Masters*.

116. For the metaphor of hunting to discover nature and peer into its secrets, which characterized many early modern scientific inquiries, see, among others, Paolo Rossi, *Philosophy, Technology, and the Arts in the Early Modern Era* (New York: Harper and Row, 1970), 42.

117. Pratt situates this moment around the year 1735, when Carl Linnaeus's *Systema Naturae* was published and the first inter-European (French and British) scientific expedition was launched to chronicle the earth's exact

shape. See Mary Louise Pratt, *Imperial Eyes: Travel Writing and Transculturation* (New York: Routledge, 1992), 15. But in a more general sense, from the very beginning the conquest of the new world defined a superior European self. One has just to look at the proliferation starting in late sixteenth century of costume books meant at separating "us" from "them," as in the immensely popular Cesare Vecellio's *Habiti antichi et moderni di diverse parti del mondo* (1589 and 1598), recently published with the original thorough commentary by Margaret F. Rosenthal and Ann Rosalind Jones, *The Clothing of the Renaissance World: Europe, Asia, Africa, the Americas* (London: Thames and Hudson, 2008).

118. Taking an actuarial stance, Marcobruno tells Vincenzo on October 25, 1611, of the extent of the Spanish fleet's wealth in a vocabulary nonchalantly mixing Italian with Spanish: "En la flota di questo ano hano levato li galloni nove milloni et sei ciento et quinze mil et novanta pesos da otto reali per cada pesos, de questi tiene sua Maestà doi milioni et sinquanta otto mil et tresiento setanta pesos el restante e de mercanti." In ASM, AG, busta 610, fol. 604r.

119. Galileo Galilei, *Sidereus Nuncius* (Milan: Unaluna, 2010).

120. Maca, for example, has many true believers today. To wit, an Italian obstetrician and gynecologist, Giovanni Menaldo, recently revealed to the media that he uses maca in his clinic in Turin to increase fertility in men by maturing spermatozoa, and in women by stimulating the production of mature ovocites. See *Oggi*, March 30, 2005, 75–79, at 75. Menaldo also experiments with the *Huanarpo macho*, the *Draconium loretense*, and the *Camu camu*.

121. See Ostino, "L'avventuroso viaggio al Perú," 20–21.

122. Scansani cites the story—told by A. Seitz, a butterfly specialist—of an Amazonian woman who was stung by the *Megalopyge orsilochus* and developed an inflammatory reaction in the upper part of her body plus fever. See Scansani, *L'amor morto*, 231–232. Scansani's novelistic rendering of Vincenzo's problems is a good read but historically unreliable.

123. José López Piñero, "La 'nuevas medicinas' americanas en la obra de Nicolas Monardes," *Asclepio* 42.1 (1990): 3–67, at 46: "Vienen a ser del grandor de una naranja."

124. Dr. Romero's research is financed by a grant of $970,000. His team hopes to be able to patent the drug at the end of a three-year study, and already a pharmaceutical company, Laboratorio Silesia, has invested in the project. See B. Wigmore, "Venom 'Viagra,'" *Mirror*, News Section (2003): 31. I would also like to thank Celia Cussen, from the University of Santiago, and Dr. Beltrán Mena for guiding me in this reading.

125. This two-year study was presented at the 2007 annual meeting of the American Physiological Society by the team of Romulo Leite. The news was also carried by the BBC on May 4, 2007, and then all over the Internet. Now a team of neurologists and sexual health specialists headed by

Dr. Gruenwald of Haifa's Rambam Hospital in Israel plans to study three types of spiders originating in South America and Africa, including the black widow and most probably the Brazilian wandering spider. This last information comes from *Ynetnews.com* of April 12, 2007.

126. To sense the visual importance of the scorpion for the House of Gonzaga, one has to look at Raphael's portrait of Elisabetta Gonzaga (1504), now at the Uffizi in Florence, in which the duchess is portrayed with a scorpion on her forehead. On the scorpion in the Gonzaga coat of arms, see Paola Goretti, "Limatura della luna argentea: La scienza dei magnifici apparati fra malinconia, vestiario e vaghezze d'antico," in *Gonzaga: La Celeste Galeria*, ed. Morselli, 185–211, at 197–198.

Epilogue

1. The architect of what has since been called "The Maze" room was Antonio Maria Viani, the prefect of the Gonzaga building sites.
2. Claudio Gallico, *"Forse che si forse che no" tra poesia e musica* (Mantua: Istituto Carlo d'Arco per la Storia di Mantova, 1961).
3. Vincenzo Errante, "'Forse che sì, forse che no': La terza spedizione del duca Vincenzo Gonzaga in Ungheria alla guerra contro il turco (1601) studiata su documenti inediti," *Archivio storico lombardo* 42.1 (1915): 15–114, at 82.
4. Maria Bellonci, *Segreti dei Gonzaga* (Milan: Mondadori, 2000), 232.
5. "Tutta la città umiliò preci pubbliche e fervorose a Dio per la salute dell'ottimo suo sovrano. . . . Il Duca, in vedendosi restabilito, ne rese grazie a Sua Divina Maestà, e per compiere un voto da lui fatto nella sua malattia, si vestì di colore bigio simile a quello de' Francescani." In Amadei, *Cronaca universale della città di Mantova* (Mantua: CITEM, 1954), 3:279.
6. "A primavera pensava di andarsene in Alemagna alla dieta," wrote Lelio Arrivabene to Duke Francesco Maria II Della Rovere, on February 17, 1612. In ASF, *Urbino*, fol. 241, c. 964v.
7. "Al terzo proferire che fece il dolcissimo nome di Gesù, spirò l'anima verso le ore due di notte delli 18 febbraio. Fu imbalsamato il di lui cadavero . . . e con questo funebre accompagnamento transferironlo alla basilica di S. Andrea." In Amadei, *Cronaca universale della città di Mantova*, 3:279.
8. The information is in the letter that Lelio Arrivabene wrote on May 22, 1612, to Francesco Maria II Della Rovere. In ASF, *Urbino*, fol. 241, c. 995r–v.
9. For a study of Renaissance techniques regarding the preparation of the ruler's body for entombment, see Giovanni Ricci, *Il principe e la morte: Corpo, cuore, effigie nel Rinascimento* (Bologna: Il Mulino, 1998). Ricci studies in particular the burial of the Este dukes in Ferrara. We have detailed information regarding the preparation for burial of Vincenzo's own son,

Guglielmo Lungaspada, whose young body was not embalmed but was instead set on the catafalque surrounded by tons of flower bouquets to mask any decomposing odor. See Giancarlo Malacarne, *Splendore e declino: da Vincenzo I a Vincenzo II (1587–1627)* (Modena: Il Bulino, 2007), 186–191.

10. "Maiestas Dei in principibus extra apparet in utilitatem subditorum, sed intus remanet quod humanum est." In Pierre Grégoire (Gregorio Tholosano), *De republica libri sex et viginti* (Lyon: Pillehotte, 1609), cited also in Ernst H. Kantorowicz, *The King's Two Bodies: A Study in Mediaeval Political Theology* (Princeton: Princeton University Press, 1957), 422.

Selected Bibliography

Manuscript Sources

Andreasi, Lodovico. "Memorie dei quattro ultimi duchi di Mantova." Cod. 162, Fondo D'Arco, Archivio Storico, Mantua.

Anon. "Racconto delle cose successe in Genova dall'anno 1600 fino al 1610." Ms. Seventeenth century, fol. 1373, July 6, 1607. In Archivio del Comune, Genoa, Fondo Brignole Sale, 109. D. 4.

Archivio di Stato di Mantova (ASM), Archivio Gonzaga (AG)

    Buste 168, 201, 202, 203, 330, 388, 465, 546, 609, 610, 611, 745, 975, 1091, 1126, 1161, 1164, 1166, 1168, 1379, 1380, 1381, 1513, 1534, 1540, 1701, 1735, 2096, 2155, 2210, 2269, 2615, 2645, 2665, 2699, 2702, 2712, 3106

    Mandati, vol. 98, busta 47

    E. XI.3, buste 574, 575

    E. XLV.3, busta 1540

    E. XXI.3, busta 777

Archivio di Stato di Firenze (ASF), Mediceo del Principato (MDP) http://bia.medici.org/DocSources/Home.do

    MDP 211, DocID 8868

    MDP 627, DocID 10868

    MDP 2646, DocID 5204

    MDP 2940, DocID 4566

    MDP 2941, DocID 4837

    MDP 2942, DocIDs 4968, 4991, 4996, 4998, 16315

    MDP 2943, DocIDs 5011, 5014, 5019, 16223

    MDP 2944, DocIDs 5074, 5097, 5099, 5114

    MDP 2945, DocID 4788

    MDP 2951, DocIDs 5428, 5542

    MDP 3255, DocIDs 10760, 10834, 11140

    MDP 3263, DocID 19030

MDP 4255, DocID 25843
MDP 4256, DocID 23079
MDP 4796, DocID 2945
MDP 5046, DocID 16148
MDP 5109, DocIDs 17625, 17646, 17660
MDP Person ID 9335

Archivio di Stato di Firenze (ASF), *Urbino*
Archivio di Stato di Venezia, Provveditori alla Sanità, Notatorio 765
Mancini, Giulio. *Della sanità*. Biblioteca Apostolica Vaticana, Barb. Lat. 4315
———. *Del Disonore*. Biblioteca Apostolica Vaticana, Barb. Lat. 4314

Newspapers and Magazines

La Repubblica. December 4, 2007
Marie Claire. January 20, 2010, online blog
New York Times. May 27, 2010, E3
Oggi. March 30, 2005, 75–79

Primary Printed Sources

Acosta, José de. *Historia natural y moral de las Indias*. Seville: de Leon, 1590. Translated into Italian as *Historia naturale, e morale delle Indie*. Venice: Basa, 1596.

Africanus, Leo (Leone Africano). "Della descrittione dell'Africa et delle cose notabili che ivi sono." In Giovanni Battista Ramusio, *Navigationi et viaggi*. 3 vols. Venice: Giunti, 1565.

Aldrovandi, Ulisse. *Ornithologiae, hoc est de avibus historiae . . . libri XII*. Bologna: Fraciscum de Franciscis, 1599.

Anania, Giovanni Lorenzo d'. *L'universale fabrica del mondo, overo cosmografia*. Venice: Muschio, 1596.

Anguillara, Lampridio. *Vaticinio et avertimenti per conservare la sanità, et prolongar la vita humana*. Ferrara: Vittorio Baldini, 1589.

Aranzi, Giulio Cesare. *De humano foetu libellus*. Bologna: Ioannis Rubii ad insigne Mercurii, 1564.

Augenio, Orazio. *Epistolarum et consultationum medicinalium alterius tomi libri XII*. Venice: Zenarium, 1592.

Avisi particolari delle Indie di Portugallo. Rome: Dorico and Bressani, 1552.

Bacci, Andrea. *De thermis*. Venice: Valgrisi, 1571.

Bartholin, Caspar. *Anatomicae institutiones corporis humani*. Oxford: Turner, 1633.

Bartholin, Thomas. *Bartolinus Anatomy, Made from the Precepts of His Father, and from Observations of All Modern Anatomists, Together with His Own*. London: John Streater, 1668.

Bauhin, Caspar. *Pinax theatri botanici*. Basel: Ludovici Regi, 1623.

Bertioli, Antonio. *Delle considerazioni . . . sopra l'olio di scorpioni dell'eccellentissimo Matthioli.* Mantua: Francesco Osanna, 1585.

Campanella, Tommaso. *De sensu rerum et magia. Libri quatuor.* Frankfurt: Apud Emmelium, 1620.

Cervio, Vincenzo. *Il trinciante.* Rome: Nella stampa del Gabbia, 1593.

Chauliac, Guy, de. *Cyrurgia Guidonis de Cauliaco.* Venice: Octaviani Scoti, 1498.

Clusius, Carolus (Charles de l'Ecluse). *Exoticorum libri decem.* Leiden: Raphelenghi, 1605.

———. *Rariorum aliquot stirpium per Hispanias observatarum historia.* Antwerp: Piantini, 1576.

Codronchi, Giovan Battista. *De morbis qui Imolae.* Bologna: Battista Bellagamba, 1603.

Colombo, Realdo. *De re anatomica libri XV.* Venice: Bevilacqua, 1559.

Colonna, Fabio. *Phytobasanos sive plantarum aliquot historia: in qua describuntur diversi generis plantae veriores.* Naples: Carlinum et Pacem, 1592.

Culpeper, Nicholas. *A Directory for Midwives; or, A Guide for Women in Their Conception, Bearing, and Suckling Their Children.* London: Cole, 1651.

Della Croce, Giovanni Andrea. *Della cirurgia libri sette.* Venice: Ziletti, 1574.

Della Porta, Giambattista. *Phytognomonica seu methodus nova facillimaque qua plantarum ac rerum omnium vires ex solo faciei inspection assignatur.* Naples, 1583.

Diversi avisi particolari dall'Indie di Portogallo, ricevuti dall'anno 1551 sino al 1558 dalli reverendi padri della Compagnia di Giesù. Venice: Tramezzino, 1565.

Donati, Marcello. *De variolis et morbillis tractatus . . . Eiusdem De radice purgante qua mechiocan vocant.* Mantua: Philoterpsem et Philoponos, 1569.

Du Chesne, Joseph (Quercetanus, Giuseppe). *Pharmacopoea dogmatorum restituta.* Paris: Morellus, 1607.

Du Laurens, André. *Historia anatomica.* Frankfurt: Rhodius, 1600.

Durante, Castore. *Herbario Nuovo . . . con figure che rappresentano le vive piante che nascono in tutta Europa, et nelle indie orientali et occidentali.* Rome: Bonfadino et Diani, 1585.

———. *Il tesoro della sanità: nel quale si da il modo da conservar la sanità, et prolungar la vita, et si tratta della natura de' cibi ed de' rimedij de' nocumenti loro.* Mantua, 1590.

———. *A Treasure of Health.* London: William Crook, 1685.

Fabrici d'Acquapendente (Fabricius ab Aquapendente), Girolamo. *De formatione ovi et pulli.* Padua: Antonij Meglietti, 1621.

———. *Opera chirurgica in duas partes divisas.* Venice: apud Robertum Megliettum, 1619.

Falloppio, Gabriele. *Observationes anatomicae.* 2 vols. Venice: Viman, 1561.

———. *Opera genuina omnia, tam practica quam theorica.* Venice: De Franciscis, 1606.

———. *Secreti diversi e miracolosi.* Venice: Imberti, 1640.

———. *De thermalibus aquis atque de fossilibus,* edited by Andrea Marcolini. Venice: Ziletti, 1564.

―――. *De ulceribus*. Venice: Bertelli, 1563.

Fioravanti, Leonardo. *Il tesoro della vita humana. Dell'Eccellente dottore e cavaliere M. Leonardo Fioravanti Bolognese. Diviso in quattro libri*. Venice: Sessa, 1570.

Fragoso, Juan. *Discursos de las cosas aromaticas*. Madrid: Yuañez, 1572.

Franco, Giacomo. *Effigie naturali dei maggior principi et più valorosi capitani di questa età con l'arme loro. Raccolte et con diligenza intagliate da Giacomo Franco*. Venice: Apud Iacobum Francum, 1596.

Giunta, Tomaso, ed. *De balneis omnia quae extant apud Graecos, Latinos, et Arabas*. Venice: Giunta, 1553.

Giusti, Vincenzo. *Irene*. Venice: Gio. Battista Somasco, 1588.

Glisson, Francis. *De rachitide, sive morbo puerili*. London: Sadler and Beaumont, 1650.

Gradi, Basilio. *Trattato della verginità et dello stato verginale: molto à proposito delle vergini che desiderano farsi grate al celeste sposo, et à tutti quelli che vogliono menar vista casta, et viver lieti et contenti nel servitio di Dio*. Rome: Bonfadino et Diani, 1584.

Grégoire, Pierre. *De republica libri sex et viginti*. Lyon: Pillehotte, 1609.

Guazzo, Stefano. *La civil conversatione del signor Stefano Guazzo*. Venice: Salicato, 1575.

Harvey, William. *Exercitationes de generatione animalium. Quibus accedunt quaedum de partu: de membranis ac humoribus uteri et de conceptione*. London: Typis Du Gardinis, 1651.

Hernández, Francisco. *Rerum medicarum Novae Hispaniae thesaurus*. Rome: Mascardi, 1651.

Marinello, Giovanni. *Gli ornamenti delle donne scritti per M. Giovanni Marinello. Et divisi in Quattro Libri*. Venice: Valgrisio, 1574.

―――. *Le medicine partenenti alle infermità delle donne*. Venice: Valgrisio, 1574.

Mattioli, Pietro. *Del modo di distillare le acque da tutte le piante*. Venice: Valgrisi, 1581.

Mazzella, Scipione. *Opusculum de Balneis Puteolanum Baiarum et Pithecusarum*. Naples: Ex typographia Stelliolae, 1593.

Mercuriale, Girolamo. *De decoratione*. Venice: Apud Paolum Meietum, 1585.

Mercurio, Girolamo. *La commare o riccoglitrice*. Venice: Ciotti, 1596.

Minadoi, Giovanni Tommaso. *De arthritide*. Padua: Bolzetta, 1602.

―――. *De humani corporis turpitudinibus cognoscendis et curandis libri tres*. Padua: Bolzetta, 1600.

Minardo, Ventura. *De balneis Calderii in agro veronensi* and *Compendio delle regole contenute ne gli Eccellentissimi Autori, che de' bagni di Caldiero nel territorio veronese hanno scritto del modo di usar dette acque e fango*. Venice: Ad instantiam Alexandri F. Thomae de Salodiis, 1571.

Monardes, Nicolás. *Delle cose che vengono portate dall'Indie Occidentali, pertinenti all'uso della medicina*. Venice: Ziletti, 1575.

Nuovi avisi dell' Indie di Portogallo. Venice: Tramezzino, 1562.

Oviedo, Gonzalo Fernández de. *Libro secondo delle Indie Occidentali . . . Summario della naturale et generale historia dell'Indie occidentali, composta da Gonzalo*

Ferdinando del Oviedo. In Giambattista Ramusio, *Terzo volume delle Navigationi et viaggi.* Venice: Giunti, 1556.

Paré, Ambroise. *Les Oevvres d'Ambroise Paré.* Paris: Gabriel Buon, 1585.

———. *Opera chirugica.* Frankfurt: Apud Johannen Feyrabend, 1594.

———. *The Workes of That Famous Chirurgion Ambrose Parey.* Translated by Thomas Johnson. London, 1638.

Persia, Ferrante. *Relatione de' ricevimenti fatti in Mantova alla Maesta della Regina di Spagna Dal Sereniss. Sig. Duca, Anno MDXCVIII del Mese di Novembre.* Ferrara: Baldini, 1598.

Ramusio, Giovanni Battista. *Navigationi et viaggi.* 3 vols. Venice: Giunti, 1565.

Rosaccio, Gioseppe. *Il mondo e le sue parti cioe Europa, Africa, Asia, et America.* Florence: Tosi, 1595.

Savonarola, Michele. *De balneis et thermis naturalibus omnibus Italiae,* in *De balneis omnia quae extant apud Graecos, Latinos, et Arabas,* edited by Tomaso Giunta. Venice: Giunta, 1553.

———. *Practica major.* Venice: Giunta, 1547.

Sydenham, Thomas. *Methodus curandi febres, propriis observationibus superstructa.* London: Crook, 1666.

Tordesillas, Antonio de Herrera y. *Historia general de los hechos de los castellanos en las islas y tierrafirme de el mar Oceano.* Madrid: Emplenta Real, 1601–1615.

Valerini, Adriano. *La celeste galeria di Minerva.* Verona: Appresso Girolamo Discepolo, 1588.

Varoli, Costanzo. *Anatomiae, sive de resolutione corporis umani libri IIII.* Frankfurt: Wechel and Fischer, 1591.

Vesalius, Andreas. *Anatomicarum Gabrielis Falloppii observationum examen.* Venice: Francesco de' Franceschi da Siena, 1564.

———. *Epistola rationem modumque propinandi radicis Chynae decocti* ("Letter on the China Root"). Brussels: Johannes Oporinus, 1546.

———. *De humani corporis fabrica.* Basilea: Johannes Oporinus, 1543.

———. (pseudo Vesalius). *Chirurgia magne,* edited by Prospero Borganucci. Venice: Valgrisi, 1568.

Zacchia, Paolo. *Quaestiones medico-legales.* 7 vols. Rome: Brugiotti, 1621–1635.

Selected Secondary Sources

Acosta, José de. *Natural and Moral History of the Indies,* edited by Jane Mangan. Durham: Duke University Press, 2002.

Adelman, Janet. "Making Defect Perfection: Shakespeare and the One-Sex Model." In *Enacting Gender on the English Renaissance Stage,* edited by Viviana Comensoli and Anne Russell, 23–52. Urbana: University of Illinois Press, 1999.

Ademollo, Alessandro. *La bell'Adriana ed altre virtuose del suo tempo alla corte di Mantova: Contributo di documenti per la storia della musica in Italia nel primo quarto del Seicento.* Città di Castello: Lapi, 1888.

Albertus Magnus. *De animalibus libri 26.* Munster: Aschendorff, 1916–1922.

Alden, John, ed. *European Americana: A Chronological Guide to Works Printed in Europe Relating to the Americas, 1493–1776.* With the assistance of Dennis C. Landis. 6 vols. New York: Readex, 1980–1988.

Alighieri, Dante. *Il Convivio,* translated by Richard Lansing. New York: Garland, 1990.

———. *Inferno,* edited and translated by Charles Singleton. Princeton: Princeton University Press, 1970.

Altieri Biagi, Maria Luisa, Clemente Mazzotta, Angela Chiantera, and Paola Altieri, eds. *Medicina per le donne nel Cinquecento. Testi di Giovanni Marinello e di Girolamo Mercurio.* Turin: UTET, 1992.

Amadei, Federico. *Cronaca universale della città di Mantova.* 3 vols. Mantua: CITEM, 1953.

Ambrose. *De institutione virginis.* In *Verginità e vedovanza,* edited by Franco Gori. 2 vols. Rome-Milan: Città nuova editrice, 1989.

Ambrosini, Federica. *Paesi e mari ignoti: America e colonialismo europeo nella cultura veneziana (secoli XVI–XVII).* Venice: Deputazione Editrice, 1982.

Anderson, Frank. *An Illustrated History of the Herbals.* New York: Columbia University Press, 1977.

Aquinas, Thomas. *Summa theologica.* Paris: Blot, 1926.

Arber, Agnes. *Herbals: Their Origin and Evolution; A Chapter in the History of Botany, 1470–1670.* Cambridge: Cambridge University Press, 1912.

Aretino, Pietro. *Lettere,* edited by Paolo Procaccioli. 6 vols. Rome: Salerno, 1997–2002.

Ariosto, Ludovico. *Orlando furioso,* edited by Marcello Turchi. Milan: Garzanti, 1974.

Bargagli, Marzio. *Storia di Caterina che per ott'anni vestì abiti da uomo.* Bologna: Il Mulino, 2014.

Barrera-Osorio, Antonio. *Experiencing Nature: The Spanish American Empire and the Early Scientific Revolution.* Austin: University of Texas Press, 2006.

Barilli, Arnaldo. *Studi farnesiani.* Parma: La Bodoniana, 1958.

Barosky, Paul. *Michelangelo's Nose: A Myth and Its Maker.* University Park: Penn State University Press, 1990.

Bellonci, Maria. *Segreti dei Gonzaga.* Milan: Mondadori, 1947.

Bellù, Adele. "Margherita Farnese, sposa mancata di Vincenzo Gonzaga." *Archivi per la storia* 1–2 (1988): 381–420.

Benassi, Enrico. *I consulti medici di Giambattista Morgagni.* Bologna: Cappelli, 1934.

Benedek, Thomas. "The Changing Relationship between Midwives and Physicians during the Renaissance." *Bulletin of the History of Medicine* 51 (1977): 550–564.

———. "The History of Gold Therapy for Tuberculosis." *Journal of the History of Medicine and Allied Sciences* 59.1 (2004): 50–89.

Benedek, Thomas, and Gerald Rodnan. "Petrarch on Medicine and the Gout." *Bulletin of the History of Medicine* 37 (1963): 397–416.
Benedetti, Alessandro. *Anatomice, sive Historia corporis humanis,* edited and translated by Giovanna Ferrari. Florence: Giunti, 1998.
Benedicenti, Alberico. *Malati, medici e farmacisti: storia dei rimedi traverso i secoli e delle teorie che ne spiegano l'azione sull'organismo.* 2 vols. Milan: Hoepli, 1924.
Bertelli, Paolo. "Appunti sulla ritrattistica di Vincenzo I Gonzaga." In *Scritti per Chiara Tellini Perina,* edited by Daniela Ferrari and Sergio Marinelli. 229–249. Mantua: Arcari, 2011.
Bertolotti, Antonino. *Le arti minori alla corte di Mantova nei secoli XV, XVI e XVII.* Bologna: Forni, 1974.
Bevacqua, Vincenzo. "L'ospedale del Brolo." *La Ca' Granda* 45.2 (2004): 30–37.
Biagioli, Mario. "Galileo's System of Patronage." *History of Science* 28 (1990): 1–61.
Bicks, Catherine. *Midwiving Subjects in Shakespeare's England.* Aldershot: Ashgate, 2003.
Bleichmar, Daniela. "Books, Bodies, and Fields: Sixteenth-Century Transatlantic Encounters with the New World *Materia Medica.*" In *Colonial Botany: Science, Commerce, and Politics in the Early Modern World,* edited by Londa Schiebinger and Claudia Swan, 83–99. Philadelphia: University of Pennsylvania Press, 2005.
Bloom, Virginia. *Flesh Wounds: The Culture of Cosmetic Surgery.* Los Angeles: University of California Press, 2003.
Boccaccio, Giovanni. *L'elegia di Madonna Fiammetta.* Florence: Moutier, 1829.
Boggione, Walter, and Giovanni Casalegno. *Dizionario storico del lessico erotico italiano.* Milan: Longanesi, 1996.
Botallo, Leonardo. *I doveri del medico e del malato,* edited by Leonardo Carerj and Anita Bogetti Fassone. Turin: UTET, 1981.
Bourgain, Pascale, ed. *Ademari Cabannensis Chronicon.* Corpus Christianorum Continuatio Mediaevalis 129. Brepols: Turnhout, 1999.
Braglia, Riccardo. *I Gonzaga: Il mito, la storia.* Cerese di Virgilio: Rossi, 2002.
Brockliss, L. W. B. "The Development of the Spa in Seventeenth-Century France." *Medical History,* Supplement 10 (1990): 23–47.
Brunori (da Meldola), Camillo. *Il medico poeta, ovvero la medicina esposta in versi, e prose italiane.* Fabriano: Gregorio Marriotti, 1726.
Burattelli, Claudia. *Spettacoli di corte a Mantova tra Cinque e Seicento.* Florence: Le Lettere, 1999.
Butler, Samuel. *Hudibras,* edited by John Wilders. London: Clarendon Press, 1967.
Cadden, Joan. *Meanings of Sex Difference in the Middle Ages: Medicine, Science, and Culture.* Cambridge: Cambridge University Press, 1993.
Calvi, Giulia. "A Metaphor for Social Exchange: The Florentine Plague of 1630." *Representations* 13 (1986): 139–163.

Calvino, Italo. "The Silver Nose." In *Italian Folktales*. London: Penguin, 2000.
Camporesi, Piero. *The Anatomy of the Senses: Natural Symbols in Medieval and Early Modern Italy*, translated by Allan Cameron. Cambridge: Polity Press, 1995.
———. *I balsami di Venere*. Milan: Garzanti, 1989.
———. *Bread of Dreams: Food and Fantasy in Early Modern Europe*, translated by David Gentilcore. Chicago: University of Chicago Press, 1989.
———. *Camminare il mondo: Vita e avventure di Leonardo Fioravanti medico del Cinquecento*. Milan: Garzanti, 1997.
———. *The Incorruptible Flesh: Bodily Mutation and Mortification in Religion and Folklore*, translated by Tania Croft-Murray. New York: Cambridge University Press, 1988.
———. "Speziali e ciarlatani." In *Cultura popolare nell'Emilia Romagna: Medicina, erbe e magia*, edited by Giuseppe Adani and Gastone Tavagnini. Milan: Silvana, 1981.
Canepa, Giuseppe. *Osteopatologia infantile: manuale-atlante di ortopedia per pediatri*. Padua: Piccin, 1996.
Capelluti, Rolando. *La chirurgia di Mo. Rolando da Parma detto dei Capezzuti. Riproduzione del Codice Latino n. 1382 della R. Biblioteca Casanatense di Roma*. Rome: Istituto Nazionale Medico Farmacologico Serono, 1927.
Capparoni, Pietro. "Le vicende della tomba di Gaspare Tagliacozzi." Rome: Istituto Nazionale Medico Farmacologico Serono, 1933. Reprint from *Bollettino dell'Istituto Storico Italiano dell'Arte Sanitaria* 32.4 (July–August 1933): 1–11.
Carletti. Francesco. *Ragionamenti del mio viaggio intorno al mondo*, edited by Gianfranco Silvestro. Turin: Einaudi, 1958.
Caro, Annibal. *La nasea*, in *Commento di ser Agresto da Ficaruolo sopra la prima ficata del padre Siceo*. Bologna: Romagnoli, 1961.
Carpue, Joseph Constantine. *An Account of Two Successful Operations for Restoring a Lost Nose from the Integuments of the Forehead*. London: Longman, Hurst, Rees, Orme, and Brown, 1816.
Carter, Tim. *Monteverdi's Musical Theatre*. New Haven: Yale University Press, 2002.
Castiglione, Baldesar. *The Book of the Courtier*, translated by George Bull. New York: Penguin, 1967.
Celsus, Aulus Cornelius. *De medicina*, translated by G. W. Spencer. Cambridge: Harvard University Press, 1935–1938.
Cermenati, Mario. "Ulisse Aldrovandi e l'America." *Annali di Botanica* 4 (1906): 313–366.
Cey, Galeotto. *Viaggio e relazione delle Indie, 1539–1553*, edited by Francesco Surdich. Rome: Bulzoni, 1992.
Chambers, David S. "Federico Gonzaga ai bagni di Caldiero." *Civiltà mantovana*, n.s. 4 (1984): 45–61.

Chrysostom, John. *On Virginity, Against Remarriage*. Translated by Sally Rieger Shore, with an introduction by Elizabeth A. Clark. Lewiston: Mellen Press, 1983.

Cipolla, Carlo. *Fighting the Plague in Seventeenth Century Italy*. Madison: University of Wisconsin Press, 1981.

———. *Miasmi e umori*. Bologna: Il Mulino, 1989.

Cipolla, Costantino, and Giancarlo Malacarne. *El più soave et dolce et dilectevole et gratioso bochone: Amore e sesso al tempo dei Gonzaga*. Milan: Franco Angeli, 2006.

Clark, Elizabeth. "Sex, Shame and Rhetoric: En-gendering Early Christian Ethics." *Journal of the American Academy of Religion* 59.2 (1991): 221–245.

Clough, C. H. "The Library of the Gonzaga of Mantua." *Librarium* 15 (1972): 50–63.

Cocco, Sean. *Watching Vesuvius: A History of Science and Culture in Early Modern Italy*. Chicago: University of Chicago Press, 2012.

Columbus, Christopher. *Textos y documentos completos: Relaciones de viajes, cartas, y memoriales*, edited by Consuelo Varala. Madrid: Allianza, 1982.

Compagni, Dino. *Cronica*, edited by Davide Cappi. Rome: Istituto Palazzo Borromini, 2000.

———. *Dino Compagni's Chronicle of Florence*, translated by Daniel Bornstein. Philadelphia: University of Pennsylvania Press 1986.

Coniglio, Giuseppe. *I Gonzaga*. Milan: Dall'Oglio, 1967.

Corradi, Alfonso. "Dell'antica autoplastica italiana." In *Memorie del Regio Istituto Lombardo di Scienze e Lettere. Classe di Scienze Matematiche e Naturali*. Ser. 3. 13 (1883): 225–275.

Cortese, Isabella. *I secreti della signora Isabella Cortese ne' quali si contengono cose minerali, medicinali, arteficiose, e alchemiche*. Milan: La vita felice, 1995.

Costa, Margherita. *Li buffoni*. In *Commedie dell'Arte*. Vol. 2, edited by Siro Ferrone. Milan: Mursia, 1986.

Crisciani, Chiara. "Oro potabile fra alchimia e medicina: due testi in tempo di peste." In *Convegno nazionale di storia e fondamenti della chimica: L'Aquila, 8–11 Ottobre 1987*, edited by Franco Calascibetta, 83–93. Rome: Accademia Nazionale delle Scienze, 1997.

Cruz, Martín de la. *The Badianus Manuscript (Codex Barberini, Latin 241), Vatican Library: An Aztec Herbal of 1552*, translated by Emily Walcott Emmart. Baltimore: Johns Hopkins University Press, 1940.

Dacome, Lucia, "Balancing Acts: Picturing Perspiration in the Long Eighteenth Century." *Studies in History and Philosophy of Biological and Biomedical Science* 43 (2012): 379–391.

Dall'Osso, Eugenio. "Giulio Cesare Aranzio e la rinoplastica." *Annali di medicina navale e tropicale* 61 (1956): 617–627.

D'Ancona, Alessandro. *Origini del teatro italiano*. 2 vols. Turin: Loescher, 1891.

Darmstaedter, Ernst. "Per la storia dell'*aurum potabile*." *Archivio di Storia della Scienza* 5.3 (1924): 251–271.

Davanzo Poli, Doretta. "La moda ai bagni di moda." In *Alle fonti del piacere,* edited by Nelli-Elena Vanzan Marchini, 77–99. Milan: Leonardo Arte, 1999.

David, Alfred. "An Iconography of Noses: Directions in the History of a Physical Stereotype." In *Mapping the Cosmos,* edited by Jane Chance and R. O. Wells Jr. Houston: Rice University Press, 1985.

Davis, Robert. *Christian Slaves, Muslim Masters: White Slavery in the Mediterranean, the Barbary Coast, and Italy, 1500–1800.* New York: Palgrave Macmillan, 2003.

Dean, Trevor, and K. J. P. Lowe, eds. *Marriage in Italy, 1300–1650.* Cambridge: Cambridge University Press, 2002.

De Asua, Miguel, and Roger French. *A New World of Animals: Early Modern Europeans on the Creatures of Iberian America.* Aldershot: Ashgate, 2005.

Della Casa, Giovanni. *Galateo, a Renaissance Treatise on Manners,* edited and translated by Konrad Eisenbicher and Kenneth B. Bartlett. Toronto: CMRS, 1994.

Della Porta, Giambattista. *Della fisionomia dell'uomo,* edited by Mario Cicognani. Milan: Longanesi, 1971.

———. *Magiae naturalis.* Palermo: Il Vespro, 1979.

De Martino, Ernesto. *La terra del rimorso: Contributo a una storia religiosa del sud.* Milan: Saggiatore, 1961.

De Renzi, Silvia. "Witnesses of the Body: Medico-Legal Cases in Seventeenth-Century Rome." *Studies in History and Philosophy of Science* 33 (2002): 219–242.

Dieffenbach, Johann Friedrich. *Surgical Observations on the Restoration of the Nose and on the Removal of Polypi and Other Tumours from the Nostrils.* London: Highley, 1833.

Donesmondi, Ippolito. *Dell'historia ecclesiastica di Mantova.* 2 vols. Bologna: Forni, 1977.

Eamon, William. "Science and Popular Culture in Sixteenth-Century Italy: The Professors of Secrets and Their Books." *Sixteenth Century Studies* 16 (1985): 471–485.

Eisenberg, I. "A History of Rhinoplasty." *South African Medical Journal* 62 (August 21, 1982): 286–292.

Ellman, Philip, and J. Stewart Lawrence. "Gold Therapy in Rheumatoid Arthritis." *British Medical Journal* 2 (1940): 314–316.

Errante, Vincenzo. "'Forse che sì, forse che no': La terza spedizione del duca Vincenzo Gonzaga in Ungheria alla guerra contro il turco (1601) studiata su documenti inediti." *Archivio storico lombardo* 42.1 (1915): 15–114.

Estes, J. Worth. "The Reception of American Drugs in Europe, 1500–1650." In *Searching for the Secrets of Nature: The Life and Works of Dr. Francisco Hernandez,* edited by Simon Varey, Rafael Chabrán, and Dora Weiner, 111–121. Stanford: Stanford University Press, 2000.

Fabrici d'Acquapendente, Girolamo. *L'opere cirurgiche del signor Fabritio d'Acquapendente . . . divise in due parti. Nella prima si tratta de' tumori, ferite, vicere, rotture, e slogature. Nella seconda dell'operationi principali di cirugia.* Bologna: Stamperia del Longhi, 1709.

Facio, Bartolomeo. *De viris illustribus liber.* Florence: Giovanelli, 1745.

Falloppio, Gabriele. *Observationes anatomicae,* edited by Gabriella Righi Riva and Pericle Di Pietro. 2 vols. Modena: Mucchi, 1964.

Favaro, Antonio. *Galileo Galilei e lo studio di Padova.* 2 vols. Florence: Le Monnier, 1966.

Favaro, Giuseppe. "Girolamo Fabrici d'Acquapendente e la medicina pratica." *Bollettino dell'Istituto Storico Italiano dell'Arte Sanitaria* 7.1 (1927): 1–10.

Fenlon, Iain. *Music and Patronage in Sixteenth-Century Mantua.* 2 vols. Cambridge: Cambridge University Press, 1980.

Ferraro, Joanne. *Marriage Wars in Late Renaissance Venice.* New York: Oxford University Press, 2001.

Ficino, Marsilio. *Commentary on Plato's Symposium on Love,* translated by Sears Jayne. Dallas: Spring Publications, 1985.

Filarete, Antonio. *Treatise on Architecture,* edited and translated by John R. Spencer. New Haven: Yale University Press, 1965.

Filippini, Nadia Maria. "Levatrici e ostetricanti a Venezia tra sette e ottocento." *Quaderni storici* 58 (1985): 149–180.

Findlen, Paula. *Possessing Nature: Museums, Collecting, and Scientific Culture in Early Modern Italy.* Berkeley: University of California Press, 1994.

Finucci, Valeria. "The Italian Memorialist: C. Faà Gonzaga." In *Women Writers of the Seventeenth Century,* edited by Katia Wilson and Frank Warner, 121–128. Athens: University of Georgia Press, 1989.

———. *The Manly Masquerade: Masculinity, Paternity, and Castration in the Italian Renaissance.* Durham: Duke University Press, 2003.

———. "Re-membering the 'I': Faà Gonzaga's Storia (1622)." *Italian Quarterly* 28 (1987): 21–32.

Fischer, Arpad. "Rapporti tecnico-chirurgici in rinoplastica tra i Branca-Vianeo e Giulio Cesare Aranzio." *Coll. Pag. Storia Med.* 22 (1969): 79–90.

Fissell, Mary. "Introduction: Women, Health, and Healing in Early Modern Europe." *Bulletin of the History of Medicine* 82 (2008): 1–17.

Fornaciari, Gino, Angelica Vitiello, Sara Giusiani, Valentina Giuffra, Antonio Fornaciari, and Natale Villari. "The Medici Project: First Anthropological and Paleopathological Results." In http://www.paleopatologia.it/articoli/aticolo.php?recordID=18.

Fracastoro, Girolamo. *De contagionibus, morbisque contagiosis et eorum curatione. Libri tres.* In *Hieronymous Fracastorius and His Poetical and Prose Works on Syphilis,* edited and translated by William Riddell. Toronto: Canadian Social Hygiene Council, 1928.

Franchini, Dario, Renzo Margonari, Giuseppe Olmi, Rodolfo Signorini, Attilio Zanca, and Chiara Tellini Perina. *La scienza a corte: Collezionismo eclettico, natura e immagine a Mantova fra Rinascimento e Manierismo.* Rome: Bulzoni, 1979.

Freud, Sigmund. *The Complete Letters of Sigmund Freud to Wilhelm Fliess, 1887–1904,* edited and translated by Jeffrey Moussaieff. Cambridge: Harvard University Press, 1985.

———. "Fragment of an Analysis of a Case of Hysteria." In *The Standard Edition of the Complete Psychological Works of Sigmund Freud,* edited and translated by James Strachey. Vol. 7. London: Hogarth Press, 1953.

———. "The Taboo of Virginity." In *The Standard Edition of the Complete Psychological Works of Sigmund Freud,* edited and translated by James Strachey. Vol. 11. London: Hogarth Press, 1957.

Furlotti, Barbara. "Università, scienza e arte: Uno sguardo generale e alcuni esempi della corrispondenza bolognese." In Furlotti, *Le collezioni Gonzaga: Il carteggio tra Bologna, Parma, Piacenza e Mantova (1563–1634).* Milan: Silvana Editoriale, 2000–2003.

Furlotti, Barbara, and Guido Rebecchini. *The Art and Architecture of Mantua: Eight Centuries of Patronage and Collecting.* New York: Thames and Hudson, 2008.

Gadebush Bondio, Mariacarla. "I pericoli della bellezza 'mangonica.' Aspetti del dibattito su protesi, trucchi e chirurgia estetica tra '500 e '600." *Micrologus: natura, scienza e società medievali* 15 (2007): 425–449.

Galilei, Galileo. *Sidereus Nuncius.* Milan: Unaluna, 2010.

Gallico, Claudio. *"Forse che sì forse che no" tra poesia e musica.* Mantua: Istituto Carlo d'Arco per la Storia di Mantova, 1961.

Garber, Marjorie. "The Insincerity of Women." In *Desire in the Renaissance: Psychoanalysis and Literature,* edited by Valeria Finucci and Regina Schwartz, 19–38. Princeton: Princeton University Press, 1994.

Gerbi, Antonello. *La natura delle Indie Nove: Da Cristoforo Colombo a Gonzalo Fernandez de Oviedo.* Milan: Ricciardi, 1975.

Ghedino, Paolo. "'Dilettose venete fonti': Le terme di Abano, Montegrotto, Battaglia, Galzignano e Teolo." In *Alle fonti del piacere: la civiltà termale e balneare fra cura e svago,* edited by Nelli-Elena Vanzan Marchini, 102–117. Milan: Leonardo Arte, 1999.

Gibson, Thomas. "The Prostheses of Ambroise Paré." *British Journal of Plastic Surgery* 8 (1955–1956): 3–8.

Gilman, Sander. "The Jewish Nose: Are Jews White? Or, the History of the Nose Job." In *Encountering the Other(s): Studies in Literature, History and Culture,* edited by Gisela Brinker-Gabler, 149–182. New York: SUNY Press, 1995.

———. *Making the Body Beautiful: A Cultural History of Aesthetic Surgery.* Princeton: Princeton University Press, 1999.

Glaser, Gabriella. *The Nose: A Profile of Sex, Beauty, and Survival.* New York: Simon and Schuster, 2002.

Glassman, Nina. *Lettere proibite: I 'cimenti' del principe Vincenzo Gonzaga.* Ravenna: Longo, 1991.

Gnudi, Martha Teach, and Jerome Pierce Webster. *The Life and Times of Gaspare Tagliacozzi, Surgeon of Bologna (1545–1599).* New York: Reichner, 1950.

Goretti, Paola. "Limatura della luna argentea: La scienza dei magnifici apparati, tra malinconia, vestiario e vaghezze d'antico." In *Gonzaga: La Celeste Galeria, L'esercizio del collezionismo,* edited by Raffaella Morselli, 185–211. Milan: Skira, 2002.

Graefe, Carl Ferdinand von. *Rhinoplastik.* Berlin: Reimer, 1818.

Green, Monica. "Bodies, Gender, Health, Disease: Recent Work on Medieval Women's Medicine." *Studies in Medieval and Renaissance History,* 3rd ser. 2 (2005): 6–12.

———. "The Development of the *Trotula.*" *Revue d'Histoire des Textes* 26 (1996): 118–203.

———. "Women's Medical Practice and Health Care in Medieval Europe." *Signs* 14 (1989): 434–473.

Greene, Roland. "Petrarchism among the Discourses of Imperialism." In *America in European Consciousness, 1493–1750,* edited by Karen Ordhal Kupperman, 130–165. Chapel Hill: University of North Carolina Press, 1995.

Grendler, Paul. *The University of Mantua, the Gonzaga and the Jesuits.* Baltimore: Johns Hopkins University Press, 2009.

Groeber, Valentin. *Defaced: The Visual Culture of Violence in the Late Middle Ages.* New York: Zone, 2004.

Gurunlouglu, Raffi, and Aslin Gurunlouglu. "Giulio Cesare Arantius (1530–1589), a Surgeon and Anatomist: His Role in Nasal Reconstruction and Influence on Gaspare Tagliacozzi." *Annals of Plastic Surgery* 60.6 (2008): 717–722.

Hacke, Daniela. *Women, Sex, and Marriage in Early Modern Venice.* Aldershot: Ashgate, 2004.

Haiken, Elizabeth. *Venus Envy: A History of Cosmetic Surgery.* Baltimore: Johns Hopkins University Press, 1999.

Hanke, Stephanie. "Bathing 'all'antica': Bathrooms in Genoese Villas and Palaces in the Sixteenth Century." *Renaissance Studies* 20.5 (2006): 674–700.

Haring, Clarence Henry. *Trade and Navigation between Spain and the Indies.* Cambridge: Harvard University Press, 1918.

Harrán, Don. "Madama Europa, Jewish Singer in Late Renaissance Mantua." In *Festa Musicologica: Essays in Honor of George J. Buelow,* edited by Thomas Mathiesen and Benito Rivera, 197–230. Stuyvesant: Pendragon Press, 1995.

———. *Salamone Rossi: Jewish Musician in Late Renaissance Mantua.* Oxford: Oxford University Press, 2003.

Harvey, Elizabeth. "Anatomies of Rapture: Clitoral Politics/Medical Blazons." *Signs* 27 (2001): 315–346.
Hassig, Debra. "Transplanted Medicine: Colonial Mexican Herbals of the Sixteenth Century." *Res: Anthropology and Aesthetics* 17/18 (1989): 30–53.
Henke, Robert. *Performance and Literature in the Commedia dell'Arte*. Cambridge: Cambridge University Press, 2002.
Hernández, Francisco. "The Antiquities of New Spain." In *The Mexican Treasury: The Writings of Dr. Francisco Hernández*, edited by Simon Varey. Stanford: Stanford University Press, 2000.
———. *Historia natural de Nueva España*. 2 vols. México: Universidad Nacional de México, 1959.
Hildebrand, Otto. *Die Entwicklung der plastischen Chirurgie*. Berlin: Hirschwald, 1909.
Hitchings, Henry. *Defining the World: The Extraordinary Story of Dr. Johnson's Dictionary*. New York: Farrar, Straus and Giroux, 2005.
Hodges, Nathaniel. *Loimologia; or, An Historical Account of the Plague in London in 1665*. London: Bell and Osborn, 1720.
Hugo, Victor. *Le Roi s'amuse / The Prince's Play*. London: Faber and Faber, 1996.
Hunter, Dianne. *Seduction and Theory: Readings of Gender, Representation, and Rhetoric*. Urbana: University of Illinois Press, 1989.
Iasiello, Italo. "Vincenzo I e il Regno di Napoli." In *Gonzaga: La Celeste Galeria, L'esercizio del collezionismo*, edited by Raffaella Morselli, 357–362. Milan: Skira, 2002.
Impy, Oliver, and Arthur MacGregor, eds. *The Origins of Museums: The Cabinets of Curiosities in Sixteenth- and Seventeenth-Century Europe*. Oxford: Oxford University Press, 1986.
Infelise, Mario. "From Merchants' Letters to Handwritten *Avvisi:* Notes on the Origins of Public Information." In *Cultural Exchange in Early Modern Europe: 1400–1700*, edited by Francisco Bethencourt and Florike Edmond, 33–52. New York: Cambridge University Press, 2006.
Intra, G. B. "Una pagina della giovinezza del principe Vincenzo Gonzaga." *Archivio storico italiano* 18 (1886): 197–230.
Jacquart, Danielle, and Claude Thomasset. *Sexuality and Medicine in the Middle Ages*. Princeton: Princeton University Press, 1988.
Jankowski, Theodora. *Pure Resistance: Queer Virginity in Early Modern English Drama*. Philadelphia: University of Pennsylvania Press, 2000.
Johnson, Virginia, and William Masters. *Human Sexual Response*. Toronto: Bantam, 1966.
Joubert, Laurent. *Popular Errors*, translated by Gregory David de Rocher. Tuscaloosa: University of Alabama Press, 1989.
Kantorowicz, Ernst H. *The King's Two Bodies: A Study in Mediaeval Political Theology*. Princeton: Princeton University Press, 1957.
Kauffmann, C. M. *The Baths of Pozzuoli: A Study of the Medieval Illuminations of Peter of Eboli's Poem*. Oxford: Bruno Cassirer, 1959.

Keller, Eve. "The Subject of Touch: Medical Authority in Early Modern Midwifery." In *Sensible Flesh: On Touch in Early Modern Culture*, edited by Elizabeth Harvey, 62–83. Philadelphia: University of Pennsylvania Press, 2003.

Kelly, Kathleen Coyne. *Performing Virginity and Testing Chastity in the Middle Ages*. New York: Routledge, 2000.

Kelly, Kathleen Coyne, and Marina Leslie, eds. *Menacing Virgins: Representing Virginity in the Middle Ages and Renaissance*. London: Associated University Presses, 1999.

Kinsey, Alfred. *Sexual Behavior in the Human Female*. Philadelphia: Saunders, 1953.

Kirshner, Julius. "The Morning After: Collecting Monte Dowries in Renaissance Florence." In *From Florence to the Mediterranean and Beyond: Essays in Honor of Anthony Molho*, edited by Diego Ramada Curto, Eric R. Dursteler, Julius Kirshner, and Francesca Trivellato, 29–61. Florence: Olschki, 2009.

Klestinec, Cynthia. "Medical Education in Padua: Students, Faculty and Facilities." In *Centres of Medical Excellence? Medical Travel and Education in Europe, 1500–1789*, edited by Ole Peter Grell, Andrew Cunningham, and Jon Arrizabalaga, 193–210. Aldershot: Ashgate, 2010.

———. "Private Anatomies and the Delights of Technical Expertise." In *Theaters of Anatomy: Students, Teachers, and Traditions of Dissection in Renaissance Venice*. Baltimore: Johns Hopkins University Press, 2011.

Kuriyama, Shigehisa. "The Forgotten Fear of Excrement." *Journal of Medieval and Early Modern Studies* 38 (2008): 413–442.

Laqueur, Thomas. "Amor Veneris, Vel Dulcedo Appelletur." In *Zone: Fragments for a History of the Human Body*, part 3, edited by Michael Feher, 90–131. New York: Zone, 1989.

———. *Making Sex: Body and Gender from the Greeks to Freud*. Cambridge: Harvard University Press, 1990.

———. "Sex in the Flesh." *Isis* 94.2 (2003): 300–306.

Lascaratos, J. C., J. V. Segas, C. C. Trompoukis, and D. A. Assimakopoulos. "From the Roots of Rhinology: The Reconstruction of Nasal Injuries in Hippocrates." *Annals of Otology, Rhinology, and Laryngology* 112.2 (2003): 159–162.

La Torre, Felice. *L'utero attraverso i secoli: da Erofilo ai giorni nostri*. Città di Castello: Unione Arti Grafiche, 1917.

Lavater, Johann Caspar. *Essays on Physiognomy: For the Promotion of the Knowledge and the Love of Mankind*. Boston: Spotswood and West, 1794.

Lavaud, B. "The Interpretation of the Conjugal Act and the Theology of Marriage." *Thomist* 1 (1939): 360–380.

Lee, Y. T., C. M. Lee, S. C. Su, C. P. Liu, and T. E. Wang. "Psoas Abscess: A 10 Year Review." *Journal of Microbiology, Immunology and Infection* 31, no. 1 (1999): 40.

Lemay, Helen. "Human Sexuality in Twelfth- through Fifteenth-Century Scientific Writings." In *Sexual Practices and the Medieval Church*, edited by Vern Bullough and James Brundage, 187–205. Buffalo: Prometheus Books, 1982.

———. "William of Saliceto on Human Sexuality." *Viator* 12 (1981): 165–181.

Levin, Carole. "Power, Politics, and Sexuality: Images of Elizabeth I." *Sixteenth Century Essays and Studies* 12 (1989): 95–110.

Litta, Pompeo. *Celebri famiglie italiane*. 11 vols. Milan: Giusti, 1919–1985.

Lochrie, Karma. *Heterosyncrasies*. Minneapolis: University of Minnesota Press, 2005.

López Piñero, José, and José Pardo. "The Contribution of Hernández to European Botany and *Materia Medica*." In *Searching for the Secrets of Nature: The Life and Works of Dr. Francisco Hernández*, edited by Simon Varey, Rafael Chabrán, and Dora Weiner, 122–137. Stanford: Stanford University Press, 2000.

López Terrada, Maria Luz, and José Pardo-Tomás. *La primeras noticias sobre plantas americanas en las relaciones de viajes y crónicas de Indias (1493–1553)*. Valencia: Instituto de Estudios Documentales, 1993.

Loughlin, Marie H. *Hymeneutics: Interpreting Virginity in the Early Modern Stage*. London: Associated University Presses, 1997.

Lower, Richard. *De catarrhis*, edited by Richard Hunter and Ida Macalpine. London: Dawsons of Pall Mall, 1963.

Luzio, Alessandro. *La Galleria dei Gonzaga venduta all'Inghilterra nel 1627–28: Documenti degli archivi di Mantova e Londra raccolti ed illustrati*. Milan: Cogliati, 1913.

Machiavelli, Niccolò. *Mandragola*, edited by Nino Borsellino. Rome: Newton and Compton, 1996.

———. *Mandragola/Clizia*. Milan: Feltrinelli, 1995.

———. *The Mandrake Root*. In *Five Comedies from the Italian Renaissance*, edited and translated by Laura Giannetti and Guido Ruggiero. Baltimore: Johns Hopkins University Press, 2003.

MacKinney, Loren. "Animal Substances in *Materia Medica*: A Study in the Persistence of the Primitive." *Journal of the History of Medicine and Allied Sciences* 1 (1946): 149–170.

Maclean, Ian. *The Renaissance Notion of Woman: A Study in the Fortunes of Scholasticism and Medical Science in European Intellectual Life*. Cambridge: Cambridge University Press, 1980.

MacLeod, Roy. "Spain and America: The Atlantic Trade, 1492–1720." In *Cambridge History of Latin America*, vol. 1. New York: Cambridge University Press, 1984.

MacNeil, Anne. "The Nature of Commitment: Vincenzo Gonzaga's Patronage Strategies in the Wake of the Fall of Ferrara." *Renaissance Quarterly* 16, no. 3 (2002): 392–403.

Magnaghi, Alberto. *Amerigo Vespucci*. Rome: Treves, 1926.

Malacarne, Giancarlo. *Le feste del principe: giochi, divertimenti, spettacoli a corte.* Modena: Il Bulino, 2002.

———. *La luna rotta: Racconti mantovani.* Mantua: Rossi, 1997.

———. *Splendore e declino: da Vincenzo I a Vincenzo II (1587–1627).* Vol. 4 of *I Gonzaga di Mantova: Una stirpe per una capitale europea.* Modena: Il Bulino, 2007.

Malizia, Enrico. *Ricettario delle streghe: Incantesimi, prodigi sessuali e veleni.* Rome: Edizioni Mediterranee, 1992.

Maltz, Maxwell. *Evolution of Plastic Surgery.* New York: Froben Press, 1946.

Mancall, Peter C. "Tales Tobacco Told in Sixteenth-Century Europe." *Environmental History* 9.4 (2004): 648–678.

Marinello, Giovanni, *Le medicine partenenti alle infermità delle donne.* In *Medicina per le donne nel Cinquecento: Testi di Giovanni Marinello e Girolamo Mercurio,* edited by Maria Luisa Altieri Biagi et al. Turin: UTET, 1992.

Marinozzi, Silvia. "The Vianeo and Gaspare Tagliacozzi: The Development of Rhinoplasty in the XV Century." *Medicina nei secoli* 11.3 (1999): 603–610.

Maron, R., D. Levine, T. E. Dobbs, and W. M. Geisler, "Two Cases of Pott Disease Associated with Bilateral Psoas Abscesses: Case Report." *Spine* 31 (2006): E561.

Marotti, Ferruccio, and Giovanna Romei, eds. *La commedia dell'arte e la società barocca: La professione del teatro.* Rome: Bulzoni, 1991.

Martín Martín, Carmen, and José Luis Valverde. *La farmacia en la América colonial: El arte de preparar medicamentos.* Granada: Universidad de Granada, 1995.

Masino, Cristoforo, and Giuseppe Ostino. "Le forniture di medicinali e 'robbe vive' alla corte di Mantova nel mese di dicembre del 1587." In *Mantova e i Gonzaga nella civiltà del Rinascimento,* edited by Accademia Nazionale dei Lincei, 375–379. Mantua: Accademia Virgiliana, 1977.

Mathes, Bettina. "As Long as a Swan's Neck? The Significance of the 'Enlarged' Clitoris for Early Modern Anatomy." In *Sensible Flesh: On Touch in Early Modern Culture,* edited by Elizabeth D. Harvey, 104–124. Philadelphia: University of Pennsylvania Press, 2003.

Mattioli, Donatella. "Fiamminghi a Mantova tra Cinque e Seicento." In Germano Mulazzani et al., *Rubens a Mantova.* Milan: Electa, 1977, 68–86.

Mattioli, Pietro Andrea. *Discorsi . . . ne' sei libri di Pedacio Dioscoride Anazarbeo della materia medicinale.* Venezia, 1744.

Mazzoldi, Leonardo. "Vita cittadina del primo '600: Lettere inedite dell'Archivio Gonzaga." *Bollettino Storico Mantovano* 3 (1956): 200–213.

Mazzoldi, Leonardo, Renato Giusti, and Rinaldo Salvatori, eds. *Mantova: La storia, le lettere, le arti.* 9 vols. Mantua: Istituto Carlo d'Arco per la Storia di Mantova, 1963.

McCarthy, John. "The Marriage Capacity of the *Mulier excisa.*" *Ephemerides Iuris Canonici* 3.2 (1947): 261–285.

McClintock, Anne. *Imperial Leather: Race, Gender, and Sexuality in the Colonial Conquest.* New York: Routledge, 1995.
McDowell, Frank. *The Source Book of Plastic Surgery, Compiled and Edited by Frank McDowell.* Baltimore: Williams and Wilkins Company, 1977.
McGee, Timothy J. "Pompeo Caccini and *Euridice*: New Biographical Notes." *Renaissance and Reformation* 26.2 (1990): 81–99.
McLaren, Angus. *Impotence: A Cultural History.* Chicago: University of Chicago Press, 2007.
McVaugh, Michael *The Rational Surgery of the Middle Ages.* Florence: Edizioni del Galluzzo, 2006.
Mina, Gabriele. "Una costruzione melanconica: Il primo dibattito sul tarantismo." In *Il morso della differenza: Antologia del dibattito sul tarantismo fra il XIV e il XVI secolo,* edited by Gabriele Mina. Nardò: Besa, 2000.
Mondeville, Henri de. *Chirurgie de Maitre Henri de Mondeville, chirurgien de Philippe Le Bel, roi de France, composée de 1306 à 1320,* edited by E. Nicaise. Paris: Baillière et Cie, 1893.
Monga, Luigi. "Odeporica e medicina: I viaggiatori del Cinquecento e la rinoplastica." *Italica* 69 (1992): 378–393.
Montaigne, Michel de. *Journal de voyage de Michel de Montaigne . . . en Italie . . . en 1580 et 1581.* Rome and Paris: Le Jay, 1774.
———. "On the Power of the Imagination." In *The Complete Essays,* translated by M. A. Screech. London: Penguin, 1993.
Moretti, Maria Rosa. *Musica e costume a Genova: Tra Cinquecento e Seicento.* Genoa: Pirella, 1990.
Morselli, Raffaella. *L'elenco dei beni del 1626–27.* Milan: Silvana Editoriale, 2000.
———, ed. *Gonzaga: La Celeste Galeria, Le raccolte.* Milan: Skira, 2002.
Moss, Jean Dietz. "The Promotion of Bath Waters by Physicians in the Renaissance." In *Rhetoric and Medicine in Early Modern Europe,* edited by Stephen Spender and Nancy Struever. Aldershot: Ashgate, 2012, 61–82.
Mozzarelli, Cesare. *Mantova e i Gonzaga dal 1382 al 1707.* Turin: UTET, 1987.
Murray, Jacqueline. "On the Origins and Role of 'Wise Women' in Causes of Annulment on the Grounds of Male Impotence." *Journal of Medieval History* 16 (1990): 235–249.
Navarrini, Roberto. "La guerra chimica di Vincenzo Gonzaga." *Civiltà mantovana* 4 (1969): 43–47.
Neri, Achille. "Il duca di Mantova a Genova nel 1592." *Archivio storico lombardo* 13 (1886): 113–126.
———. "Il duca di Mantova a San Pier D'Arena." *Giornale ligustico* 13 (1886): 160–164.
Olmi, Giuseppe. *L'inventario del mondo: Catalogazione della natura e luoghi del sapere nella prima età moderna.* Bologna: Il Mulino, 1992.
O'Malley, Charles D. *Andreas Vesalius of Brussels.* Berkeley: University of California Press, 1964.

Orlando, Filippo. "Altri documenti inediti sul parentado fra la principessa Eleonora de' Medici e il principe Don Vincenzo Gonzaga e i cimenti a cui fu costretto il detto principe per attestare la sua potenza virile." In *Giornale di erudizione: corrispondenza letteraria, artistica e scientifica*, edited by Filippo Orlando. Florence, 1893.

Orlando, Filippo, and Giuseppe Baccini. "Il parentado fra la principessa Eleonora de' Medici e il principe Don Vincenzo Gonzaga ed i cimenti a cui fu costretto il detto principe per attestare come egli fosse abile alla generazione. Documenti inediti tratti dal Regio Archivio di Stato di Firenze." In *Bibliotechina Grassoccia: Capricci e curiosità letterarie inedite o rare*, no. 5. Florence, 1886. Reprinted in *Una prova di matrimonio*. Rome, 1961.

Ostino, Giuseppe. "L'avventuroso viaggio al Perú di Evangelista Marcobruno, speziale mantovano, nei primi anni del '600 alla ricerca di una curiosa droga." *La farmacia nuova* 24.8–9 (1968): 3–22.

Oviedo, Gonzalo Fernández de. *Historia General y Natural de las Indias*. Madrid: Nabu Press, 2010.

———. *Naturale e generale historia dell'Indie*. In Giovanni Battista Ramusio, *Navigazioni et viaggi*, edited by Marica Milanesi. Vol. 5. Turin: Einaudi, 1985.

———. *Sommario della naturale e generale istoria dell'Indie occidentali di Gonzalo Ferdinando d'Oviedo*. In Giovanni Battista Ramusio, *Navigazioni e viaggi*, edited by Marica Milanesi. Vol. 5, 207–339. Turin: Einaudi, 1985.

Pagliari, Irma. "'Una libreria che in Italia non v'era una simile ne' anco a Roma': La biblioteca dei Gonzaga." In *Gonzaga: La Celeste Galeria: L'esercizio del collezionismo*, edited by Raffaella Morselli, 111–125. Milan: Skira, 2002.

Palmer, Richard. "Pharmacy in the Republic of Venice in the Sixteenth Century." In *The Medical Renaissance in the Sixteenth Century*, edited by A. Wear, R. K. French, and I. M. Lonie, 99–117. Cambridge: Cambridge University Press, 1985.

Pardo-Tomás, José. *Oviedo, Monardes, Hernández: El tesoro natural de America; Colonialismo y ciencia en el siglo XVI*. Madrid: Nivola, 2002.

Park, Katharine. "Cadden, Laqueur, and the One-Sex Body." *Medieval Feminist Forum* 46.1 (2010): 96–100.

———. "Natural Particulars: Medical Epistemology, Practice, and the Literature of Healing Springs." In *Natural Particulars: Nature and the Disciplines in Renaissance Europe*, edited by Anthony Grafton and Nancy Siraisi, 347–367. Cambridge: MIT Press, 1999.

———. "The Rediscovery of the Clitoris." In *The Body in Parts: Fantasies of Corporeality in Early Modern Europe*, edited by David Hillman and Carla Mazzio, 171–193. New York: Routledge, 1997.

———. *Secrets of Women: Gender, Generation, and the Origins of Human Dissection*. New York: Zone Books, 2006.

Park, Katharine, and Robert Nye. "Destiny Is Anatomy." *New Republic* 204 (February 18, 1991): 53–57.

Parrott, David. "The Mantuan Succession, 1627–31: A Sovereignty Dispute in Early Modern Europe." *English Historical Review* 112 (1997): 20–65.

Paschetti, Bartolomeo. *Del conservare la sanità, et del vivere de' Genovesi*. In *Del conservare la sanità di Bartolomeo Paschetti*, edited by Gino Fravega. Pisa: Tip. Giradini, 1964.

Pastore, Alessandro. *Il medico in tribunale: La perizia medica nella procedura penale d'antico regime*. Bellinzona: Edizioni Casagrande, 1998.

Pazzini, Adalberto. "La medicina alla corte dei Gonzaga a Mantova." In *Mantova e i Gonzaga nella civiltà del Rinascimento*, edited by Accademia Nazionale dei Lincei, 291–351. Mantua: Accademia Virgiliana, 1977.

Pelizza, Andrea. *Riammessi a respirare l'aria tranquilla: Venezia e il riscatto degli schiavi in età moderna*. Venice: Istituto Veneto di Lettere, Scienze ed Arti, 2012.

Perocco, Daria. *Viaggiare e raccontare: Narrazione di viaggio ed esperienze di racconto tra Cinque e Seicento*. Alessandria: Edizioni dell'Orso, 1997.

Petrarca, Francesco. *De remediis utriusque fortunae libri II*. In *In Our Image and Likeness: Humanity and Divinity in Italian Humanist Thought*, edited by Charles Trinkaus. Notre Dame: University of Notre Dame Press, 1955.

Peyrefitte, Roger. *The Prince's Person*. London: Panther, 1964.

Phillips, Carla Rahn. "The Growth and Composition of Trade in the Iberian Empires, 1450–1750." In *The Rise of Merchant Empires: Long-Distance Trade in the Early Modern World, 1350–1750*, edited by James Tracy, 34–101. New York: Cambridge University Press, 1990.

Piccinelli, Roberta. "Le *facies* del collezionismo artistico di Vincenzo Gonzaga." In *Gonzaga: La Celeste Galeria, L'esercizio del collezionismo*, edited by Raffaella Morselli, 341–347. Milan: Skira, 2002.

———, ed. *Le collezioni Gonzaga: Il carteggio tra Firenze e Mantova (1554–1626)*. Milan: Silvana Editoriale, 2002.

———, ed. *Le collezioni Gonzaga: Il carteggio tra Milano e Mantova (1563–1634)*. Milan: Silvana Editoriale, 2003.

Pigafetta, Antonio. *Viaggio atorno il mondo fatto e descritto per messer Antonio Pigafetta vicentino*, in Giovanni Battista Ramusio, *Navigazioni et Viaggi*, edited by Marica Milanesi. Vol. 2. Turin: Einaudi, 1985.

Piñero, José López. "La 'nuevas medicinas' americanas en la obra de Nicolas Monardes." *Asclepio* 42.1 (1990): 3–67.

Pinto-Correia, Clara. *The Ovary of Eve: Egg and Sperm and Preformation*. Chicago: University of Chicago Press, 1997.

Pirrotta, Nino. *Music and Culture in Italy from the Middle Ages to the Baroque*. Cambridge: Harvard University Press, 1984.

Pomata, Gianna. *Contracting a Cure: Patients, Healers, and the Law in Early Modern Bologna*. Baltimore: Johns Hopkins University Press, 1998.

Porter, Roy. "The Patient's View: Doing Medical History from Below." *Theory and Society* 14 (1985): 175–198.

———. "The Rise of Physical Examination." In *Medicine and the Five Senses*, edited by Roy Porter and William Bynum, 79–97. Cambridge: Cambridge University Press, 2003.

———, ed. *Patients and Practitioners: Lay Perspectives of Medicine in Pre-industrial Society*. Cambridge: Cambridge University Press, 1985.

Porter, Roy, and G. S. Rousseau, *Gout: The Patrician Malady*. New Haven: Yale University Press, 1998.

Portioli, Attilio. *I Gonzaga ai bagni di Petriolo presso Siena nel 1460–61*. Mantua: Eredi Segna, 1870.

Porzio, Camillo. *L'istoria d'Italia nell'anno 1547 e la descrizione del regno di Napoli*. Naples: Tramater, 1839.

Pratt, Mary Louise. *Imperial Eyes: Travel Writing and Transculturation*. New York: Routledge, 1992.

Puccinotti, Francesco. "Della rachitide." In *Opere complete edite ed inedite*. Naples: Pellerano, 1858.

Putelli, Raffaello. *Il duca Vincenzo I Gonzaga e l'interdetto di Paolo V a Venezia*. Venice: Istituto Veneto di Arti Grafiche, 1911.

Quondam, Amedeo. *Il naso di Laura. Lingua e poesia lirica nella tradizione del classicismo*. Modena: Panini, 1991.

Rabelais, Francois. *Gargantua and Pantagruel*. In *Oeuvres completes*. Paris: Editions du Seuil, 1995.

Ramazzini, Bernardino. *La salute dei principi ovvero come difendersi dalle malattie e dai medici*, edited by Francesco Carnevale. Florence: Tosca, 1992.

Ramusio, Giambattista. *Navigationi et viaggi*, edited by with an introduction by F. R. A. Skelton and George Parks. 3 vols. Amsterdam: Theatrum Orbis Terrarum, 1967–1970.

———. *Navigazioni e viaggi*, edited by Marica Milanesi. 6 vols. Turin: Einaudi, 1978–1988.

Redi, Francesco. *Esperienze intorno alla generazione degli insetti*. In *Scienziati del Seicento*, edited by Maria Luisa Altieri Biagi and Bruno Basile, 314–463. Milan: Ricciardi, 1980.

Ricci, Giovanni. *Il principe e la morte: Corpo, cuore, effigie nel Rinascimento*. Bologna: Il Mulino, 1998.

Rippa Bonati, Maurizio, and José Pardo-Tomás, eds. *Il teatro dei corpi: Le pitture colorate d'anatomia di Girolamo Fabrici d'Acquapendente*. Milan: Mediamed, 2004.

Risse, Guenter. "Medicine in New Spain." In *Medicine in the New World: New Spain, New France, and New England*, edited by Ronald Numbers, 12–63. Knoxville. University of Tennessee Press, 1987.

———. "Transcending Cultural Barriers: The European Reception of Medicinal Plants from the Americas." In *Botanical Drugs of the Americas in the Old and New Worlds*, edited by Wolfgang-Hagen Hein, 31–42. Stuttgart: Wissenschaftliche Verlagsgesellschaft, 1984.

Riva, Alessandro. *Flesh and Wax: The Clemente Susini's Anatomical Models in the University of Cagliari.* Nuoro: Ilisso Edizioni, 2007.

Rocke, Michael. *Forbidden Friendships: Homosexuality and Male Culture in Renaissance Florence.* New York: Oxford University Press, 1996.

Rogers, Blair O. "Nasal Reconstruction 150 Years Ago: Aesthetic and Other Problems." *Aesthetic Plastic Surgery* 5 (1981): 283–327.

Rollo, Franco, M. Mascetti, and R. Cameriere. "Titian's Secret: Comparison of Eleonora Gonzaga della Rovere's Skull with the Uffizi Portrait." *Journal of Forensic Sciences* 50.3 (May 2005): 602–607.

Rosenthal, Margaret F. and Ann Rosalind Jones. *The Clothing of the Renaissance World: Europe, Asia, Africa, the Americas.* London: Thames and Hudson, 2008.

Rossi, Paolo. *Philosophy, Technology, and the Arts in the Early Modern Era.* New York: Harper and Row, 1970.

Rubens, Peter Paul. *Correspondance de Rubens et documents épistolaires concernant sa vie et ses oeuvres.* 6 vols. Anvers: Veuve de Backer, 1887–1909.

Ruggiero, Guido. *The Boundaries of Eros: Sex Crime and Sexuality in Renaissance Venice.* New York: Oxford University Press, 1985.

Sahagún, Bernardino de. *Florentine Codex: A General History of the Things of New Spain,* edited and translated by Arthur Anderson and Charles Dibble. 13 vols. Santa Fe and Salt Lake City: School of American Research and University of Utah, 1950–1983.

Samaden, Lucia. "Giovanni Tommaso Minadoi (1548–1615): da medico della 'nazione' veneziana in Siria a professore universitario a Padova." *Quaderni per la storia dell'università di Padova* 31 (1998): 91–164.

Samonà, Carmelo. "La letteratura dell'esperienza vissuta: I cronisti delle 'Indie.'" In *La letteratura spagnola dei secoli d'oro,* edited by Carmelo Samonà, Guido Mancini, Francesco Guazzelli, and Alessandro Martinegro, 100–134, Florence: Sansoni, 1973.

Sandei, F., M. Rippa Bonati, G. Leoni, and G. Reginato. "Le fistole dell'ano. Cenni storici." *Rivista italiana di colon-proctologia* 7.1 (1988): 34–41.

Scansani, Stefano. *L'amor morto.* Milan: Mondadori, 1991.

Schiesari, Juliana. "The Face of Domestication: Physiognomy, Gender Politics and Humanism's Others." In *Women, Race, and Writing in the Early Modern Period,* edited by Margot Hendricks and Patricia Parker, 55–70. New York: Routledge, 1994.

Schulenburg, Jane Tibbetts. "The Heroics of Virginity: Brides of Christ and Sacrificial Mutilation." In *Women in the Middle Ages and the Renaissance: Literary and Historical Perspectives,* edited by Mary Beth Rose, 29–72. Syracuse: Syracuse University Press, 1986.

Schwarz, Kathryn. "The Wrong Question: Thinking through Virginity." *differences* 13.2 (2002): 1–34.

Segarizzi, Arnaldo, ed. *Relazioni degli ambasciatori veneti al Senato.* 3 vols. Bari: Laterza, 1912–1916.

Serafin, Silvana. *La natura del Perù nei cronisti dei secoli XVI e XVII.* Rome: Bulzoni, 1988.

Sermidi, Michaela. "Vanità, lusso, arte e scienza: Il collezionismo onnivoro di Vincenzo I Gonzaga a Venezia." In *Le collezioni Gonzaga: Il carteggio tra Venezia e Mantova (1588–1612),* edited by Michaela Sermidi, 13–72. Milan: Silvana Editoriale, 2003.

———, ed. *Le collezioni Gonzaga: Il carteggio tra Venezia e Mantova (1588–1612).* Milan: Silvana Editoriale, 2003.

Seward, Desmond. *Prince of the Renaissance: The Life of François I.* London: Constable, 1973.

Sforza, Caterina. *Experimenti de la Ex.ma S.ra Caterina da Furlj matre de lo Inllux. mo Signor Giovanni de Medici,* edited by Desiderio Pasolini. Imola: Tip. d'Ignazio Galeati, 1894.

Shakespeare, William. *Timon of Athens,* edited by Anthony Dawson and Gretchen Minton. London: Arden Shakespeare, 2008.

Shemek, Deanna. "Aretino's *Marescalco:* Marriage Woes and the Duke of Mantua." *Renaissance Studies* 16.3 (2002): 366–380.

Silvestri, Alfonso. "Gaspare Tagliacozzi a Mantova." *Archiginnasio* 32 (1937): 89–100.

Simon, Kate. *I Gonzaga: Storia e segreti.* Rome: Newton-Compton, 1990.

Simons, Patricia. "Alert and Erect: Masculinity in Some Italian Renaissance Portraits of Fathers and Sons." In *Gender Rhetorics: Postures of Dominance and Submission in History,* edited by Richard C. Trexler, 162–186. Binghampton: MRTS, 1994.

———. *The Sex of Men in Premodern Europe: A Cultural History.* Cambridge: Cambridge University Press, 2011.

Simonsohn, Shlomo. *History of the Jews in the Duchy of Mantua.* Jerusalem: Kiryath Sepher, 1977.

Sissa, Giulia. "La verginità materiale: Evanescenza di un soggetto." *Quaderni storici* 25 (1990): 739–756.

Sogliani, Daniela, ed. *Le collezioni Gonzaga: Il carteggio tra Venezia e Mantova (1563–1587).* Milan: Silvana Editoriale, 2002.

Stallybrass, Peter. "Patriarchal Territory: The Body Enclosed." In *Rewriting the Renaissance: The Discourses of Sexual Difference in Early Modern Europe,* edited by Margaret Ferguson, Maureen Quilligan, and Nancy J. Vickers, 123–142. Chicago: University of Chicago Press, 1986.

Sterzi, Giuseppe. "Giulio Casserio, anatomico e chirurgo (c. 1552–1616)." *Nuovo archivio veneto,* ser. 3, 18 (1909): 207–278; 18 (1910): 25–111.

Stolberg, Michael. "The Decline of Uroscopy in Early Modern Learned Medicine, 1500–1650." *Early Science and Medicine* 12 (2007): 313–336.

———. "A Woman Down to Her Bones: The Anatomy of Sexual Difference in the Sixteenth and Early Seventeenth Centuries." *Isis* 94.2 (2003): 274–299.

Strainchamps, Edmond. "The Life and Death of Caterina Martinelli: New Light on Monteverdi's 'Arianna.'" *Early Music History* 5 (1985): 155–186.

Strocchia, Sharon. "Taken into Custody: Girls and Convent Guardianship in Renaissance Florence." *Renaissance Studies* 17.2 (2003): 177–200.

Sundt, Halfdan. "The Diagnosis and Frequency of Tuberculous Disease of the Knee." *Journal of Bone and Joint Surgery* 13 (1931): 740–758.

Tagliacozzi, Gaspare. *La chirurgia plastica per innesto di Gaspare Tagliacozzi*, edited and translated by Werner Vallieri. Bologna: Montaguti, 1964.

———. *De curtorum chirurgia per insitionem*, translated by Joan H. Thomas, with an introduction by Robert M. Goldwyn. New York: Gryphon Editions, 1996.

Talbot, Charles. "America and the European Drug Trade." In *First Images of America: The Impact of the New World on the Old*, edited by Fredi Chiappelli, 833–844. Berkeley: University of California Press, 1976.

Tasso, Torquato. "Canzone 10." In *Scelta di poesie liriche dal primo secolo della lingua al Novecento*. Florence: Le Monnier, 1839.

Taton, René, ed. "Las Ciencias in la America Colonial." In Taton, *Historia general de las ciencias*, translated by Manuel Sacristán. Vol. 2, *La ciencia moderna*, 791–822. Barcelona: Ediciones Destino, 1972.

Taviani, Ferdinando, and Mirella Schino. *Il segreto della Commedia dell'Arte: La memoria delle compagnie italiane del XVI, XVII, e XVIII secolo*. Florence: Usher, 1986.

Terpstra, Nicholas. *Lost Girls: Sex and Death in Renaissance Florence*. Baltimore: Johns Hopkins University Press, 2010.

Thompson, Charles. *The Mystic Mandrake*. New York: University Books, 1968.

Traub, Valerie. "The Psychomorphology of the Clitoris or, the Reemergence of the *Tribade* in English Culture." In *Generation and Degeneration: Tropes of Reproduction in Literature and History from Antiquity to Early Modern Europe*, edited by Valeria Finucci and Kevin Brownlee, 153–186. Durham: Duke University Press, 2001.

Treadwell, Nina. "'Simil combattimento fatto da Dame': The Musico-Theatrical Entertainments of Margherita Gonzaga's *Balletto delle donne* and the Female Warrior in Ferrarese Cultural History." In *Gender, Sexuality and Early Music*, edited by Todd Borgerding, 27–40. New York: Routledge, 2002.

Tripodi, Domenico. "Sull'arte di acconciare i nasi: i Vianeo e la 'Magia Tropaensium.'" *Valsalva* 44 (1968): 54–56.

Turner, Daniel. *Syphilis: A Practical Dissertation on the Venereal Disease*. London: Walthoe et al., 1732.

Van Eickels, Klaus. "Gendered Violence: Castration and Binding as Punishment for Treason in Normandy and Anglo-Norman England." *Gender and History* 16.3 (2004): 588–602.

Vasari, Giorgio. *The Lives of the Most Excellent Painters, Sculptors and Architects*, edited by George Bull. New York: Penguin, 1965 and 1971.

Veneziani, Sabrina. "Le lezioni dermatologiche di Girolamo Mercuriale." In *Girolamo Mercuriale: Medicina e cultura nell'Europa del Cinquecento*, edited by Alessandro Arcangeli and Vivian Nutton, 203–215. Florence: Olschki, 2008.

Venturini, Elena. "Il vestibolo dell'imperatore: Vicende di collezionismo artistico nelle relazioni tra Gonzaga e Asburgo." In *Le collezioni Gonzaga: Il carteggio tra la Corte Cesarea e Mantova (1559–1636)*, edited by Elena Venturini, 15–134. Milano: Silvana Editoriale, 2002.

———. ed. *Le collezioni Gonzaga: Il carteggio tra la Corte Cesarea e Mantova (1559–1636)*. Milan: Silvana Editoriale, 2002.

Verdi, Giuseppe. *Rigoletto*. New York: Riverrun Press, 1982.

Vesalius, Andreas. *The Epitome of Andreas Vesalius*, translated by L. R. Lind. New York: Macmillan, 1949.

Vespucci, Amerigo. "Sommario di Amerigo Vespucci Fiorentino di due sue navigationi al Magnifico M. Piero Soderini Gonfalonier della Magnifica Republica di Firenze." In Giovanni Battista Ramusio, *Navigationi et viaggi*, edited with an introduction by F. R. A. Skelton and George Parks. 3 vols. Amsterdam: Theatrum Orbis Terrarum, 1967–1970.

Vigilio, Giovanni Battista. *La insalata. Cronaca mantovana dal 1561 al 1602*, edited by Daniela Ferrari and Cesare Mozzarelli. Mantua: Gianluigi Arcari Editore, 1992.

Virgil. *Aeneid*, translated by Robert Fagues. London: Penguin, 2006.

Voltaire. *Oeuvres completes*. Paris: Imprimerie de la Société Littéraire Typographique, 1785.

Wachtel, Nathan. *The Vision of the Vanquished: The Spanish Conquest of Peru through Indian Eyes, 1530–1570*. New York: Barnes and Noble, 1977.

Warren, Jonathan Mason. "Rhinoplastic Operation." *Boston Medical and Surgical Journal* 16 (1837): 69.

Webster, Jerome Pierce, and Martha Teach Gnudi. "Documenti inediti intorno alla vita di Gaspare Tagliacozzi." In *Studi e memorie per la storia dell'Università di Bologna*, vol. 13. Bologna: Istituto per la Storia dell'Università, 1935.

Wigmore, B. "Venom 'Viagra.'" *Mirror*, News Section (2003): 31.

Williamson, Susan, and Rachel Novak. "The Truth about Women." *New Scientist*, August 1, 1998, 1–5.

Zanca, Attilio. *Notizie sulla vita e sulle opere di Marcello Donati da Mantova (1538–1602), medico, umanista, uomo di stato*. Pisa: Tip. Editrice Giardini, 1964.

Zanca, Attilio, and Adriano Galassi. "Saggio di bibliografia medica mantovana rinascimentale." In *Mantova e i Gonzaga nella civiltà del Rinascimento*, edited by Accademia Nazionale dei Lincei, 399–421. Mantua: Accademia Virgiliana, 1977.

Zuccolo, Simeon (Zuccolo da Cologna). *La pazzia del ballo*. Bologna: Forni, 1969.

Acknowledgments

Many years ago I was unable to participate in a discussion group of graduate students and faculty due to a last-minute fender bender that kept me away. The topic was Torquato Tasso, the Renaissance Italian epic and lyric poet whom many know today because he was famously imprisoned in a madhouse in Ferrara by the Duke of Este as a result of his persecution mania. The following day I asked a friend how the discussion went. The reunion was pathetic, he admitted, because rather than concentrating on Tasso's apologetic rewriting of his chivalric romance—the subject of the day—the group took time to lament the fact that Vincenzo Gonzaga, then a young prince in the Duchy of Mantua, could have done more in securing his beloved poet's quick transfer from Ferrara to Mantua, that is, from prison to a sheltered court life, but did nothing. Naively, I asked why. He was too preoccupied with personal problems at the time, my friend answered. That was all—and I knew nothing about these problems.

For reasons that I have still been unable to process but that must have been deeply psychological, from that moment on Vincenzo's personal problems began to have a fascination of their own for me. What stirred my curiosity was not the well-known narrative of a charismatic leader notorious for his licentious and disastrously reckless life—the glitzy, honeyed existence that Giuseppe Verdi felt to be relevant enough to play up with visceral emotion in *Rigoletto* almost three centuries later. Rather, it was the aesthetic inquisitiveness; the gifted mind; and specifically the inner turmoil, the physical annoyances, and the health troubles of an impetuous yet sensible Renaissance prince that gave me food for thought. Here was a complex, restless, and eclectic "modern" man, who time and again found that there were too few hours in a day. Thus I started my research.

There have been a number of friends and colleagues who have kindly provided occasions to test my thoughts or offered patient ears to my updates. I would like to thank first of all Giuseppe Gerbino for giving me, unwittingly, the impetus to write this book; Maurizio Rippa Bonati for instructing me thoroughly on the medical part of my inquiry and for so freely spreading around his time, energy, and immense erudition; Elizabeth Clark for the many conversations at dinner over the subject and for having graciously critiqued the entire manuscript; Ronald Witt and Mary Ann Frese Witt for their generous friendship; David Aers, Renzo Derosas, Paul Grendler, Margaret Humphreys, Michael McVaugh, Albert Rabil, and Alessandro Riva for their invaluable advice; and I Tatti Studies series editors Edward Muir and Kate Lowe for believing that my study merited publication. I would also like to thank Marina Brownlee, Andrea Carlino, Dino Cervigni, Stanley Chojnacki, Michael Cornett, Celia Cussen, William Eamon, Joanne Ferraro, Norman Fiering, Eileen Gillooly, Martin Marafioti, Kent Mullikin, Giuseppe Ongaro, Mary Pardo, José Pardo-Tomás, Gianna Pomata, Richard Powell, Guido Ruggiero, Nicholas Terpstra, and Susan Zimmerman for their advice during this long-gestating project.

Needless to say, I owe heartfelt gratitude to the chairs of my department, Roberto Dainotto, Margaret Greer, and Michèle Longino, for their support, and to deans George MacLendon and Gregson Davis for granting me sabbatical leaves and a Dean's Leave at crucial times during the writing of this book. I am also indebted to my Italian "crew" for their cheerful, supportive, and generous hospitality—Annamaria Ferrarotti, Gianfranco Finucci, Luciano Donato, Elisabetta Graziosi, and Sandra Trevisan. Marco Callegari and Paola Modesti helped in surmounting bureaucratic hassles, and Rosamaria Preparata, Carmen Mullin, Julie Linehan, Beatrice Litt, Franca Dotti, Paula Breedlove, and Mariella Bacigalupo were unstinting in their good-humored approval. Mark Sosower was for many years my sounding board, and I am still reeling from his untimely loss. Finally, I thank the two anonymous readers of my manuscript for their generous critiques and for their expertise, as well as Ian Stevenson at the Press, who guided me through the last stages of publication with solicitude and a good sense of humor. Jamie Thaman and Kimberly Giambattisto were generous clarity-seeking manuscript and production editors, and I am most grateful for their excellent suggestions. This book is dedicated to Haig Khachatoorian, who came late in the process of writing—and stayed with joyful enthusiasm.

A number of colleagues and friends offered the occasion for me to reflect on the material I explore in this work by inviting me to share it in a variety of venues in places as diverse as the Università di Padova, the Università di Bologna, the Université de Genéve, Brown University, Columbia University, New York University, Princeton University, the University of Maryland, the University of Miami, the University of Pennsylvania, CUNY Graduate Center, and of course Duke University. The responses and candid comments I received from each audience were extremely helpful, and I took them all to heart.

I also benefited through the years from a number of grants that allowed me to concentrate fully on my initial archival research and later on subsequent writings and rewritings. I would like to thank the directors and staffs at the Franklin Center at Duke University, the John Carter Brown Library at Brown

University, and the National Humanities Center in North Carolina. I also profited from grants by the Trent Foundation and the Faculty Research Council at Duke University. Finally, given the documentary nature of this book, I would like to thank the staffs at Duke University Library and Brown University Library, as well as the staffs at the Marciana Library in Venice, the State Archives in Venice and Mantua, and the Biblioteca Civica in Padua.

Some aspects of Chapter 1 were developed in two earlier articles, "The Virgin's Body and Early Modern Surgeons," in *Masculinities, Childhood, Violence: Attending to Early Modern Women—and Men,* ed. Amy E. Leonard and Karen L. Nelson (Newark: University of Delaware Press, 2011), 195–221; and "Devianza sessuale e imperativi genealogici: Il caso di Margherita Gonzaga," in *Acta Histriae* 15.2 (2007): 385–98 (in Italian and Slovenian). I had the opportunity to discuss topics presented in Chapter 4 in "'There's the Rub': Searching for Sexual Remedies in the New World," in "The Diseased Body in Premodern Europe: Ideology and Representation," ed. Susan Zimmerman, special issue, *Journal of Medieval and Early Modern Studies* 38.3 (2008): 523–557.

Index

Acosta, José de, 137, 142
Africanus, Leo, 132
Albertus Magnus, 34
alchemy, alchemical concoctions, 16, 101, 116, 133–135, 145
Aldrovandi, Ulisse, 64, 130, 134
Alençon, Anne d', 8
Alighieri, Dante, 98, 121
Alvarez, Marcelo, 21
Anania, Giovanni Lorenzo d', 138
Andreini, Giovanni Battista, 16
Andreini, Isabella, 16
Anguillara, Lampridio, 108
Antwerp, 122
aphrodisiacs, 122, 130–132, 135–136; use of animals, 130–132, 136–137, 139–140
Aquinas, Thomas, 85–86
Aranzi, Giulio Cesare, 41, 42, 44, 46, 77
Aretino, Pietro, 125
Ariosto, Lodovico, 85
Arrivabene, Lucio, 60
arthritis, "rheumatism," rheumatoid arthritis, 7, 23, 24, 99, 100–112, 114, 115, 117, 142, 147. *See also* catarrh; gout; rickets; tuberculosis
Augenio, Orazio, 36
Augustine, 46, 110
Averroes, 34
Avicenna, 34
Avisi, 138

Barcelona, 121, 127, 143, 145
Barlaymonte, Gioan de, 127
Bartholin, Caspar, 58
Bartholin, Thomas, 57
Basile, Adriana, 20, 72

Bauhin, Caspar, 133
Beato Gabriele, 49
Bellonci, Maria, 60, 126, 150
Berengario da Carpi, Jacopo, 33
Bertioli, Antonio, 143
Bimini, 120
Blandin, Philippe, 91
blood, 33, 34, 38, 84, 91, 100, 102, 104, 105, 107, 108, 126, 132, 142, 144, 148, 153; bloodletting, 108; menstrual blood, 35, 36, 40, 45, 54
Boccaccio, Giovanni, 115
Bocchi, Zanobio, 134
Boccone, Paolo, 142
Boi, Antonio Francesco, 58
Bolivia, 25, 122, 147
Bologna, 24, 41, 64, 65, 75, 77, 91, 92, 105, 134
Bonatti, Celliero, 127, 128, 144, 145
Borgarucci, Prospero, 76
Borro, Diomede, 44
Borromeo, Carlo, 43, 45, 46, 47, 48, 56, 60, 89
Borromeo, Federico, 60
Bragadin, Marcantonio, 86
Brahe, Tycho, 88–89
Branca, Gian Paolo, 7
Branca-Minuti, Gustavo, 74, 75, 91
Brasavola, Antonio, 138
Brazil, 25, 136, 139, 148
Briceño, Ramon, 147
Brussels, 13, 111, 113
Butler, Samuel, 93

Cádiz, 121, 143
Caimo, Zaccaria, 44, 45, 46

Index

Callao, 122, 143
Calvino, Italo, 86
Campanella, Tommaso, 93
Camporesi, Piero, 141
Canali, Giuseppe, 43
Canissa, 96, 97, 114, 150
Capello, Bianca, 50
Capelluti, Rolando, 74
Cara, Marchetto, 150
Carletti, Francesco, 140
Caro, Annibal, 89
Carpue, J. C., 90
Cartagena, 121, 143, 144
Casale, 13, 116
Castiglione, Baldesar, 70
Catania, 74
catarrh, "fluxes," 25, 103–105, 106, 117, 118. *See also* arthritis; knee pain
Catullus, 116
Cavriani, Cesare, 44
Cei, Galeotto, 140
Celsus, Aulus Cornelius, 45, 74
Cesi, Bishop of Casale, 49
Charlemagne, 3
Charles I, King of England, 13
Charles V, Holy Roman Emperor, 28, 152
chastity, 31, 47; signs of, 32; for church canonists, 32, 56. *See also* virginity
Chauliac, Guy de, 74
Chiabrera, Gabriello, 16
Chieppio, Annibale, 60, 70, 111, 112, 127
Chiut, Giovan Battista, 127
Chrichton, James, 9
Christine de Lorraine, 111
Chrysostom, John, 32
Chuquiabo, 122, 128, 144, 145
Church of Santa Barbara, 3
Church of Sant'Andrea, 2, 153, 154
Cieza de Léon, 138
Cimenes, Emanuel, 122, 127
Clement VIII, Pope, 18, 43, 44, 46, 47, 59, 60
clitoris, 34, 56; debates on its presence and size, 56–59
Codronchi, Giovan Battista, 141
Colmar, 63, 64
Colombo, Realdo, 36, 42, 57
Colonna, Fabio, 137
Columbus, Christopher, 102, 130, 135, 141
Compagni, Dino, 89
Contarini, Francesco, 13
Contrayerba, 144

Cornaro, Giacomo Alvise, 68, 101, 116
Corradi, Alfonso, 90
Cortese, Isabella, 132
Costa, Filippo, 135
Costa, Margherita, 86
court performances (plays, pastorals, music), 15, 16, 18, 26, 60, 63, 72, 108, 117
Cranach, Lucas the Elder, 119
Crusades, 13, 19, 62, 63, 96, 111, 150
Cueva, 142
Culpeper, Nicholas, 36
cura del legno. See *Guaiacum*
Cuzco, 122, 144
Cyprus, 86, 131

dall'Armi, Francesco, 65
D'Annunzio, Gabriele, 151
d'Argellata, Pietro, 74
d'Aviz, Maria (of Portugal), 28
Del Carretto, Agnese, 19
Delfino, Tiberio, 43
Della Casa, Giovanni, 88; *Galateo,* 88
Della Croce, Giovanni Andrea, 90
Della Porta, Giambattista, 23, 32, 89, 131
Della Rovere, Duchess Eleonora Gonzaga of Urbino, 85
Della Rovere, Duke Francesco Maria, 60
De Rossi, Salamone, 15, 18
Dieffenbach, Johann Friedrich, 91
Dioscorides, 133
Donati, Marcello, 9, 29–31, 42, 43, 45, 46, 56, 102, 104, 132
dowry, 41, 45, 50, 52, 54. *See also* marriage
Du Laurens, André, 59
Durante, Castore, 132, 138

East Indies, 127, 146
Ebreo, Leon, 18
Elizabeth I, Queen of England, 4, 41
erysipelas, skin rash, 23, 63, 64, 68, 94, 101, 110, 113, 142. *See also* nose; tuberculosis
Este, Cesare d', 51
Este, Duke Alfonso II d', 6, 51
Este, Marchioness Isabella d', 101, 150
examination of pudenda: female, 31, 40–46; male, 48–49

Fabrici d'Acquapendente, Girolamo, 30, 31, 38, 40, 42, 43, 44, 46, 56, 58, 59, 76, 118

Falloppio, Gabriele, 35, 38, 43, 57, 58, 71, 76, 110
Famagusta, 86
Farnese, Duke Alessandro, 29
Farnese, Duke Ottavio, 41, 42, 43, 52
Farnese, Duke Ranuccio, 60
Farnese, Margherita, 10, 22, 28–31, 41–50, 55–61, 63, 101
Fedeli, Compagnia de', 72
Ferdinand I, Holy Roman Emperor, 6
Ferdinand I, King of Sicily, 74
Ferdinand II, Archduke of Austria, 6, 10
Ferrara, 9, 46, 60, 63
fever, 1, 5, 7, 21, 25, 26, 42, 63, 97, 100, 101, 102, 103, 104, 115, 128, 141, 145, 147, 148, 153
Ficino, Marsilio, 70
Filarete, Antonio, 107
Fioravanti, Leonardo, 75, 76, 77, 138
fistula (psoas abscess), 8, 43, 48, 55, 100, 101, 107. *See also* tuberculosis
Flanders, 3, 13, 24, 28, 29, 97, 111, 114
Fliess, Wilhelm, 90
Florence, 19, 35, 51, 57, 58, 89, 113, 122
Fracastoro, Girolamo, 87
Fragoso, Juan, 137
Franchetti, Giuditta, 18
Freud, Sigmund, 23, 59, 60, 90

Gadebush Bondio, Mariacarla, 71
Galen, Galenic medicine, 7, 54, 56, 74, 93, 98, 104, 105, 129, 130, 132, 133, 134, 138, 152
Galilei, Galileo, 5, 7, 16, 72, 101, 118, 128, 146
Galletti, Piero, 55
Garda, 116
Genoa, 12, 103, 110, 117, 118, 121, 128, 141
Gentile da Foligno, 105
Gilman, Sander, 90, 93
Giulia, orphan from Pietà, 52–54
Gnudi, Martha Teach, 66, 68, 78
gonorrhea, 94, 101, 126. *See also* syphilis
Gonzaga, Archduchess Anna Caterina of Innsbruck, 6, 97
Gonzaga, Archduchess Consort Eleonora of Habsburg, 10
Gonzaga, Bishop Francesco, 20, 115
Gonzaga, Duchess Leonora of Austria, 6, 9, 110
Gonzaga, Duchess Margherita of Ferrara, 6, 9

Gonzaga, Duchess Margherita of Lorraine, 10
Gonzaga, Duchess Margherita of Savoy, 126
Gonzaga, Duchess Maria of Monferrato, 8, 10
Gonzaga, Duke Carlo, 8
Gonzaga, Duke Federico II, 3, 100, 108, 110, 116
Gonzaga, Duke Ferdinando, 10, 16, 72, 145
Gonzaga, Duke Francesco III, 3, 7
Gonzaga, Duke Francesco IV, 3, 10, 96, 110, 125–126, 134, 145, 153
Gonzaga, Duke Vincenzo: as art collector, 2, 13, 14, 18, 26, 71–72, 135, 151–152; as patron of literature/theater, 15, 16, 18, 71–72; as patron of music, 13, 15, 18, 20, 35, 63, 117, 150
Gonzaga, Duke Luigi of Nevers, 8
Gonzaga, Duke Vincenzo II, 10, 112
Gonzaga, Francesco, 19
Gonzaga, Guglielmo Domenico (Lungaspada), 3, 10
Gonzaga, Marquess Francesco II, 4, 96, 101, 102, 110
Gonzaga, Marquis Ludovico III, 100, 110
Gonzaga, Scipione, 65, 68
Gonzaga, Silvio, 20
Gonzaga Duke Guglielmo I, 3, 6, 7, 8, 9, 11, 28, 29, 31, 42, 43, 44, 45, 49, 50, 51, 76, 100, 102, 110
Gonzaga-Nevers, 8, 41, 61, 118
Gonzaga of Guastalla, 41, 112
gout, 7, 101–104, 105, 107, 115. *See also* arthritis; catarrh; knee pain
Gradi, Basilio, 47
Graefe, Carl Ferdinand von, 90–91
Grégoire, Pierre, 154
Gregory XIII, Pope, 46
Griffon, Jean, 73
Guadalupe, 143
Guaiacum, 68
Guarini, Giovanni Battista, 15, 72
Guglielmo da Saliceto, 33
Gusano, 25, 126–129, 135, 139, 144–148. *See also* worms, bugs, spiders
Gutiero, Andrés, 75

headache, 21, 101, 112, 116, 141, 142
Hellman, Carlo, 127
Henry II, Duke of Lorraine, 10
Henry III, King of France, 112, 116

Henry IV, King of France, 18, 118
Henry VIII, King of England, 111–112
herbs, herbals, herbalists, 1, 16, 33, 131, 132–136, 137, 138, 146; holistic cures with herbs, 16, 26, 109, 101, 130–132, 135–136, 144. *See also* aphrodisiacs
Hernández, Francisco, 137
Herrera, Antonio de, 120
Hildebrand, Otto, 86
Hippocratics, 56, 104
Hugo, Victor, 21
Hungary, 2, 19, 62, 63, 64, 96, 123
Hutson, John, 58
hymen and hypertrophic hymen, 22, 30, 31, 34–36, 38, 40–43, 45–47, 49–50, 51, 53, 54–59; illustration, 38–40; surgical interventions (hymenectomy), 38, 40, 41, 43, 45

Iberti, Annibale, 103, 117, 125
Innsbruck, 24, 97, 111
Iseo, 110, 113

Jackson, Michael, 94
Jeanne de France, 44
Jewish: community, 18, 90, 93; music, 14
Johnson, Virginia, 23, 53
Joubert, Laurent, 33, 35–36, 38, 89

kidney stones, 106, 110, 117
Kinsey, Alfred, 23, 53
knee pain, osteoarticular tuberculosis, 7, 97, 99, 100, 103, 111, 116, 117. *See also* arthritis; catarrh; gout
Kuriyama, Shigehisa, 104
Kurtz, Joacob, 134

Lanfranco of Milan, 74
Langosca, Maria Teresa, 44
Lavater, Johann Caspar, 74
Leite, Romulo, 148
Leroux, Gaston, 87
Lima, 122, 143, 144
López de Gomara, 138
Loreto, 103, 118
Louis XII, King of France, 44
Lower, Richard, 105
Lucan, 110

Machiavelli, Niccolò, 53, 106, 130; *Clizia*, 110; *Mandragola*, 106, 131
MacMillan, Clara, 53
Madonna Antonia, 44

Madrid, 121, 127
Magli, Giovanni Gualberto, 15
Malatesta, Paola, 110
Mancini, Giulio, 32, 87
Manta, 122, 143
Mantegna, Andrea, 13, 100
Mantua, 7, 8, 9, 11, 12, 15, 16, 17, 18, 20, 22, 29, 48, 49, 61, 72, 100, 134, 142, 150, 151, 153; Peaceful University of, 16, 72
Manzoni, Alessandro, 61; *I promessi sposi*, 61
Marcobruno, Giuseppe, 127
Marcobruno, Evangelista, 24, 121, 123, 127–129, 135, 137–139, 142, 143–148
Marcolini da Fano, Andrea, 43, 46
Margaret of Habsburg, Duchess of Parma, 29
Marinello, Giovanni, 84, 131
marriage, 10, 22, 28, 30, 34, 49, 50, 52, 55, 60, 61, 86, 88, 99, 118; dissolution, 22, 46, 48; lack of consummation, 29, 30, 41, 42–43, 46, 49, 53, 54. *See also* dowry
Marseille, 143
Martinelli, Caterina, 20
Massa, Niccolò, 58
Masters, William, 23, 53
Mattioli, Pietro, 132, 133, 138
Maura Lucenia, nun, 47, 61
McClintock, Anne, 140
McVicar, David, 21
Medici, Grand Duchess Johanna of Austria de', 10
Medici, Granduke Cosimo I de', 86
Medici, Granduke Cosimo II de', 89
Medici, Granduke Ferdinando de', 17, 19, 50, 103, 111, 117, 145
Medici, Granduke Francesco de', 10, 50, 51, 53
Medici, Queen Maria of France de', 18, 118
Medici Gonzaga, Duchess Caterina of Mantua, de', 10, 61, 89
Medici Gonzaga, Duchess Eleonora of Mantua de', 2, 10, 12, 15, 18, 26, 50, 55, 60, 97, 113, 118, 142, 145, 150
Meravaglia, Margherita, 44
Mercuriale, Girolamo, 71, 76, 77
Mercurio, Girolamo, 36
Mexico, 127, 135, 136, 137
Michelangelo, 85
Milan, 13, 18, 43, 44, 46, 48, 49, 60, 102, 103

Minadoi, Giovanni Tommaso, 71, 104–105
Minardo, Ventura, 107
Moletti, Giuseppe, 7, 72
Monardes, Nicolás, 137, 142, 144, 147
Mondeville, Henri de, 74
Mondino de Luzzi, 34
Monferrato, 8, 13, 116, 154
Montaigne, Michel de, 21, 29, 110
Montecatini, Ugolino da, 105–106
Monteczuma, 147
Monteverdi, Claudio, 15, 20, 63
Morgagni, Giambattista, 142
Moro, Benedetto, 118
Morosini, Francesco, 17, 19, 125
Mozart, Wolfgang, 32

Namur, 29
Naples, 2, 17, 19, 20, 71, 72, 114, 115
nose: cutting off (*denasatio*), 23, 87; as esthetically important, 70–73, 78, 84–85, 89, 94; as sexual metaphor, 23, 33, 86–88, 90; surgery, 23, 66, 73–78, 90–94; as symptom or metaphor for disease, 23, 68, 87–88, 104; unguents or treatments for the nose, 65, 75, 110. *See also* erysipelas; syphilis
Nunes, Kenia Pedrosa, 48

O'Connell, Helen, 58
Ocsko, Wojcieck, 77
Order of the Golden Fleece, 13
Order of the Redeemer, 20, 123
Osanna, Francesco, 72
Ostino, Giuseppe, 147
Ottomans (Turks), 12, 62, 63, 96, 123
Oviedo, Gonzalo Fernández de, 120, 133, 138, 141, 142

Padua, 16, 68, 72, 101, 105, 110; University of, 7, 30, 31, 34–38, 58, 68, 71, 75, 76, 104
Paleologo, Margherita, 63
Pallavicino, Eufrosina, 44
Panama, 122, 143
Panigarola, Teodora, 44
Paracelsus, Paracelsian, 132
Paré, Ambroise, 36, 76, 76, 104
Park, Katharine, 105
Parma, 10, 22, 28, 29, 30, 40, 42–45, 47, 60, 61
Pasha, Mustafa, 86
Paul V, Pope, 18, 20
Pazzini, Adalberto, 68

Pendasio, Cesare, 41, 45
Pendasio, Federico, 64
Persia, Ferrante, 111, 112
Peru, 25, 122, 127, 128, 129, 130, 136, 137, 138, 143, 144, 145, 147, 148
Peter of Eboli, 114–115
Petrarca, Francesco and Petrarchism, 71, 85, 102, 126
Petrozzani, Tullio, 64
pharmacy, pharmacists, 33, 127, 138, 143, 146
Philip II, King of Spain, 13, 28, 52
Philip III, King of Spain, 3, 114, 129
Piacenza, 41
Pieno, Benedetto, 118
Pierce, Jerome, 66, 68, 78
Pisa, 35, 72
plague, 8, 133
Pliny the Elder, 106, 111, 131
Plowden, Edmund, 4
Pomponazzi, Aurelio, 9
Ponce de Leon, 119, 120
Porter, Roy, 5, 99
Portobelo, 121, 143
Portugal, 3, 28, 114
Porzio, Camillo, 75
Potosí, 121, 128, 143, 144
Pott's Disease, hunchback, 6, 35, 42, 100, 110. *See also* rickets; tuberculosis
Pourbus, Frans the Younger, 13, 20, 31, 71, 115, 123
Pozzuoli. *See* thermal baths
Prague, 18, 71
Pratt, Mary Louise, 146
prostate, 58

Ramazzini, Bernardino, 4, 113
Ramponi, Virginia, 15
Ramusio, Giovanni Battista, 138
Raphael, 13
Rasi, Francesco, 15, 117
Redi, Francesco, 141
Reggio, 55, 60
relics, 2, 17, 63; Most Precious Blood, 2, 63
religious orders: Hospitallers, 18; Theatine, 17
Rhazes, 34
rickets, 99–100
Rigoletto, 20–21, 125
Rome, 13, 43, 65, 86, 138
Romero, Fernando, 147
Rosaccio, Gioseppe, 138
Roswrun, Hermann, 96

Rousseau, G. S., 5
Roxane, 23
Rubens, Peter Paul, 3, 13, 14, 71, 114
Rudolph II, Holy Roman Emperor, 18, 71
Ruggiero, Guido, 87
Ruscelli, Girolamo, 138

Sack of Mantua, 16, 61, 87
Salando, Fernando, 142
Salerno, 33
Sampierdarena, 103, 110, 117, 118
Sanseverino, Barbara, 19
Sassonia, Ercole, 36
Savonarola, Michele, 35, 106
Sbaraglia, Girolamo, 92
Scansani, Stefano, 147, 148
seawater cures, 103, 110, 117–118. *See also* thermal baths
Segovia, 121, 128
Seville, 121, 128, 143, 144, 145
sexual performance: interview about it, 45, 52–54, 55; supervised, 50, 51–53
Sforza, Caterina, 33, 131
Shakespeare, William, 23, 88, 134, 154
Simons, Paricia, 125
Sixtus V, Pope, 86
skin pathologies (lupus, scrofula, erysipelas), 23, 63, 64, 68, 94, 98, 101, 106, 110. *See also* syphilis; thermal baths; tuberculosis
Soles, Fipippo, 145
Solimei, Giovanni Battista, 65
Soranus of Ephesus, 34, 106
Spa (Belgium). *See* thermal baths
Spanish fly, 126, 142, 144. *See also* worms, bugs, spiders
spiders. *See* worms, bugs, spiders
Spini, Iacopo, 122
Stratford-upon-Avon, 154
Striggio, Alessandro, 97
surgery: genital, 38, 40, 43, 45–46, 59; sedation, 78
surgery, plastic. *See* nose
Sushura, Hindi medicine, 74, 90
Susini, Clemente, 58
Sydenham, Thomas, 102–103
syphilis, syphilitic, 4, 23, 24, 48, 66, 68, 87–88, 93, 94, 98, 101, 102, 106, 110, 112, 126, 133, 136, 139, 140

Tagliacozzi, Gaspare, 23, 57, 66, 73, 74, 76–78, 84, 87, 90–94, 101, 110; accuses following his method, 76, 90–94; sympathetic nose, 92–93; visits to Mantua, 64–66, 70. *See also* nose; skin pathologies (lupus, scrofula, erysipelas)
Tasso, Torquato, 12, 16, 19, 71; *Gerusalemme Liberata*, 19, 71
testicles, 55, 89, 131, 132, 139; female testicles (ovaries), 56, 59
thermal baths: as fountain of youth, 119–120; healing therapies, 105–109; reason for thermal sojourns, 97–99; structure of baths, 107, 114–115; as vacation spots, 98–99, 115, 117–118, 119; Baths: Abano/Montegrotto, 56, 105, 109, 110, 116; Acqua, 107; Acqui, 111; Aix-la-Chapelle, 115; Baden-Baden, 119; Boario, 110, 113; Caldiero, 107, 108, 110, 116; Lucca, 107, 110; Petriolo, 107, 110; Porretta, 24, 105, 106; Pozzuoli/Agnano (Campi Flegrei), 24, 107, 113–115, 117; Roman Empire baths, 105, 107, 114; San Filippo, 106; Sirmione, 116; Spa (Belgium) 6, 24, 97, 103, 108, 110, 111–113, 116–117, 118; Vichy, 115; Villa, 24, 65, 106, 110; Viterbo, 98–99. *See also* seawater cures
Titian, 13, 84, 85, 152
Tornatore, Giovanni Pietro, 103
Tossignano, Pietro, da, 105
Tropea, 75, 93
tuberculosis, 5, 7, 24, 52, 65, 68, 70, 94, 99, 100, 103, 126, 133

urine, 32, 35, 75, 104, 111, 131, 144
uterus, 38, 46, 59, 106, 109

Valerini, Adriano, 72
Varoli, Costanzo, 57
Vasari, Giorgio, 70
Venice, 7, 13, 18, 45, 51, 52, 87, 123, 152
Verdi, Giuseppe, 20, 125
Vesalius, Andreas, 35, 36, 56, 57, 58, 71, 76, 152
Vespucci, Amerigo, 25, 139, 148
Viagra, 25, 121–122, 132, 147–148. *See also* worms, bugs, spiders
Vianeo Pietro and Paolo, 75, 77, 93
Vienna, 64
Vinta, Belisario, 53, 54, 111
Virgil, 87, 114
virginity: fake claims, 33; as physical condition, 32, 35, 56; recipes, 33–34; taboo, 59–60; tests, 32–34. *See also* chastity

Visconti, Galeazzo, 102
Visegrád, 62
Vitruvius, 106
Voltaire, 93

Warren, Jonathan Mason, 91
West Indies, 127, 128, 135, 140, 146
worms, bugs, spiders: as aphrodisiac, 25, 127–128, 139–141, 147, 148; curative, 134, 138, 142–143, 148; infestation, 140–142; as metaphor of fear and decadence, 140–141; as poisonous, 128, 134, 141, 144, 148. See also *Gusano*; Spanish fly

Zacchia, Paolo, 76
Zárate, Agustín de, 138
Zibramonti, Aurelio, 41, 46, 48, 58